Overcoming Anxiety
A Five Areas Approach

Dr Chris Williams MBChB BSc MMedSc MD MRCPsych,
Senior Lecturer and Honorary Consultant Psychiatrist,
Division of Community-based Sciences,
Section of Psychological Medicine,
University of Glasgow Medical School,
Glasgow, UK

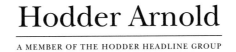
Hodder Arnold
A MEMBER OF THE HODDER HEADLINE GROUP

First published in Great Britain in 2003 by
Hodder Arnold, an imprint of Hodder Education and a member of the Hodder Headline
Group, an Hachette Livre UK Company, 338 Euston Road, London NW1 3BH

http://www.hoddereducation.com

Distributed in the United States of America by
Oxford University Press Inc.,
198 Madison Avenue, New York, NY10016
Oxford is a registered trademark of Oxford University Press

Whilst the advice and information in this book are believed to be true and
accurate at the date of going to press, neither the author nor the publisher
can accept any legal responsibility or liability for any errors or omissions
that may be made. In particular (but without limiting the generality of the
preceding disclaimer) every effort has been made to check drug dosages;
however, it is still possible that errors have been missed. Furthermore,
dosage schedules are constantly being revised and new side-effects
recognised. For these reasons the reader is strongly urged to consult the
drug companies' printed instructions before administering any of the drugs
recommended in this book.

British Library Cataloguing in Publication Data
A catalogue record for this book is available from the British Library

Library of Congress Cataloging-in-Publication Data
A catalog record for this book is available from the Library of Congress

ISBN: 978 0 340 81005 7

6 7 8 9 10

Commissioning Editor: Serena Bureau
Development Editor: Layla Vandenbergh
Project Editor: Zelah Pengilley
Production Controller: Deborah Smith
Cover Design: Ian Hughes
Indexer: Laurence Errington

Typeset in 11 on 15pt Sabon by Phoenix Photosetting, Chatham, Kent
Printed and bound by Antony Rowe

What do you think about this book? Or any other Arnold title?
Please send your comments to www.hoddereducation.com

Overcoming Anxiety
A Five Areas Approach

Contents

Forewords

Acknowledgements

Introduction

Part 1   Understanding anxiety: initial self-assessment

Part 2   *Overcoming Anxiety*: self-management workbooks and worksheets

Part 3 Using the *Overcoming Anxiety* materials: advice for health care practitioners and self-help support groups

Index

Forewords
A user-group viewpoint

We all get anxious at times – parents worry about children, students worry about exams. We all worry at times about our health, about money or the lack of it, about the world political or environmental situation – the list is endless.

Most people cope with these worries, work through them and move on, but for a considerable minority of people, anxiety in various forms takes a hold and gets progressively worse, leading to distress and reduced functioning in all areas of life.

Cognitive behaviour therapy (CBT) is well researched and a known effective approach to overcoming the problems of anxiety disorders. Unfortunately, there are not enough CBT practitioners available to meet the tremendous need for services. The development over the last few years of structured self-help groups run by voluntary organisations, such as Triumph Over Phobia, has gone some way to help support anxiety sufferers in their own self-treatment. Again, limited resources mean that there will probably never be enough of these groups to meet demand.

The workbooks of *Overcoming Anxiety* will, I am sure, contribute greatly to filling gaps in such services. They could be used by the anxiety sufferer with limited practitioner support (at primary as well as at secondary level) and they could also be used as a resource in self-help groups.

Because of the stigma still attached to mental health problems, some people prefer to by-pass the mental health services – and group work is not for everyone, so these books are also ideal for working through alone.

What I like about *Overcoming Anxiety* is the very practical, step-by-step approach, constant reference to consolidating on successes and to making sure people 'walk before they run'. The language is straightforward and jargon-free, and the reader is encouraged to work at 'bite-sized chunks'. People are helped to think through their physical symptoms and unhelpful behaviours and to make graded progress. Explanations and suggestions are offered at every stage. The workbooks are delightfully illustrated with amusing but relevant cartoons.

Overcoming Anxiety will surely be a tremendous practical resource for practitioners, self-help groups and individuals alike.

Joan Bond
Former National Development Officer of the charity Triumph over Phobia

A clinical psychologist's viewpoint

The anxiety disorders are among the most common problems reported by people of all ages. They can prevent people from leading full, productive lives and place a heavy burden on society. However, anxiety disorders can respond very well to appropriate treatment. Since the mid-eighties, cognitive behaviour therapy (CBT) for anxiety disorders has developed rapidly. It has moved from moderately effective approaches for coping with the signs of anxiety disorders to more focused treatment packages for each of the forms that anxiety disorders can take. These treatment packages, each based on a clear understanding of the particular form of anxiety, use specific techniques to address the thoughts and behaviours that keep people 'stuck' in vicious circles. As a psychologist involved in clinical research, I have been involved in developing and testing some of these packages. Even though we know that they work, it does not mean that they are immediately available. It can take years for the packages to become widely known. The information about anxiety, the techniques, and the exercises found in *Overcoming Anxiety* are based on treatment packages that have been shown to be effective in numerous trials. Indeed, the focused treatments on which much of this book is based have revolutionised the treatment of anxiety. By providing important parts of these treatments in simple language and in a structured format, those helping people with anxiety will now have greater access to credible tools.

An important part of my work is training health workers in CBT. At the Newcastle Cognitive and Behaviour Therapies Centre we offer a wide range of training. For over a decade the Centre has been providing a year-long course in CBT that addresses a range of problems, including the anxiety disorders. Although the core ideas of CBT are easy to understand, it takes a great deal of time, effort, and training to become an effective therapist for a wide range of problems. We know that we cannot train enough therapists to the level of expertise required to deliver focused and individualised treatments for all the people who would benefit from a CBT approach for anxiety.

The challenge then is how to make these treatments more available without losing the key parts of the therapy. In other words, can we scale them down rather than watering them down? Can we package these treatments so that they can be used safely and effectively by a wide range of people working with people with common mental health problems? Can we make the essential ingredients of these treatments easily understood and easy to use? This book seeks to meet this challenge. It is well grounded in current CBT approaches for anxiety, the information is easily accessible for people in a helping role who may not have specialised knowledge of CBT, and the material is presented in a practical, structured format.

We know that it is common for people to have more than one form of anxiety. Likewise, it is also common for people with anxiety to also suffer from low mood and depression. The approach developed here by Chris Williams follows his previous work in the field of depression. Indeed, one of the strengths of this book is that it fits with *Overcoming Depression*. A common language and a common format in the different sections of this book as well as in the previous book means that people working with common mental health problems can 'mix and match' the worksheets to fit the inevitable mixture of presenting problems.

In conclusion, I believe that this book will contribute to more people receiving timely CBT for anxiety. Those who are trying to make psychological therapies more accessible for common mental health problems will welcome it. It succeeds in striking a balance. On the one hand, important parts of the focused treatments for the different forms of anxiety can be found throughout the book. On the other hand, the book builds increasing familiarity with common principles through a standard presentation style. In this way, people with anxiety and those that seek to help them can develop a high degree of understanding. For trainers, service developers, helpers and those with anxiety alike, I believe *Overcoming Anxiety* will be warmly welcomed as a credible and accessible approach to the cognitive behavioural treatment of anxiety disorders.

Professor Mark Freeston
Director of Research and Training
Newcastle Cognitive and Behavioural Therapies Centre
Newcastle-upon-Tyne, UK

A nurse's viewpoint

Overcoming Anxiety: A Five Areas Approach, like its companion guide *Overcoming Depression: A Five Areas Approach*, published in 2001, provides a comprehensive self-help package presented in an interactive, user-friendly format. The text uses a practical, problem-solving approach to dealing with anxiety-based problems in a style which is both engaging and accessible to the reader. Overall the most convincing aspect of the book is that its content speaks for itself in that it has clearly been developed in the real world of mental health practice by a clinician who knows what he is talking about.

What is especially impressive is that the content of each workbook is based on empirically validated CBT interventions incorporating the most up to date CBT treatment models. This represents a significant advance in the field of self-help literature for anxiety disorders. Similarly the comprehensive content of the book, including a workbook on medication and its use in conjunction with CBT interventions, reflects current best practice principles for the treatment of anxiety disorders. The book also gives consideration to the commonly encountered, but frequently disregarded phenomenon of the co-morbidity between depression and anxiety disorders and the implications of this for treatment.

Overcoming Anxiety will be an invaluable resource both to those who suffer with anxiety based problems and the clinicians who endeavour to help them. This book is a must buy for any health professional aspiring to use CBT to treat anxiety disorders. Breaking down the global problem of anxiety into its constituent disorders provides an educational component which can only advance the understanding and treatment of anxiety disorders in everyday clinical practice.

In this book Chris Williams has increased accessibility to an intervention of proven efficacy in the treatment of anxiety disorders. Standing alongside *Overcoming Depression: A Five Areas Approach* this publication comes highly recommended for individuals seeking a useful self-help guide, as well as for integration into service protocols for the treatment of anxiety disorders across health care settings.

Anne Garland
Nurse Consultant in Psychological Therapies and President-elect of the
British Association for Behavioural and Cognitive Psychotherapies
(BABCP www.BABCP.com), Nottingham Psychotherapy Unit

A psychiatrist's viewpoint

Dr Chris Williams is a gifted clinician and trainer who is also a nationally recognised expert in cognitive behaviour therapy. He has particular expertise in the management of common mental disorders in primary care and has developed a well-known series of book and computer-based self-help materials. He has a strong commitment to developing self-help materials that are accessible and jargon-free. In the development of *Overcoming Anxiety*, a range of practitioners and service users have been invited to comment upon the content of the materials. The success of this process is seen within the text. Each workbook is structured with practical use in mind. The five areas CBT model provides a step-by-step way of identifying current problems. The page layout helpfully uses pictures, illustrations and text to promote effective use. Dr Williams also clearly knows his subject. The text shows his ability to engage the reader so that they interact with the content rather than just passively reading it. He writes clearly and simply. This is I believe the first self-help book to formally publish its readability scores (see Part 3) and this is to be welcomed. He has made great efforts to ensure that the text is readily accessible. At the same time the materials are never patronising and manage to maintain a balance between being informative, encouraging and helpful. The evidence base for the effectiveness of self-help materials that utilise the cognitive behaviour therapy model is significant, and it is to be expected that *Overcoming Anxiety* will also prove effective as a training tool for practitioners and an essential resource for service users and self-help groups.

This companion volume to the well-received *Overcoming Depression: A Five Areas Approach* uses the same workbook format to address all the key presentations seen in anxiety. Each workbook uses modern educational techniques to guide the reader through the process of self-assessment and then on to self-management. Key workbooks include self-assessment of generalised anxiety, panic and phobias, obsessive-compulsive problems, and health anxiety and responding to physical problems. The challenge of health anxiety – often ignored in self-help approaches – is addressed, as is the important issue of how people respond in the face of physical health problems. The book contains insights that will prove invaluable to those facing physical health problems such as chronic fatigue, pain and other longer-term physical illness.

The remainder of the workbooks cover a series of focused topics including problem solving, assertiveness, identifying and challenging anxious or obsessive thinking, overcoming avoidance and reducing unhelpful behaviours. These are also fully compatible and interchangeable with the linked workbooks in *Overcoming Depression*. The style of the workbooks continues to avoid much of the jargon of the CBT model. Helpful worksheets encourage readers to try out the key skills in their everyday lives. They communicate key clinical points succinctly and encourage the reader to put what they have learned into practice.

In Part 3 of the book, there are some helpful notes addressing the issue of how to use a self-help approach. A clear definition of self-help is provided, together with a summary of the evidence base for self-help. A particularly useful section addresses how to deliver such self-help materials within clinical and user group settings – a topic again often ignored. These guide the reader through issues such as how to set up a self-help room, and how to best select, introduce and monitor the use of self-help materials.

This book offers a well-written, accessible resource that will prove invaluable to practitioners and service users alike. It offers an ideal way to start to tackle some of the most common problems experienced by people in the western world.

Professor Jan Scott
Institute of Psychiatry, Denmark Hill, London

A general practitioner's viewpoint

Virtually every patient attending a doctor's surgery is likely to be experiencing a degree of anxiety. In most cases this emotional response will be appropriate and helpful. Without it many patients would ignore potentially serious symptoms and fail to look after their health.

However, like every form of emotion, anxiety can be excessive or unhelpful, leading to great suffering amongst patients in terms of distressing and frightening thoughts and feelings, spiralling physical symptoms and, sometimes, unhelpful behaviours, as so effectively described in this text.

As well as causing patient suffering, excessive anxiety can place a great strain upon health care systems and health professionals, including those in primary care. Patient anxiety often leads to increasing demands for help. This raises the issue of how to offer something effective within the limited time and resources available within primary care. Unfortunately, conventional attempts to 'cure' the problem may prove unhelpful. This may lead not only to potential difficulties with drug dependence but escalating dependence upon professionals, as we try ever harder to reassure patients and eliminate symptoms.

Is there a practical alternative approach? The evidence for the effectiveness of cognitive behavioural therapy in the treatment of the anxiety disorders is now beyond dispute and, for example, for panic disorder it is the treatment of choice. However, trained CBT therapists remain a very scarce resource so how can we 'plug the gap'? The companion to this volume, *Overcoming Depression: A Five Areas Approach*, has already proved to be an effective means of offering this form of therapy to patients in a structured self-help format with relatively little input from health care professionals.

I believe *Overcoming Anxiety: A Five Areas Approach* will prove to be just as effective in its impact. The highly structured form of the book provides a sense of security for patients, whilst its interactive nature emphasises the essential need for active involvement in dealing with the problem of anxiety rather than avoiding the problem by seeking an external 'cure'. An essential theme of *Overcoming Anxiety* is the effective and compassionate way in which it deals with the central issue of avoidance in anxiety – a trap we can all fall into when we come under pressure to provide quick fixes and easy cures.

Overcoming Anxiety builds upon the user-friendly Five Areas Assessment to provide clear explanations of the different anxiety disorders and to help patients to understand their own difficulties. The same approach is then used within a series of workbooks to provide structured, active approaches to treatment based upon proven cognitive and behavioural techniques with a strong emphasis upon a pragmatic problem-solving approach. A final benefit of *Overcoming Anxiety* is that anxiety and depression very commonly coexist and this volume is designed to interact and integrate with its companion volume *Overcoming Depression* in a powerful and consistent way.

Practitioners who have *Overcoming Anxiety* available on their bookshelves are likely to experience not only the direct benefits to their patients but an improvement in the quality of their own professional lives.

Dr Steve Williams MRCP MRCGP
General Practitioner, The Garth Surgery, Guisborough, Cleveland

Acknowledgements

I wish to thank my various colleagues both in Glasgow and Leeds who have helped comment on these self-help materials as they were written, especially Mumtaz Ahmad, Nick Bell, Joe Bouch, Frances Cole, Alan Davidson, Mark Freeston, Judith Halford, Julie Hickson, Dale Huey, Sandra Johnston, Anne Joice, Catriona Kent, Sandra Kinnear, Kathryn Mainprize, Willie Munro, Liz Rafferty, Eileen Riddoch, Julie Tiller, Graeme Whitfield, Alison Williams and Stephen Williams. In particular I would like to thank my colleagues and fellow trustees at Triumph over Phobia: Joan Bond, Susan Shaw and Celia Scott-Warren for their helpful comments.

Although their names are not on the front of the workbooks, many others have contributed their insights and clinical experience in ways that have enriched the content. I also wish to thank the various people experiencing problems of anxiety and depression who I have worked with clinically over recent years, and who have used the various worksheets and workbooks. Their inputs have helped shape and refine what you find included here.

The cartoon illustrations in the workbooks have been produced by Keith Chan (kchan75@hotmail.com) and are copyright of Media Innovations Ltd. Keith has been working as a freelance illustrator since leaving Wolverhampton University with a BA Hons degree in illustration. His varying and adaptable style means he has produced work in the fields of greetings cards, children's story books, comic books and magazines.

Finally, I wish to thank my wife Alison who has supported me during the writing of this book and also our daughter Hannah who is always a source of light in my life.

Chris Williams,
September 2003

Introduction: Using the Overcoming Anxiety materials

Problems of anxiety and depression are common difficulties that can affect anyone at some stage in their lives. At any one time, around one in ten people experience levels of anxiety that affect them at such a level as to be defined by doctors as an anxiety disorder. Anxiety can affect people in many different ways – these include worry, generalised anxiety, panic attacks, phobias and obsessive-compulsive disorder. Anxiety may also become focused upon physical health problems and can act to worsen such problems, whatever their original cause.

Overcoming Anxiety is the second book in a series and uses a similar format to the first book, *Overcoming Depression: A Five Areas Approach* (published in 2001 by Arnold). Like that book, *Overcoming Anxiety* uses the popular self-help format and has been designed to be worked through at home in the person's own time with support from a health care practitioner, self-help support group or trusted friend. The materials use modern educational techniques and the evidence-based cognitive behaviour therapy (CBT) approach to help bring about helpful change. The CBT approach has much to teach about worry, fear and panic and provides a valuable resource for those experiencing these common problems. The approach has a proven effectiveness in the treatment of anxiety disorders and also may be helpful for those facing long-term physical health problems.

The structure of the book

The book is arranged in three parts. The workbooks are contained in Parts 1 and 2 and can be used either alone or as part of a complete course. A diagrammatic overview of the course is provided on page xiv.

Part 1: *Understanding anxiety: initial self-assessment* contains Workbooks 1a to 1e, the *Understanding ...* workbooks. They are designed to help the reader to identify their current problem areas. The first, Workbook 1a: *Understanding how anxiety is affecting me*, will help the reader identify which of the other workbooks in Part 1 to read. They cover in turn the topics of *generalised anxiety/worry, panic* and *phobias, obsessive-compulsive disorder* and *how we respond to physical health problems*. Each of these workbooks will help the reader understand more about the ways that anxiety can affect them, using the Five Areas Assessment model to help identify key problem areas for change.

After reading their chosen workbooks in Part 1, the reader will have a clear idea which of the other self-help workbooks to read in Part 2.

Part 2: *Overcoming Anxiety* self-management workbooks and worksheets consists of Workbooks 2–9, which give practical guidance on key areas of self-management:
- Problem solving
- Assertiveness
- How to identify and then challenge extreme and unhelpful thinking
- Overcoming avoidance and unhelpful behaviours
- Overcoming sleep problems
- Using anti-anxiety medications

The worksheets provide information on two quite frequent features of anxiety, hyperventilation and depersonalisation, with some practical advice on possible ways to overcome these problems. Workbook 10, *Planning for the future*, helps summarise what has been learned and assists the reader in planning how to respond to any future problems of anxiety.

The reader can choose to read as many or as few of the workbooks in the course as they wish. The format also encourages dipping into the workbooks as and when they are needed.

Part 3 provides information aimed at health care practitioners and those based in self-help support groups who wish to consider ways of using this approach in their work. It includes a discussion of the self-help approach, a description of how to use self-help with individual patients/clients, and also a description of how to introduce self-help into a clinical service, including how to develop and support a self-help room.

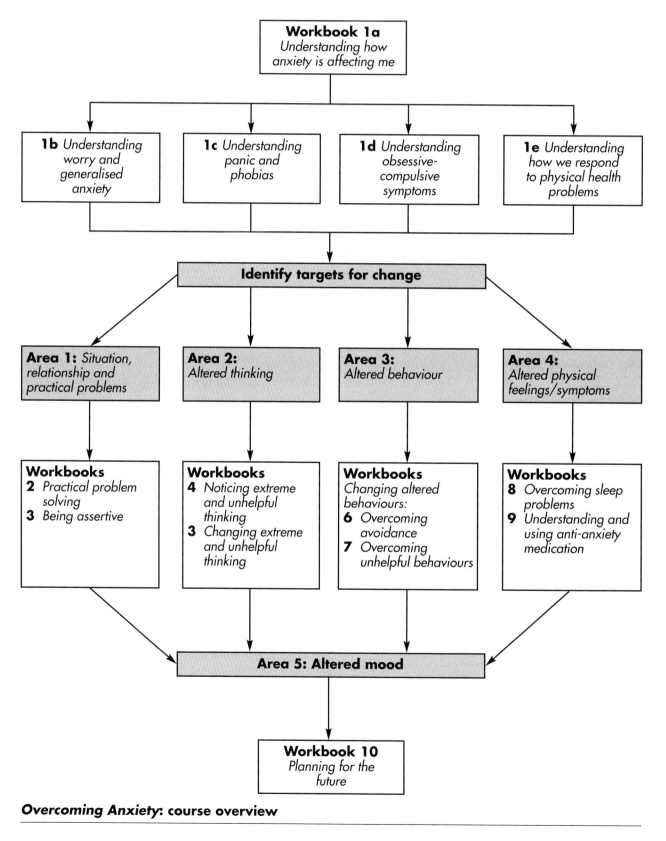

Overcoming Anxiety: course overview

A note for health care practitioners

The workbooks and worksheets in *Overcoming Anxiety* are fully compatible with the model and content of the companion volume, *Overcoming Depression*. In Part 2 the workbooks covering problem solving, assertiveness, noticing and changing extreme and unhelpful thinking, overcoming unhelpful behaviours, overcoming sleep problems and planning for the future are all fully compatible but shorter versions of those found in *Overcoming Depression*. They focus on the essentials in each area and do so concisely and clearly. This allows practitioners who use both books to provide either 'long' or 'shorter' versions of these key workbooks, thus allowing a tailored treatment plan. This is in response to feedback from clinicians that they would find shortened versions of the workbooks of great use for those who prefer a more focused approach. A balance has been struck so that the *Overcoming Anxiety* course contains the full range of key topics needed for the self-assessment and self-management of anxiety, but does so in a way that allows a flexible use of workbooks from the *Overcoming Depression* course. Two workbooks that are unique to the *Overcoming Anxiety* course are included in Part 2 of the book. These are Workbook 6: *Overcoming avoidance* and Workbook 9: *Understanding and using anti-anxiety medication*.

A note about copyright: the materials once purchased in book form may be copied by the owner as many times as required. This includes use both in clinical practice and in training.

If you yourself currently have problems of anxiety

If you are reading this book because you are currently experiencing problems of anxiety, please think about discussing what you learn from it with a few trusted people such as friends, your health care practitioner or others who normally support you – for example, members of your self-help group, church, mosque, synagogue or temple. They may be able to provide useful support for you if you get stuck or wish to ask questions about any of the workbooks. If you would prefer them not to mention your conversation to others, ask them to agree to this and choose these people carefully so that you talk to those whose confidentiality and advice you trust.

Using the workbooks

The content of this book is designed in a way so that you can easily dip in to certain workbooks if they cover particular problem areas you wish to find out about. **You might find it most helpful to read Part 1 of the book first** as this will help you to understand the causes and key areas of self-management that you can use to overcome your problems.

As you read the book, it is important to be realistic in your expectations of how quickly you will improve. Recovery from problems such as anxiety and depression may take a number of months and patience is an important part of recovery. I hope that this book will help you on the way.

As you read each workbook, try to really think about what you are reading, and in particular, consider how what you are reading might apply to you. To help you do this, each workbook is divided into clear sections. If you are feeling very anxious or depressed, you may have noticed that your energy and concentration levels are not as good as they would normally be. If this is true for you, bear it in mind when reading the book. You may find it easier to set yourself the goal of *reading just one section of a workbook at a time*. Try to be realistic as to how much you read at once. Similarly, if you think there is too much to take in at once, it is a good idea to try to read each workbook quite slowly to allow yourself thinking time so that you can get as much out of it as possible.

As you read each section:

- Try to answer all the questions asked. The process of having to **stop, think** *and* **reflect** on how the questions might be relevant to you is a crucial part of getting better.

- You will probably find that some aspects of each workbook are more useful to you at the moment than others. That is normally the case. Just try to focus on the helpful bits that apply to you. **Write down your own notes** of key points in the margins or in the *My notes* area at the end of each workbook to help you remember information that has been helpful. Plan to **review your notes regularly** to help you apply what you have learned.

- Once you have read through an entire workbook, you may find it helpful to **put it on one side and then re-read it a few days later**. It may be that different parts of it become clearer, or seem more useful, on second reading.

- Within each workbook, important areas are labelled as key points. Certain areas that are covered may not be relevant for everyone. Such areas will be clearly identified so that you can choose to skip optional material if you wish.

- Throughout the book, 'real life' examples are provided to help build understanding. All examples have been created for this book.

A note about copyright: The materials once purchased in book form may be copied by the owner as many times as required.

Other ways of accessing treatment

Other self-help materials in the same series

This book is part of a series of self-help resources that address common mental health problems. Additional printed self-help resources in the same series are:

Overcoming Depression: A Five Areas Approach by Chris Williams, published by Arnold (2001). ISBN 0–340–76383–3

I'm not supposed to feel like this: A Christian self-help approach to depression and anxiety by Chris Williams, Paul Richards and Ingrid Whitton, published by Hodder & Stoughton (2002). ISBN 0–340–78639–6.

A computerised interactive version of *Overcoming Depression* aimed at people with depression is published by Media Innovations (www.calipso.co.uk), who act on behalf of the University of Leeds.

Self-help charitable organisations

A range of excellent self-help organisations exists. They can provide a useful source of support and information. The list below is in no way exhaustive.

Triumph over Phobia (TOP UK)

A self-help voluntary organisation that is user-led. It runs self-help groups led by ex-sufferers of phobia, panic and obsessional compulsive disorder. TOP runs self-help groups throughout the UK.

Triumph over Phobia, 7a Bridge Street, Bath, BA2 4AS
Email: triumphoverphobia@compuserve.com
Web address: www.triumphoverphobia.com
Tel: 01225 311582

Obsessive Action

A national organisation for people with obsessive-compulsive disorder (OCD), their carers and interested professionals.

Obsessive Action, Aberdeen Centre, 22–24 Highbury Grove, London, N5 2EA
Email: admin@obsessive-action.demon.co.uk
Web address: www.obsessive-action.demon.co.uk
Tel: 0207 226 4000

National Phobics Society

A national charity run by sufferers and ex-sufferers of anxiety disorders. The aim is to provide information and self-help services. A wide range of anxiety disorders are covered including tranquilliser problems, phobias, obsessive-compulsive disorder, generalised anxiety and panic attacks.

National Phobics Society, Zion Community Resource Centre,
339 Stretford Road, Hulme, Manchester M15 4ZY
Email: natphob.soc@good.co.uk
Web address: www.phobics-society.org.uk
Tel: 0870 7700456

Finding help from a cognitive behaviour therapy practitioner

The first step in accessing local treatment is to discuss the problem with your health care practitioner. Many CBT practitioners work in the NHS. However, some areas still have limited resources. Also, some practitioners provide CBT privately. Your practitioner will be able to advise you on access to local resources and refer you on, if appropriate.

You can also find an accredited CBT therapist by looking at the home page of BABCP – the British Association for Behavioural and Cognitive Psychotherapies. This is the lead body for CBT in the UK. Their website provides information about CBT and free downloadable leaflets. You can obtain useful information about a range of common mental health difficulties. The website has a searchable database of accredited CBT practitioners throughout the UK. Please note that other practitioners offering CBT are also registered by other reputable bodies.

BABCP, The Globe Centre, PO Box 9, Accrington BB5 0XB

Email: info@BABCP.com

Web address: www.babcp.com

Tel: 01254 875277

A request for feedback

An important factor in the development of all the Five Areas Assessment workbooks is that the content is updated on a regular basis, using feedback from users and practitioners. If there are areas which you find hard to understand, or which seem poorly written, please let me know and I will try to improve things in future. I regret that I am unable to provide any specific replies or advice on treatment.

> **To provide feedback, please contact me via:**
> **Email:** Feedback@fiveareas.com
> **Mail:** Dr Chris Williams, Section of Psychological Medicine, Gartnavel Royal Hospital, 1055 Great Western Road, Glasgow, G12 0XH

Part 1

Understanding anxiety: initial self-assessment

Workbook 1a

Understanding how anxiety is affecting me

Dr Chris Williams

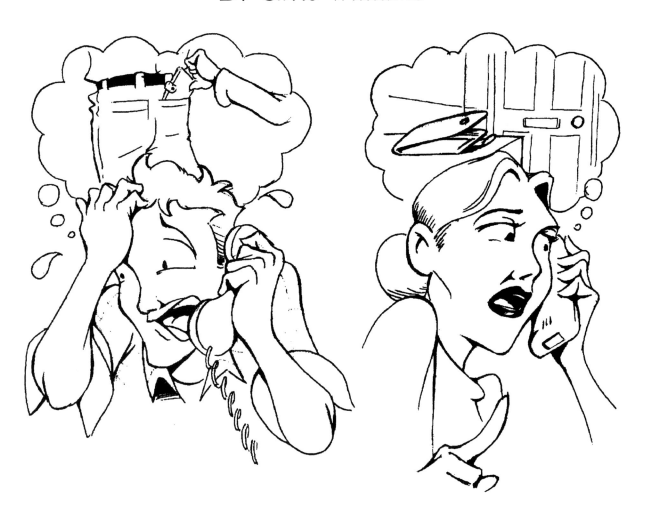

A Five Areas Approach

Section *1*   **Introduction**

How to use this workbook

This workbook is part of the *Overcoming Anxiety* course. It has been written by a practitioner who has many years experience in the Cognitive Behaviour Therapy (CBT) approach. This approach is effective for the treatment of common anxiety problems such as panic, worry, phobias and obsessive-compulsive disorder. It can also be used to provide a useful approach when you are facing problems of physical illness – especially when this has lasted for some time. Self-help treatments using CBT – such as these workbooks – help you to understand more about how your problems are affecting you. The workbooks help you to learn skills that you can use to overcome your anxiety problems.

Each workbook can be read either alone or in addition to other workbooks in the course. Each focuses on a different type of problem. These are worry, panic, phobias, obsessive-compulsive symptoms (OCD) and how you respond to physical health problems.

This first workbook will help you to identify which further workbooks to read to help you overcome your own problems of anxiety. It will cover:
● how to use the workbook most effectively;
● the different ways that anxiety can affect you;
● the Five Areas of Anxiety: the *situations, relationship and practical problems* faced, and the *altered thinking, emotional* and *physical feelings* and *behaviour* that are part of anxiety;
● which workbooks to use to find out more about your own problems of anxiety.

Don't be concerned if any of these words seem new or difficult to understand. All the terms will be described clearly as you read through the workbook.

Take time to read the workbook at your own pace. You don't have to sit down and read it in one go. You may find it most helpful to set yourself the target of reading the workbook one section at a time.
● Try to **answer all the questions** asked. The process of having to *stop, think and reflect* on how the questions might be relevant to you is crucial to getting better.
● **Write down** your own notes in the margins or in the *My notes* area at the back of the workbook to help you remember information that has been helpful. **Plan to review your notes regularly** so that you apply what you have learned.
● Once you have read through the entire workbook once, **put it on one side** and then **re-read it** a few days later. It may be that different parts of it become clearer, or seem more useful on second reading.
● Use the workbook to **build upon the help you receive in other ways,** such as from reading other helpful material, talking to friends, or attending self-help organisations and support groups.
● **Discuss the workbook** with your health care practitioner and those who give you helpful support so that you can work together on overcoming the problems.

Section 2   Understanding anxiety

What is anxiety?

Anxiety, *tension*, *stress*, and *panic* are all terms used to describe what is a widespread problem. Anxiety can affect **anyone**. At any one time, over one in ten people experience high levels of anxiety. Think back to your class at school. In an average class size of thirty, this means that typically three of your classmates will have anxiety problems at the moment. Some well-known people have experienced problems of high anxiety. You may have seen television programmes or read books about their experiences. When anxiety occurs at a high level, it affects the person's *mood* and *thinking*, creates a range of *physical symptoms* in their body, and often causes the person to alter *what they do*.

The anxiety balance

In anxiety the threat or danger being faced is often **overplayed** and built up in our mind. At the same time we usually **underplay** our own capacity to cope with the problem. We become over-sensitive to possible threats so that we can escape and avoid these.

The anxiety balance

In a situation with no anxiety we feel in balance. We know we can deal with our problems.

Threat/difficult situation   My capacity to cope
       ↓_____↓
                                         ⇑

Normally, when there is no anxiety, we feel **able to cope** with the problems we face. In anxiety this balance is upset. An unhelpful focus on problems and difficulties occurs. The problem is seen as too large or overwhelming, and we think we cannot cope. In both situations, the anxiety balance is upset, and the result is increasing distress.

Q. Do I feel in balance at the moment?   Yes ☐   No ☐

The anxiety balance has important implications. It means **that it is not the situation or problem alone that causes anxious worrying, instead it is how we interpret it**. This is not to say that practical problems and difficulties don't need to be dealt with – they do. However, anxious worrying is not an effective solution.

Can anxiety be helpful?

Some level of anxiety is a common and normal emotion, which at times is helpful even though it can feel unpleasant. For example:

- in situations of sudden danger anxiety helps us to get away as rapidly as possible;
- if you walk along a badly maintained path next to a large drop, anxiety can be life-saving, appropriate and helpful.

However, sometimes anxiety can occur inappropriately and then it becomes unhelpful. Anxiety may arise in situations that are not really dangerous at all, or the anxiety can be excessive and well beyond what is actually helpful or appropriate in the circumstances.

How our bodies react to anxiety

Your body reacts to physical danger in a set way. The **fight or flight adrenaline response** creates many different physical and emotional changes. Your heart rate and breathing both speed up so that your muscles are ready to react to defend yourself or run away. This is very useful when the danger is real. Think about a time when you have had a sudden shock – perhaps you have stepped into the road when a car was coming and didn't realise till you heard the car horn. Your body releases adrenaline, which makes your heart beat faster. The fight or flight adrenaline response causes you to pay especial attention to any potential threats around you. In the same way, your body reacts to frightening thoughts just as it would to a physical danger. You can find out more about this in the other workbooks of this course.

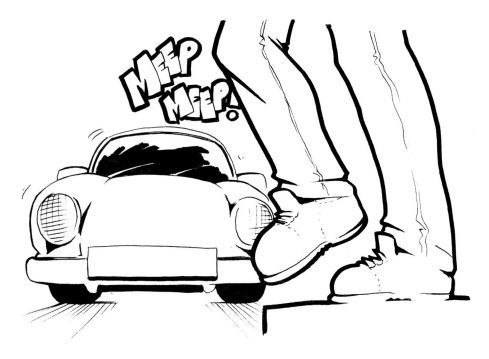

Key point: Anxiety is an uncomfortable experience. It can affect your thinking and feelings, create physical symptoms in your body, and interfere with your daily activities. Each of these changes can then act to keep anxiety going. If you are experiencing anxiety, you need to find out more about how anxiety is affecting you so that you will have a clear plan of what you need to do to overcome it.

The next section of this workbook will help you find out about the different ways in which anxiety can affect you.

Section 3 Understanding anxiety using the Five Areas Assessment approach

One helpful way of understanding the impact of anxiety on us is to consider the ways that anxiety affects different areas of our life. A **Five Areas Assessment** approach can help us to do this by examining in detail five important aspects of our lives. These are our:

- Life situation, relationships and practical problems.
- Altered thinking.
- Altered feelings (also called emotions or moods).
- Altered physical symptoms/feelings in the body.
- Altered behaviour or activity levels.

Think about how the Five Areas Assessment can help us understand the following two situations involving John and Anne.

Situation 1: John's wallet

John is going shopping. As he gets ready to leave home, he suddenly realises that he cannot find his wallet **(=life situation/practical problem)**. He jumps immediately to the very worst conclusion that his wallet and credit cards have been stolen last time he was out **(=altered thinking)**. This makes him feel very anxious and panicky. What he thinks has affected how he feels **(=altered feelings/emotions)**. He begins to notice a sick feeling in his stomach. He also feels quite sweaty and clammy and has a tense feeling in his head **(=altered physical symptoms)**. He immediately contacts his credit card agency and bank to cancel the cards **(=altered behaviour)**.

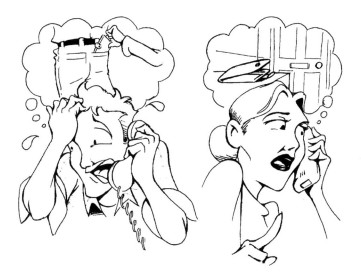

He then phones his friend Anne to tell her what has happened. She is sympathetic and encourages John to try to remember where he last saw the wallet. Anne suggests that he looks around the house to see if he can find it. John thanks her and is pleased that he has called her because he feels a little better as a result. He promises to phone Anne back that evening to let her know if he finds the wallet.

Later that day he finds the wallet in his coat pocket. He realises he had forgotten he put it there yesterday. He then tried to avoid seeing or talking to Anne because he is worried that she will think he is *'a right fool'*. He doesn't phone her back that evening to let her know he has found the wallet.

How John interpreted the situation was both *extreme* and *unhelpful.* He ended up feeling very anxious and physically unwell. He now is unable to use his credit cards as a result of his unfounded fears.

The following diagram presents the Five Areas Assessment as applied to John's situation. It links these five areas to make sense of what happens when we have strong emotions of anxiety – or of depression, anger or shame.

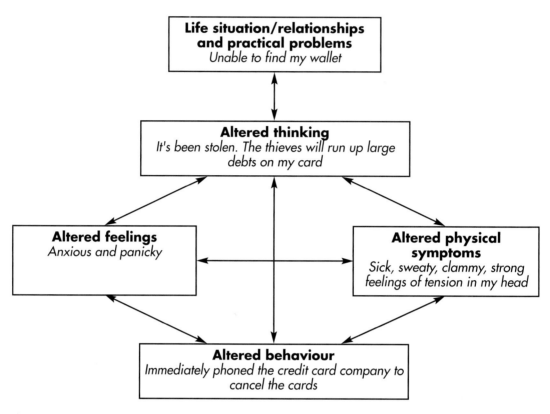

John's Five Areas Assessment

The five areas diagram shows that what we think about a situation or problem may affect how we feel physically and emotionally, and also alters what we do (behaviour or activity levels). Look at the arrows in the diagram. The five areas (*situation*, *relationship* or *practical problems*, *thinking*, *emotional* and *physical feelings*, and *behaviour* changes) are interconnected and affect one another.

Think about how well John's reactions in the diagram can be explained using this approach. You may find the diagram difficult to understand at first, or you may not be sure whether it applies to you.

How do John's *thoughts, and physical/emotional reactions* fit together? How does what he thought about the situation affect how he felt?

How do John's *thoughts and behaviour* fit together? How does what he thought about the situation affect what he did?

What do you think of his interpretation of what had happened (immediately *jumping to the very worst conclusion* that the wallet was stolen) and his prediction that Anne will think badly of him (sometimes called *mind-reading*)?

How could John have altered how he felt and what he did (immediately cancelling the cards and then failing to phone Anne after he found the wallet again)?

Situation 2: Anne fears a broken friendship

Anne is wondering why John has not phoned her back to tell her if he has found his wallet. He promised he would do so (=**life situation/relationship**). Why hasn't he? Anne begins to worry that she may have sounded irritable towards John. The fact is that he has phoned her many times in similar situations, when he has lost something important, and it usually turns up after he has searched for a while. He just doesn't look properly at first. Oh dear, thinks Anne, she must have sounded irritable towards John. She was not supportive enough, and did not behave like a true friend (=**altered thinking**). She blames herself for upsetting him and not being a good friend and feels guilty (=**altered emotions**). That night Anne can't relax (=**altered physical sensations**) and lies awake worrying that she has upset John and harmed their friendship. She decides not to phone him for a few days (=**altered behaviour**) because she is not sure how he will react if she really has upset him. Perhaps he will break off their friendship?

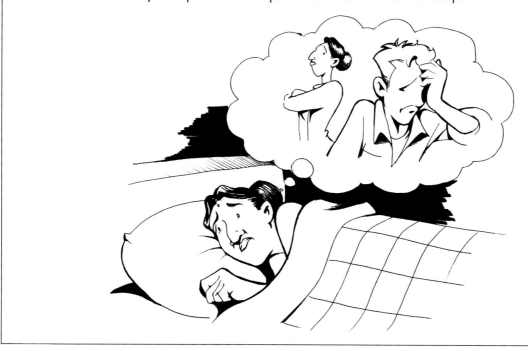

The following diagram presents Anne's Five Areas Assessment.

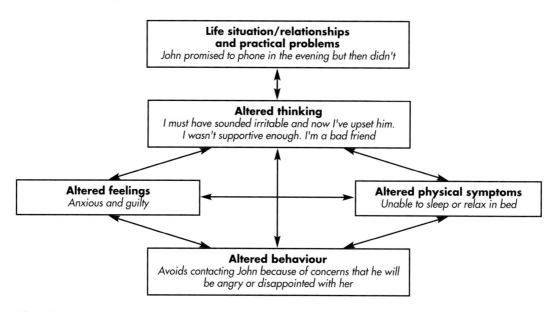

Life situation/relationships and practical problems
John promised to phone in the evening but then didn't

Altered thinking
I must have sounded irritable and now I've upset him. I wasn't supportive enough. I'm a bad friend

Altered feelings
Anxious and guilty

Altered physical symptoms
Unable to sleep or relax in bed

Altered behaviour
Avoids contacting John because of concerns that he will be angry or disappointed with her

Anne's Five Areas Assessment

How do Anne's *thoughts* and *physical/emotional reactions* fit together?

How do Anne's *thoughts* and her *behaviour* fit together?

Did her fear that she had upset John affect how she felt and what she did?   Yes ☐   No ☐

Were her thoughts that she had upset John accurate and helpful?

How did her worries alter how she felt emotionally?

How could she have checked out what John really thought?

In these two examples, the person's fears (*jumping to the very worst conclusion* and *mind-reading* what the other person thought) led them to feel more anxious. Something that took only a few minutes on the phone resulted in much worry over the following hours. It also unhelpfully affected how they behaved. In both Anne's and John's case, in spite of their worries, neither of them actually did something to check out how their friend had actually reacted. If they had done so, they would have realised quite how wrong and unhelpful their fears were.

These examples also show that it is not necessarily the events themselves that cause upset, but the **interpretation** the person makes of the event. In anxiety and depression, we tend to develop extreme, negative and unhelpful thinking styles. These thoughts can build up out of all proportion, and unhelpfully affect how we feel and what we do. This then can keep the feelings of distress going.

You will have the opportunity at the end of this workbook to begin to see whether the Five Areas approach can help you understand how anxiety is affecting you.

Section 4   The different ways anxiety can affect you

Anxiety tends to affect people in the same sort of way again and again. For example, some people always notice a headache or eyestrain when they become anxious. Others notice their anxiety in other ways. They may become prone to worry and turn things over in their minds again and again. In some their anxiety can reach a very high level and they feel panicky. Sometimes compulsive rituals enslave them and the person feels compelled to repeat a certain action over and over.

The following few pages will help you to find out more about these different ways that anxiety can affect you. It is important to realise that problems of anxiety and depression often occur together, as well as separately. Because of this you will find out more about depression as well as about the different ways anxiety can affect you.

What is depression and how can it affect anxiety levels?

Feeling fed up and low in mood is a normal part of life. When difficulties or upsetting events occur it is not unusual to feel down and stop enjoying things. Likewise when good things happen, a person may experience happiness, pleasure and a sense of really being able to achieve things in life. The reasons for low mood are usually clear. This includes a stressful situation, a relationship difficulty, feeling let down by someone, financial difficulties, unforeseen events or some other practical problem. Most of the time the drop in mood only lasts for a short period of time and then we 'bounce back'.

Occasionally, however, this 'depressed' feeling can worsen and completely dominate our life. When someone feels very low for more than two weeks, doctors call this a *depressive illness*. It is important to say that depression is very common and no one should feel ashamed if they are diagnosed with depression. The term describes a broad range of symptoms that vary from person to person but which have an unhelpful impact on their lives. Depression and anxiety often occur together – with up to one in five people noticing both problems at the same time. Depression can worsen problems such as anxiety. If this is the case for you then treatment of the depression may result in a marked improvement in your anxiety problems too.

The following checklist will help you to identify whether you have any of the common symptoms of depression.

Depression checklist

Situation, relationship and practical problems

Q. Have I had any recent significant life losses or life difficulties?   Yes ☐   No ☐

Altered thinking

Q. Have I become very much more critical of myself?   Yes ☐   No ☐

Q. Am I very negative about things in general?   Yes ☐   No ☐

Q. Am I sometimes hopeless about the future and the possibility of recovery?   Yes ☐   No ☐

Q. Am I finding it more difficult to keep my mind focused on things?   Yes ☐   No ☐

Altered feelings

Q. Do I feel depressed or weepy?   Yes ☐   No ☐

Q. Is my ability to enjoy things lower than normal?   Yes ☐   No ☐

Altered physical symptoms

Q. Has there been a change in my appetite, energy levels, or sleep?   Yes ☐   No ☐

Altered behaviour

Q. Have I begun to reduce or stop doing things that previously gave me a
sense of pleasure or achievement?   Yes ☐   No ☐

Q. Have I begun to be less socially active/staying in more?   Yes ☐   No ☐

If you have answered **Yes** to questions in most of the five areas, you are probably experiencing a depressive illness. This depression is affecting your thinking, feelings, body, behaviour and social activities to a significant extent. Talk to your health care practitioner to find out more about this. They will be able to offer you important information that will help you to work out together whether you are experiencing a depressive disorder.

Next step: Depression and anxiety often occur together. Even if you think depression may be a problem for you, you may still gain useful information from the current workbook. If you want to find out more about depression, please discuss this with your health care practitioner.

What are worry and generalised anxiety?

Worrying thoughts are common in anxiety.

> **Definition:** *In worry, we anxiously go over things again and again in a way that is unhelpful because it does not actually help us sort out the difficulties that we are worried about.*

Sometimes the worry may be out of all proportion. For example, something that originally happened in a few moments, such as something that someone has said to you, can be on your mind for much of the following days or weeks. This can add up in total to many days or even weeks of worry over the following months. You may also find that you are feeling worried without being too sure what you are worrying about.

People who worry about very many things in life are sometimes described as having problems of *generalised anxiety*. Overall, about one in twelve people have problems of generalised anxiety at any one time. This means that several people in your own road/street are likely to have problems of anxious worry at the moment.

The following checklist will help you to identify whether you have any of the common symptoms of worry.

Worry/generalised anxiety checklist

Q. Am I worried about things on most days and find it difficult to stop worrying?   Yes ☐   No ☐

Q. Am I anxiously going over things again and again in my mind in a way that hasn't actually helped me sort out my problems?   Yes ☐   No ☐

Q. Have I become over-sensitive to possible difficulties and potential threats?   Yes ☐   No ☐

Q. Am I downplaying my own ability to overcome these problems?   Yes ☐   No ☐

Q. Do anxious worries cause me to feel physically on edge and tense?   Yes ☐   No ☐

Q. Do I feel mentally and physically tired as a result of worry?   Yes ☐   No ☐

Q. Do I have problems sleeping because of worry?   Yes ☐   No ☐

Q. Have anxious thoughts caused me to reduce or stop what I do?   Yes ☐   No ☐

Q. Have worrying thoughts caused me to avoid dealing with difficult situations or people?   Yes ☐   No ☐

If you have answered **Yes** to several of these questions, then generalised anxiety is a problem for you.

Next step: Make sure you finish reading the current workbook. You should then read Workbook 1b: *Understanding worry and generalised anxiety.*

What are panic attacks?

Sometimes anxiety can be so strong, and we feel so mentally and physically tense and unwell that we stop what we are doing and try to leave or escape the situation. Sometimes we may feel paralysed into inactivity like rabbits caught in the headlamps of a car and freeze, expecting disaster to strike at any moment. This feeling of acute fear, dread or terror is called a *panic attack*. Panic attacks rarely last longer than 20–30 minutes.

During panic, there are strong beliefs that something terrible or catastrophic is happening right now. Common fears are '*I'm going to faint*', '*I'm going to suffocate*' '*I'm going to collapse*', '*I'm going to have a stroke*', or '*I'm going to have a heart attack*'. Sometimes the fear is of *going mad* or *losing control*. The fear is always immediately threatening, scary and catastrophic. We may then become overly aware of the anxious fears and quickly stop what we are doing, and hurry away from the situation.

In some cases, there isn't fear of any specific catastrophe but we still experience a panic attack.

This occurs when other upsets or fears build up and up in our minds. At least one in ten people experience a panic attack at some time in their lives.

Panic attack checklist

Q. Do I notice anxiety that rises to a peak? Yes ☐ No ☐

Q. Do I feel mentally very scared and physically unwell during the panic? Yes ☐ No ☐

Q. Do I fear that something terrible/catastrophic will happen during the panic? Yes ☐ No ☐

Q. Do I become overly aware of the things that I fear might happen during panic? Yes ☐ No ☐

Q. Am I downplaying my own ability to overcome these problems? Yes ☐ No ☐

Q. Do I stop what I am doing and try to immediately escape or leave when I feel like this? Yes ☐ No ☐

If you have answered **Yes** to several of these questions, then panic may be a problem for you. Talk to your health care practitioner about this.

Next step: Make sure you finish reading the current workbook. You should then read Workbook 1c: *Understanding panic and phobias.*

What is a phobia?

You may have friends or relatives who are very scared of creatures such as spiders, or of situations such as heights, or you yourself may have such fears. Sometimes we may become so fearful that even just thinking about the feared situation can result in strong feelings of panic. We may avoid anything to do with that situation as a result. This can lead to an increasingly restricted lifestyle, lack of confidence and additional long-term distress. When this occurs, we are described as having a **phobia**. Phobias, worry, depression and panic attacks commonly occur together.

Definition: A *phobia* describes high anxiety (often with panic attacks) that regularly occurs in a particular situation. We become overly aware of any possible threats relating to our fear and try to avoid or quickly leave any situations, people or places that cause us to feel anxious. We often know logically that the situation will not harm or kill us, yet we experience the anxiety anyway.

There are many different types of phobia:
- **Avoidance of specific situations or objects.** For example, a common phobia is a fear of heights. Almost any object can become a cause of phobic fear. Common ones are wasps, or spiders.
- **Avoidance of one-to-one and other conversations with people.** This is called *social phobia* where there is excessive shyness and very high anxiety in social situations. Sometimes there may be a more focused fear of public speaking to a large group of people. For example, a teacher may become anxious leading a class.
- **Avoidance of specific places.** You may have heard of people who have panic attacks on buses or in shops or other crowded situations where it is difficult to escape. This is called *agoraphobia* – one of the most common forms of phobia.

Virtually any situation, place or person/group can become the focus of a phobia. Each phobia has a specific name. The description above summarises the main types that occur.

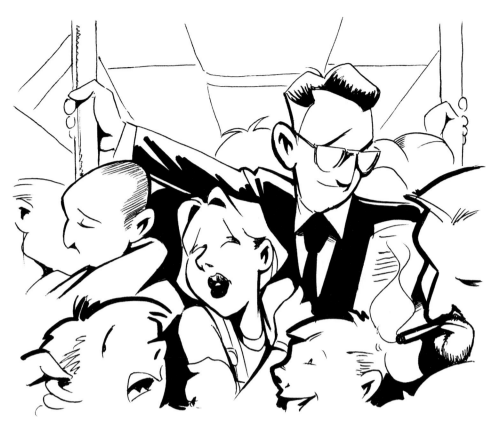

Phobia checklist

Q. Do I notice strong feelings of anxiety or panic when I face particular situations, people or places?   Yes ☐   No ☐

Q. Does even thinking about these situations, places or people make me feel nervous?   Yes ☐   No ☐

Q. Have I become overly sensitive to anything to do with the phobic fear?   Yes ☐   No ☐

Q. Am I downplaying my own ability to overcome these fears?   Yes ☐   No ☐

Q. Am I avoiding these situations, places or people?   Yes ☐   No ☐

Q. Overall, am I living an increasingly restricted lifestyle as a result?   Yes ☐   No ☐

If you have answered **Yes** to any of these questions, then you may have a phobia. Talk to your health care practitioner about this.

Next step: Make sure you finish reading the current workbook. You should then read Workbook 1c: *Understanding panic and phobias.*

What are obsessions and compulsions?

In obsessive-compulsive disorder (OCD), the main features seen are:
- obsessional thoughts;
- compulsive behaviours.

These usually occur together.

Obsessional thoughts

The term *obsessional thought* describes a situation where the person repeatedly notices that anxious or upsetting thoughts pop into mind again and again and again. A milder form of this experience is quite common in society. Many people occasionally have the experience of noticing that a tune or piece of music seems to get 'stuck' and goes round and round in their mind for a time before eventually disappearing. In most cases this is seen as either 'okay' (the person just hums along) or slightly annoying and frustrating. Eventually it stops.

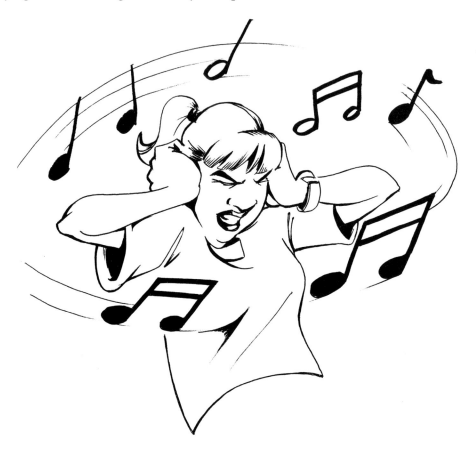

The big difference in obsessive-compulsive disorder is that the thought *continues* to go round and round for a very long time in spite of efforts by the person to stop thinking it. Because the thoughts are so distressing, the person becomes overly aware of them, and tries hard not to think the upsetting thought.

Key point: Common obsessional thoughts can include a fear of hurting or damaging others in some way, or of causing harm through not having done something. The person is worried that something really bad will happen as a result. They may know rationally that no such harm is really *likely* to occur, yet in spite of this, the worrying fears dominate their thinking. Sometimes obsessive thinking results in the person becoming crippled by doubt about a particular issue. They go round and round trying to answer the question to the very last detail, yet find it impossible to reach a conclusion.

Compulsive actions

Because obsessive thoughts are so scary and upsetting, the person with obsessive-compulsive disorder may try to avoid them or prevent harm occurring as a result. This can involve:

- trying hard to avoid thinking the obsessional thoughts in the first place;
- carrying out mental rituals such as thinking particular words, phrases or prayers in order to make the thoughts feel 'right' or 'safe';
- carrying out activities or behaviours to prevent or reverse the harmful consequence occurring: for example, repeatedly checking that the light switches are off, endlessly cleaning the house, or washing hands to an excessive extent;
- avoiding any situations that they fear may cause things to get worse.

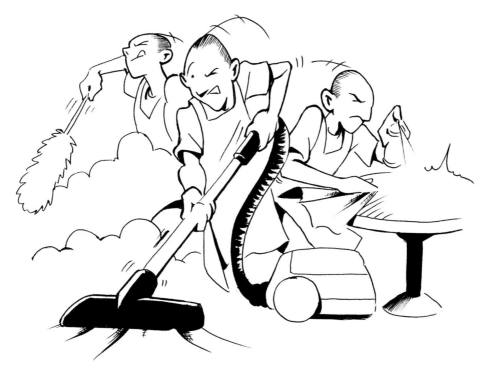

These actions might in moderation be seen as sensible and appropriate (e.g. checking the door is locked once at night before going to bed is a quite sensible and reasonable thing to do); however in obsessive-compulsive disorder things gets completely out of hand. The compulsions can dominate and lead to an increasingly restricted life.

Obsessive-compulsive checklist

Obsessive thinking

Q. Do I have thoughts, memories, impulses, images or ideas that seem to go
round and round in my mind? Yes ☐ No ☐

Q. Are these thoughts unpleasant and/or upsetting to me? Yes ☐ No ☐

Q. Do I think that I am guilty and overly responsible for bad things occurring? Yes ☐ No ☐

Q. Have I become overly sensitive to these thoughts/fears? Yes ☐ No ☐

Q. Am I downplaying my own ability to overcome these problems? Yes ☐ No ☐

Q. Do I dwell on things I have (or could have) done that *might* result in
harm to others? Yes ☐ No ☐

Q. Do I fear I *might* lose control and do something that will harm or upset others? Yes ☐ No ☐

Q. Do I worry that things I haven't done properly *might* result in harm to others? Yes ☐ No ☐

Q. Do I have doubts and go over the same questions again and again with no
chance of ever finding a solution? Yes ☐ No ☐

Compulsions

Q. Do I recurrently carry out mental rituals such as counting or deliberately
thinking 'good' thoughts/saying prayers to make things feel 'right'? Yes ☐ No ☐

Q. Do I compulsively check, clean or do things a set number of times or in
exactly the 'correct' order so as to make things 'right'? Yes ☐ No ☐

If you have answered **Yes** to several of these questions, then you may have obsessive-compulsive
disorder. Talk to your health care practitioner about this.

Next step: Make sure you finish reading the current workbook. You should then read Workbook
1d: *Understanding obsessive-compulsive symptoms (OCD)*.

Facing problems of physical illness

Physical illness affects different aspects of our lives. It creates many challenges for us as individuals.
The Five Areas approach can help us to understand the impact of physical illness on our lives. It can
also help us to identify certain actions and strategies that help us cope with illness.

Choice point: If you have problems with physical health problems, read the rest of this section of
the workbook. If you don't have physical health problems please move to the start of the next section
of the workbook.

Psychological approaches can help us to respond more effectively when we are ill. They can be useful
when you are struggling to cope with ill health. It is not surprising in such situations that there is a
psychological impact of illness, for illness affects all aspects of how we feel, not just our bodies. The
course addresses two key physical health problems: *living with the challenge of physical illness* and
also *health anxiety*.

Living with the challenge of physical illness

Physical illness has a significant impact on how we feel. Especially when symptoms are long-term, we can become demoralised, frustrated or ground down. We may have all sorts of uncertainties or fears about illness, and whether we will be able to cope. These anxieties about our symptoms can sometimes worsen how we feel.

There may be many things we can no longer do because of illness. This might include going for a walk or playing sport as well as the numerous everyday things that make up our life. In severe illness this can include core tasks such as our ability to get up, care and cook for ourselves. We may also be unable to continue to work. This can lead to a loss of income and all the positive things that work previously offered us such as a role, a structure to our day and a regular income. There are many uncertainties, doubts and fears about the future.

Illness not only affects us, it also affects those around us – family, neighbours and friends. Some may not know what to say or do to help us beyond sending initial 'Get-well' cards and flowers. Sometimes the support you first received starts to fall away. There can be a cost to those who offer us care and support. Sometimes they struggle to cope in supporting us. Occasionally, our health care practitioners may not be able to provide the type of support we need.

Illness affects our activity levels and our ability to socialise. You may find that you end up cutting down or stopping things in life that previously gave you a sense of pleasure or achievement. You may become uncertain about what activities you can safely do, and which may worsen how you feel. You may do things to improve how you feel. However, sometimes we can choose actions that actually worsen how we feel. For example, we may drink too much, or try other unhelpful behaviours that backfire and worsen how we feel. Sometimes we are so preoccupied by illness that it comes to dominate our life and other things are squeezed out.

Identifying problems in coping with longer-term physical illness: a checklist

Q. Am I currently facing the challenge of physical illness?   Yes ☐   No ☐

Q. Do I have problems coping with how I feel physically?   Yes ☐   No ☐

Q. Do I feel demoralised, frustrated or ground down at times by how I feel physically?   Yes ☐   No ☐

Q. Do I feel uncertain or anxious about the future impact of my illness?   Yes ☐   No ☐

Q. Have I had to stop or reduce doing things that previously gave me a sense of pleasure or achievement?   Yes ☐   No ☐

Q. Do I find it difficult keeping up with the core activities of life such as getting up, cooking, cleaning etc.?   Yes ☐   No ☐

Q. Is anyone I know unsure about how to best support me?   Yes ☐   No ☐

Q. Do I find that anyone who offers me support has started to drift away from me?   Yes ☐   No ☐

Q. Is my health care practitioner able to offer me the kind of supportive care I need?   Yes ☐   No ☐

Q. Is anyone I know who offers me care and support struggling to cope themselves at the moment?   Yes ☐   No ☐

If you have answered **Yes** to any of these questions, then your physical illness is having a significant impact on you or others.

Next step: Make sure you finish reading the current workbook. You should then read Workbook 1e: *Understanding how we respond to physical health problems.*

Health anxiety

Anxious worrying can sometimes focus upon how we feel physically. In health anxiety, we fear that we have one or more serious illnesses. This results in many visits to doctors or other health care practitioners because we feel ill. In health anxiety the results of all examinations and investigations show no evidence of serious illness. The health fears remain none the less and we continue to feel ill.

In health anxiety we may be reluctant to even consider the possibility that anxiety may be part of the problem. Sometimes our relatives or health care practitioners suspect the 'diagnosis' even before we recognise it ourselves. This is because in health anxiety we do actually feel physically ill. Each of the actions we do is a sensible response in the face of illness. What marks out the problem as health anxiety is the fact that anxiety exaggerates the health-seeking behaviours to an unhelpful degree. The health fears dominate our thinking and worsen how we feel. This causes us to react in ways that worsen the situation. We become overly aware of how our body feels. We may seek excessive reassurance from others, or spend all our time monitoring how we feel. This may include doing things such as looking in the mirror, or constantly checking for lumps. These actions can become part of the problem.

Health anxiety checklist

Q. Do I feel very anxious whenever I think about my physical health?   Yes ☐   No ☐

Q. Am I going to the doctor far more than I used to?   Yes ☐   No ☐

Q. Am I thinking again and again about how ill I feel, yet my doctor's tests seem to show no strong evidence of a physical illness?   Yes ☐   No ☐

Q. Am I finding it difficult accepting that the physical tests and investigations show little or no strong evidence of a physical illness?   Yes ☐   No ☐

Q. Am I constantly examining myself (e.g. taking my pulse or temperature or checking myself for lumps or looking at myself in the mirror)?   Yes ☐   No ☐

Q. Am I constantly aware of how my body feels and paying particular attention to symptoms that especially worry me?   Yes ☐   No ☐

Q. Has my own health care practitioner or someone else that I would usually trust told me that they think I am too worried about my health?   Yes ☐   No ☐

If you have answered **Yes** to several of these questions, then you may have problems of health anxiety.

Next step: Make sure you finish reading the current workbook. You should then read Workbook 1e: *Understanding how we respond to physical health problems.*

You have now been introduced to the areas covered by the workbooks contained in the course. The final section will help you review which workbooks you choose to use as part of your own plan to move forwards.

Section 5 **Next steps**

Look back at your answers to the questions in the previous section. Then use the following table to help you summarise which workbooks are right for you to read next. If you have identified several workbooks you could start with the one that is highest in the table. Read this one and then work your way through any others in order. Alternatively, choose to read the one that addresses the area that you think is causing you the most problems at the moment. You may find it helpful to discuss this with your health care practitioner or someone else whose support you find helpful.

Workbook	Plan to read	Tick when completed
1a: *Understanding how anxiety is affecting me*	✔	
1b: *Understanding worry and generalised anxiety*		
1c: *Understanding panic and phobias*		
1d: *Understanding obsessive-compulsive symptoms (OCD)*		
1e: *Understanding how we respond to physical health problems*		

Each of the workbooks will help you find out more about how anxiety is affecting you. You will also complete your own detailed Five Areas Assessment in each problem area you have identified. This will help you to identify which further steps you need to make in order to move forwards.

Summary

In this workbook you have covered:
- how to use the workbooks found in the *Overcoming Anxiety* course;
- the different ways that anxiety can affect you;
- the Five Areas of Anxiety: the *situations, relationship and practical problems* faced, and the *altered thinking, feelings/emotions, physical symptoms* and *behaviour* that are part of anxiety;
- which workbooks to use to find out more about your own problems of anxiety.

Putting into practice what you have learned

Experience has shown that you are likely to make the most progress if you are able to put into practice what you have learned in the workbook. Each workbook will encourage you to do this by suggesting certain tasks for you to carry out in the following days.

Please can you:
- Read through the current workbook again and think in detail about how anxiety is affecting your thinking, emotional and physical feelings, and behaviour. Think about which areas you want to change.

- Choose **two episodes** over the next week when you feel more anxious. If your problem is of physical illness, instead choose times when you feel physically or emotionally worse. Use the blank Five Areas Assessment sheet that follows this section to record the impact on your thinking, mood, body and behaviour at that time. Try to generate a summary of what you notice in each of the five areas (life situation, relationships and practical problems, altered thinking, feelings, physical symptoms and behaviour). Look back to the *John's wallet* example (p. 1a.5) to help you do this. Please photocopy or draw out additional copies of the assessment sheet as you need it.
- Finally, review your list of which workbook(s) you will use and in your own time move on to your first choice.

If you have difficulties with these tasks, don't worry. Just do what you can. If you have found any aspects of this workbook unhelpful, upsetting or confusing, please can you discuss this with your health care practitioner or someone else whose opinion you trust.

A request for feedback

An important factor in the development of all the Five Areas Assessment workbooks is that the content is updated on a regular basis based upon feedback from users and practitioners. If there are areas which you find hard to understand, or which seem poorly written, please let me know and I will try to improve things in future. I regret that I am unable to provide any specific replies or advice on treatment.

> **To provide feedback, please contact me via**
>
> **Email:** Feedback@fiveareas.com
>
> **Mail:** Dr Chris Williams, Department of Psychological Medicine, Gartnavel Royal Hospital, 1055 Great Western Road, Glasgow, G12 0XH

Acknowledgements

I wish to thank all those who have commented upon this workbook especially Frances Cole, Sandra Johnston, Willie Munro, Liz Rafferty, and Stephen Williams.

The cartoon illustrations in the Workbooks have been produced by Keith Chan (kchan75@hotmail.com) and are copyright of Media Innovations Ltd.

My notes

....
....
....
....
....
....
....
....
....
....
....
....
....
....
....
....
....
....
....
....
....
....
....
....
....

My notes

....

Worksheet: A Five Areas Assessment of a specific time when I feel more anxious/worse

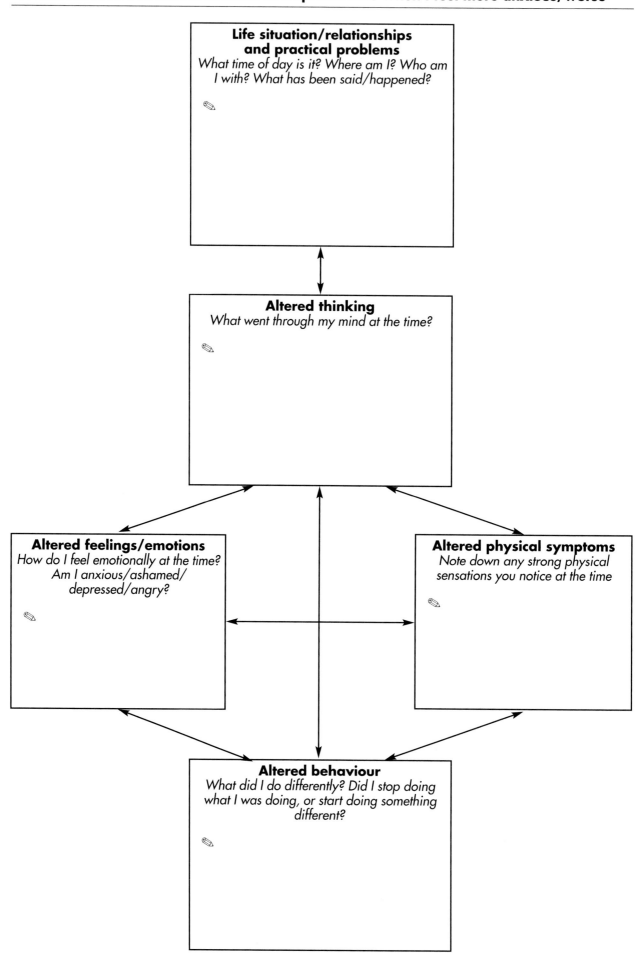

Workbook 1b
Understanding worry and generalised anxiety

Dr Chris Williams

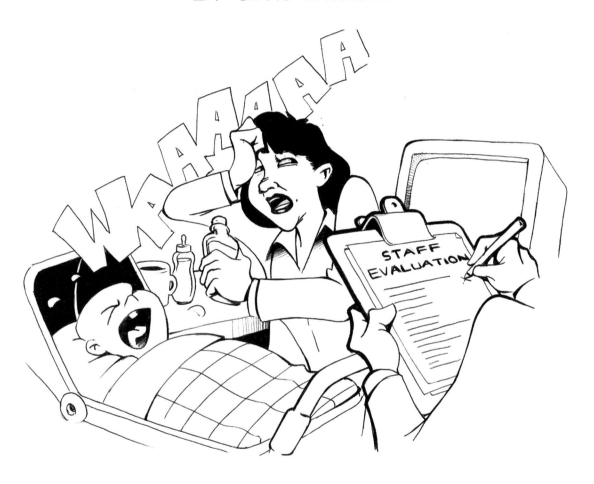

A Five Areas Approach

Section 1 **Introduction**

This workbook will cover:
- how to use the workbook most effectively;
- the key elements of worry and of generalised anxiety – so that you will understand how anxiety can affect you;
- the impact of how what you think can affect how you feel and alter what you do;
- the Five Areas of Anxiety: the *situations, relationship and practical problems* faced, and the *altered thinking, emotional* and *physical feelings* and *behaviour* that occur as part of anxiety;
- the areas you need to tackle in order to overcome your own problems of anxiety.

Don't be concerned if any of these words seem new or difficult to understand. All the terms will be described clearly as you read through the workbook.

How to use this workbook

Take time to read the workbook at your own pace. You don't have to sit down and read it in one go. You might find it most helpful to set yourself the target of reading the workbook one section at a time.
- Try to **answer all the questions** asked. The process of having to *stop, think and reflect* on how the questions might be relevant to you is crucial to getting better.
- **Write down** your own notes in the margins or in the *My notes* area at the back of the workbook to help you remember information that has been helpful. **Plan to review your notes regularly** so that you apply what you have learned.
- Once you have read through the entire workbook once, **put it on one side** and then **re-read it** a few days later. It may be that different parts of it become clearer, or seem more useful on second reading.
- Use the workbook to **build upon the help you receive in other ways**, such as from reading other helpful material, talking to friends, or attending self-help organisations and support groups.
- **Discuss the workbook** with your health care practitioner and those who give you helpful support so that you can work together on overcoming the problems.
- **Remember that although change can seem difficult at first, it is possible.**

Understanding anxiety

Anxiety, tension, stress, and *panic* are all terms that are used to describe what is a widespread problem for many people. Anxiety can affect everyone and anyone.

Can anxiety be helpful?

Anxiety is a common and normal emotion, which can be helpful even though it can feel unpleasant. For example, at lower levels it can help motivate us to prepare for events such as interviews or exams. Anxiety is also helpful in situations of sudden danger, where it helps us to respond and get away as rapidly as possible. The problem is when we feel anxious in situations that are not dangerous at all. Another problem is feeling anxious well beyond what is helpful in the circumstances. For example, being so anxious that you cannot relax or sleep.

What are worry and generalised anxiety?

Worrying thoughts are common in anxiety.

> **Definition:** *In worry, we anxiously go over things again and again in a way that is unhelpful because it does not actually help us sort out the difficulties that we are worried about.*

Worry causes us to think again and again about things that have occurred in the past. It can also focus on things in the present, or what might be in the future. This type of widespread anxious worrying is sometimes described as *generalised anxiety* – we feel generally anxious about very many things in life. Because people don't often want to talk about mental health problems you may think you are the only person to have these difficulties. This is not true. You may be surprised to learn that about one in twelve people currently experience problems of generalised anxiety. There are likely to be at least one or two people living quite near to you in your street who currently are experiencing problems with anxiety. There will also be people who have experienced problems of anxiety in the past.

In anxiety, we often overplay the threat or danger we are facing, and at the same time usually downplay our own capacity to cope with the problem. It also causes us to be overly sensitive to possible threats and difficulties. Little things that ordinarily wouldn't upset really seem to strike home. Tears may be near to the surface. A wave of anxiety can seem to carry you from worry to worry, resulting in physical and mental tension. You may think that you cannot cope with the demands you face, or the demands you place upon yourself. Things seem too much. There is no rest from the problems, nor can you stop thinking about them. Anxiety affects all aspects of your life. You may be clumsier and make more mistakes. Attempts to get things right further add to anxiety and become just one more thing to beat yourself up about. Does this sound like you?

The following checklist will help you to identify whether you have any of the common symptoms of anxious worrying:

Generalised anxiety checklist

Q. Am I worried about things on most days and find it difficult to stop worrying?   Yes ☐   No ☐

Q. Am I anxiously going over things again and again in my mind in a way that hasn't actually helped me sort out my problems?   Yes ☐   No ☐

Q. Have I become over sensitive to possible difficulties and potential threats?   Yes ☐   No ☐

Q. Am I downplaying my own ability to overcome these problems?   Yes ☐   No ☐

Q. Do anxious worries cause me to feel physically on edge and tense?   Yes ☐   No ☐

Q. Do I feel mentally and physically tired as a result of worry?   Yes ☐   No ☐

Q. Do I have problems sleeping because of worry?   Yes ☐   No ☐

Q. Have anxious thoughts caused me to reduce or stop what I do?   Yes ☐   No ☐

Q. Have worrying thoughts caused me to avoid dealing with difficult situations or people?   Yes ☐   No ☐

If you have answered **Yes** to several of these questions, then generalised anxiety is a problem for you.

Worrying thoughts can also occur mixed in with other problems

- Depression often causes anxious worrying. Here, depressing thoughts are linked in with low mood, a lack of enjoyment and reduced activity. If you think you may be depressed then you should talk to your health care practitioner about this to find out more.
- Panic attacks may occur with high levels of anxiety and fear. If you think this might apply to you, Workbook 1c: *Understanding panic and phobias* will help you find out more.
- Obsessional thoughts, which seem senseless and unwanted, may go round and round your mind and focus on fears that some harm or damage may result from something you have done or might do. Workbook 1d: *Understanding obsessive-compulsive symptoms (OCD)* addresses this.
- Problems in how to deal with ongoing physical illness and anxiety about health are both described in Workbook 1e: *Understanding how we respond to physical health problems.*

The next section of the workbook will help you to identify exactly how anxiety is affecting you.

Section 2   Understanding generalised anxiety: my own Five Areas Assessment

The Five Areas Assessment *approach* provides a clear summary of the difficulties faced by people with anxiety in each of the following areas:

1 Life situation, relationships, practical problems and difficulties (e.g. problems at home or work)
2 Altered thinking (with extreme and unhelpful thinking)
3 Altered feelings (also called mood or emotions)
4 Altered physical symptoms/feelings in the body
5 Altered behaviour or activity levels (with avoidance, or unhelpful behaviours)

The Five Areas Assessment shows that what a person thinks about a situation or problem may affect how they feel emotionally and physically. It also alters what they do. Look at the arrows in the diagram. Each of the five areas affects the others and offers possible areas of change to reduce anxiety.

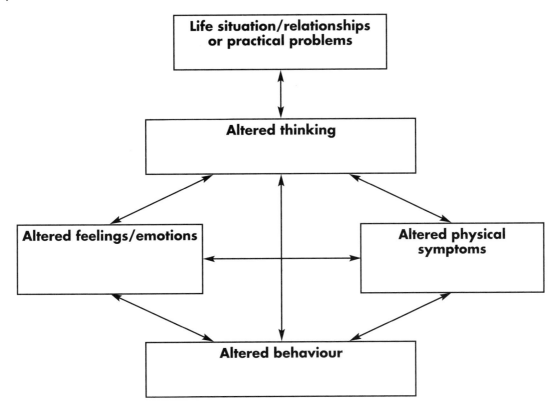

The Five Areas Assessment

The links between the areas also mean that the actions that people take when they are anxious can both improve or sometimes act to worsen or keep their symptoms of anxiety going. You will learn more about this as you read this workbook.

You will now see how this approach can help you understand your own anxiety.

> **Key point:** As you go through the Five Areas Assessment, please think about how anxiety has affected you **in the last week**. Try to answer all the questions and really think about how they apply to you. By doing this you will be able to identify possible target areas for change.
>
> In order to break down the task, areas 1–4 will be covered in this section. Area 5, altered behaviour, is covered in Section 3.

Area 1: Situation, relationship and practical problems

All of us from time to time face practical problems or difficulties in relationships. When we face a large number of problems we may begin to feel overwhelmed. Difficult situations include everyday events such as comments from family, friends or others that we take personally. Practical problems may include:

- debts, housing or other difficulties;
- problems in relationships with family, friends or colleagues;
- other difficult situations that you face, such as problems at home or work (or lack of work – for example, unemployment).

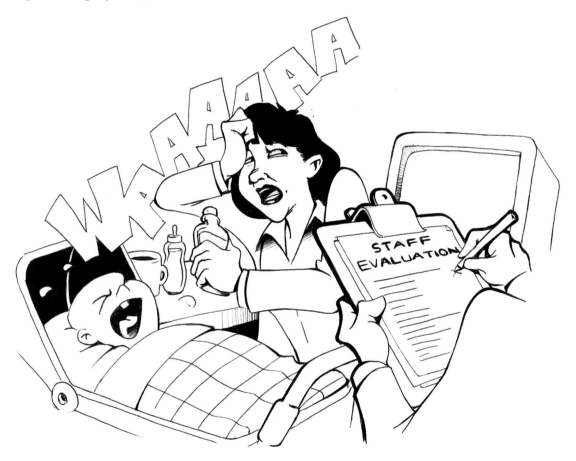

The following table refers to several common *situation*, *relationship* and *practical problems* that may be associated with anxious worrying. Are any of these relevant to you?

Situation, relationship and practical problems

I have relationship difficulties (such as arguments).	Yes ☐	No ☐
I can't really talk and receive support from my partner.	Yes ☐	No ☐
There is no one around who I can really talk to.	Yes ☐	No ☐
My children won't do what I tell them.	Yes ☐	No ☐
I have difficulties with money problems or debts.	Yes ☐	No ☐
There are problems with my flat/house.	Yes ☐	No ☐
I am having problems with my neighbours.	Yes ☐	No ☐
I don't have a job.	Yes ☐	No ☐
I have difficulties with colleagues at work.	Yes ☐	No ☐

You may notice that different situations, places or people also seem to worsen your anxiety. Write these here:

> ✎

You will find out more about this as you complete your own Five Areas Assessment.

Summary for Area 1: Situation, relationship and practical problems

Having answered these questions:

Q. Overall, do I have any problems in this area?   Yes ☐   No ☐

These difficulties are potential targets for change. You will find out more about what steps to take to tackle these in Section 4 of the workbook.

Area 2: Altered thinking in anxiety and worry

In anxiety, it is common to unhelpfully focus on difficult situations and problems. This results in anxious worrying about things such as:
- past or current problems;
- difficulties you may face in the future.

This anxious worrying does not sort out the problems. Dwelling on problems actually worsens things and quickly puts everything out of proportion.

There are several ways that anxious thinking causes problems in generalised anxiety.

The unhelpful thinking styles

Anxious thinking shows certain common themes.

- We may overlook our strengths and be very self-critical. We may have a **bias against ourselves** and think that we cannot sort out our difficulties.
- We may unhelpfully dwell on past, current or future problems. We may **put a negative slant on things** and apply a **negative mental filter** that focuses only upon difficulties and failures. When this occurs, it is almost as if we are wearing dark-tinted glasses. We see everything that happens as being bad or not good enough, and discount or overlook any achievements.
- We are prone to having a **gloomy view of the future** and get things out of all proportion. We make **negative predictions** about how things will work out.
- We may **jump to the very worst conclusion (catastrophic thinking)** that things will go very badly wrong.
- When we feel anxious we may be prone to **mind-read** and **second-guess that others think negatively of us**. We rarely check out whether these fears are true.
- We may **feel unfairly responsible** if things don't turn out well (**bear all responsibility/take all the blame**) and take things personally and to heart.
- We make **extreme statements** and have **unhelpfully high standards and rules** that are almost impossible to meet. We often use phrases like '*I should/must/ought/have to …*'. Similarly if even one thing goes wrong, we may say things such as '*Just typical – everything always messes up*'.
- Overall, in anxiety our thinking can become **extreme, unhelpful** and lacking all proportion.

By focusing on problems that are taken out of all proportion, our own strengths and ability to cope are overlooked or downplayed. Things are seen as being out of control and we can feel under great pressure.

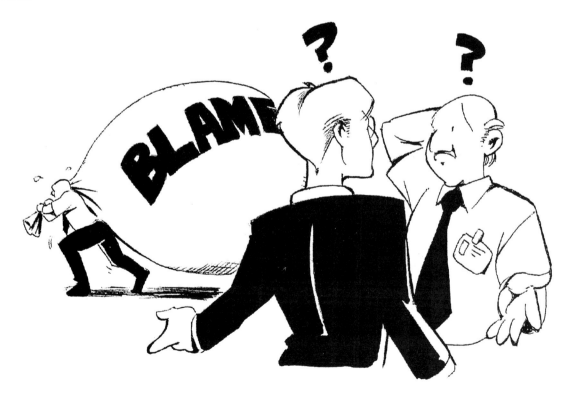

> **Key point:** It is important to realise that all the unhelpful thinking styles occur in each of us from time to time. However during times of anxiety or depression they become more frequent and are harder to dismiss from the mind.

Now, consider your own thinking over the last week:

My anxious thinking

Q1 Am I being my own worst critic *(bias against myself)*? Yes ☐ No ☐

Q2 Am I focusing on the bad in situations *(a negative mental filter)*? Yes ☐ No ☐

Q3 Do I have a gloomy view of the future *(make negative predictions)*? Yes ☐ No ☐

Q4 Am I jumping to the very worst conclusion *(catastrophising)*? Yes ☐ No ☐

Q5 Am I second-guessing that others think badly of me without actually checking *(mind-reading)*? Yes ☐ No ☐

Q6 Am I taking unfair responsibility for things that aren't really my fault *(bearing all responsibility/taking all the blame)*? Yes ☐ No ☐

Q7 Do I have unhelpfully high standards and use the words *should, must, ought* and *got to* a lot, or make statements such as *'Just typical'* when something goes wrong *(unhelpfully high standards/rules)*? Yes ☐ No ☐

If you have answered **Yes** to any of the questions it is likely that extreme anxious thoughts are adding to you problems.

Why are these unhelpful thinking styles so unhelpful?

These extreme thinking styles are unhelpful because of the impact of believing them on how you feel and on what you do.

Anxious thoughts ⟷ Feel more anxious

Anxious thoughts ⟷ Act in ways that worsen how you feel

Think about a recent time when you have felt more anxious or depressed. Were any unhelpful thinking styles present? Did they have an impact on how you felt and what you did at the time?

Read the table below to find more about the links between situations, thoughts, feelings and behaviour.

Situation, relationship or practical problem	Immediate worrying thought	Unhelpful thinking style	Emotional and/or physical impact	Behaviour change
You are asked to a party.	*'I won't have anything to say.'*	Making negative predictions about the future.	Anxiety and feel physically tense.	Lie that you are double-booked and don't go (*avoidance*).
You cannot complete one part of a task.	*'It's all gone wrong.'*	Putting a negative slant on things (*negative mental filter*).	Anxiety and physical symptoms of a faster heart rate and shallow rapid breathing when thinking of this failure.	Become very flustered. Give up trying to do it. Avoid doing it again in future.
You speak to someone and as you do so you worry what he or she thinks of you.	*'They think I'm boring and unattractive.'*	Second-guessing that others don't like you without actually checking if this is true (*mind-reading*).	Anxiety and physical symptoms, including going red and feeling hot and sweaty.	*Unhelpfully avoid* eye contact as you talk. Bring the conversation to an abrupt end. *Avoidance* of speaking to people in future, leading to isolation.

The unhelpful thinking styles can thus worsen how you feel emotionally and physically, and unhelpfully alter what you do in both the short and in the longer term.

Other thinking changes also occur in anxiety:

Becoming overly aware of things that seem scary

Anxiety causes us to pay particular attention and watch out for specific threats that are particularly scary to us. This can include difficult situations or the reactions of other people. The focus can also be inside us – such as our being very aware of our heart rate and unable to sleep as a result. Sometimes we even worry about our anxious worrying.

Allowing our minds to be dominated by anxious worrying thinking

Anxious worrying often gets out of proportion. For example, something may originally have happened in a few moments, such as something that someone has said. However, it can then dominate our thinking for much of the following days or weeks. This can add up in total to many days or even weeks of worry over the following months. The following questions will help you begin to think about this further.

Checklist: The impact of anxiety on me

How long have I had the anxiety? _____ months/years (please delete)

How intense does the anxious worrying seem at its worst?   Low ☐   Moderate ☐   Very High ☐

On average, how much of my waking day do I spend worrying? _____ hours

What does this add up to over the last month? _____ hours (approximately)

Overall, are worries and fears increasingly taking over my life?   Yes ☐   No ☐

Sometimes people try to cope with anxiety by trying not to think about it. *Is this an effective strategy?* In order to see if this works, try this practical experiment. Please try as hard as you can **not** to think about the following object. Please try very hard for the next 30 seconds not to think about a white polar bear.

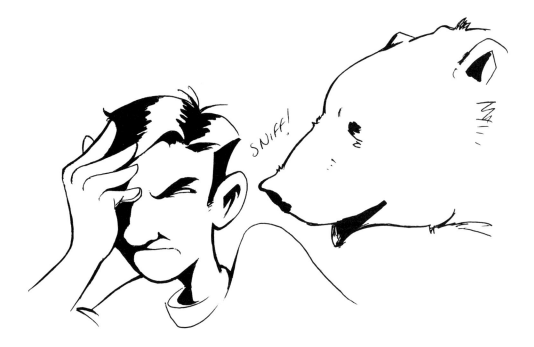

After you have done this, think about what happened. Was it easy not to think about the bear, or did it take a lot of effort? You may have noticed that trying hard not to think about it actually made it worse! Alternatively, you may have spent a lot of mental effort trying hard to think about something else such as a *black polar bear* instead. This is very like anxious worrying. We may try hard not to worry – but find this just makes things worse. Instead, we need to find new and more effective ways of identifying and then challenging our worrying thoughts.

Images and mental pictures – an important part of anxiety

Another way that we think is often in mental images. Some people (although not all) notice mental pictures or images in their mind when they become anxious and worry. Images are a form of thought and may be 'still' images (like a photograph), or be moving (like a video). Sometimes images may be in black and white, sometimes in colour. They may include a mental picture of some bad event

---

occurring. For example, it may be an image of something that has been said or done in the far past, or earlier today. As with all fears, the images add to feelings of anxiety.

Q. Am I prone to noticing upsetting images or memories? Yes ☐   No ☐

Summary for Area 2: Altered thinking

Having answered these questions:

Q. Overall, do I have any problems in this area? Yes ☐   No ☐

These difficulties are potential targets for change. You will find out more about what steps to take to tackle these in Section 4 of the workbook.

Area 3: Altered feelings/emotions in anxiety

In generalised anxiety, the following are common altered feelings:

- **Anxiety (also often called 'stress' or 'tension')**

In anxiety, the person feels troubled, unsettled and uneasy within himself or herself.

- **Anger or irritability**

Little things that normally wouldn't bother you may now seem to really irritate or upset you. Anger tends to happen when you, or someone else, break a rule that you think is important, or acts to threaten or frustrate you in some way.

- **Shame**

Feelings of shame occur when you see yourself as having undesirable qualities which if revealed to others will result in ridicule and humiliation. For example, this might be in your:
- *physical appearance (e.g. how your nose, ears, face, bottom, breasts etc. appear to others);*
- *emotions (e.g. shame at being anxious);*
- *personality (e.g. that you are not confident in everything you do);*
- *or actions (e.g. that you lied and avoided going to the party because of anxiety).*

These concerns lead to behaviours to hide these perceived 'faults' from others.

- **Low mood**

Depression may occur at the same time as generalised anxiety. It can both start and worsen anxious worrying. Common terms that people use to describe depression include feeling low/sad/blue/upset/down/miserable or fed up. You may find that you are more easily moved to tears and that things you would normally cope with really seem to strike home. Typically in severe depression the person feels excessively down and few, if any, things can cheer them up. If you feel like this, speak to your doctor or health care practitioner.

My altered feelings

Q. Do I feel anxious?　　　　　　　　　　　　　　　　　Yes ☐　　No ☐

Q. Do I get more easily angry, frustrated or irritable than previously?　　Yes ☐　　No ☐

Q. Do I feel shame about aspects of my actions or myself?　　Yes ☐　　No ☐

Q. Am I feeling depressed, upset or low in mood and no longer enjoy things
as before?　　　　　　　　　　　　　　　　　　　　　Yes ☐　　No ☐

Summary for Area 3: Altered feelings/emotions

Having answered these questions:

Q. Overall, do I have any problems in this area?　　Yes ☐　　No ☐

These difficulties are potential targets for change. You will find out more about what steps to take to
tackle these in Section 4 of the workbook.

Area 4: Altered physical sensations in anxiety

When a person becomes anxious, they may notice altered physical sensations such as feeling restless
and unable to relax. Feelings of **mental tension** can also cause **physical tension** in your muscles and
joints. This may cause feelings of shakiness, weakness, pain or tiredness. It can be surprising how
tiring anxiety can be and some people may feel completely exhausted as a result. In anxiety, your
muscles may be held tense for many weeks on end – a bit like running a marathon every day. This
muscle tension can also cause symptoms such as tension headaches, eyestrain, or stomach or chest
pains.

Other common symptoms include sickness, loose bowel movements, or a churning ('butterfly')
stomach. This can cause you to lose your appetite. Symptoms of tension may lead to difficulties
getting to sleep or staying asleep. This can be because of worries about life, or even about the fact
that you are not sleeping. You may feel hot or cold, sweaty or clammy. You may also notice that your
heart seems to be racing, or you may feel fuzzy-headed or disconnected from things.

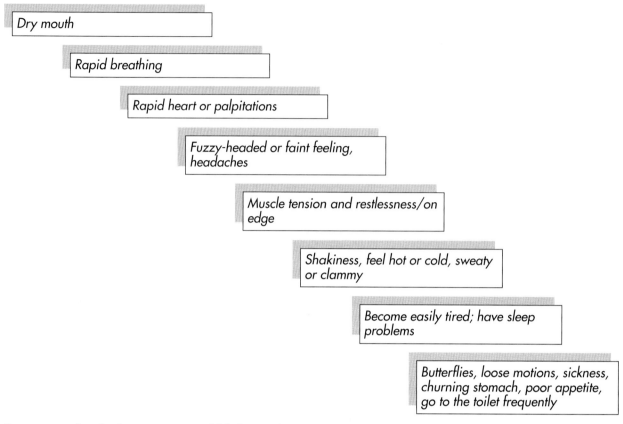

Dry mouth

Rapid breathing

Rapid heart or palpitations

Fuzzy-headed or faint feeling, headaches

Muscle tension and restlessness/on edge

Shakiness, feel hot or cold, sweaty or clammy

Become easily tired; have sleep problems

Butterflies, loose motions, sickness, churning stomach, poor appetite, go to the toilet frequently

Common physical symptoms of high anxiety

What causes these physical symptoms?

Your body reacts to extreme and unhelpful frightening thoughts just as it would to a physical danger. The **fight or flight adrenaline response** creates all of the symptoms described above. This is very useful when the danger is real. Think about a time when you have had a sudden shock – perhaps you have stepped into the road when a car was coming and didn't realise till you heard the car horn. Your body releases adrenaline which makes your heart beat faster. The purpose is to prepare the body to defend yourself or run away. Blood is pumped faster round the body so that the muscles are ready to react and breathing may speed up to allow more oxygen to get to the muscles. Sometimes rapid breathing continues long enough to cause a state of anxious over-breathing – also known as *hyperventilation.*

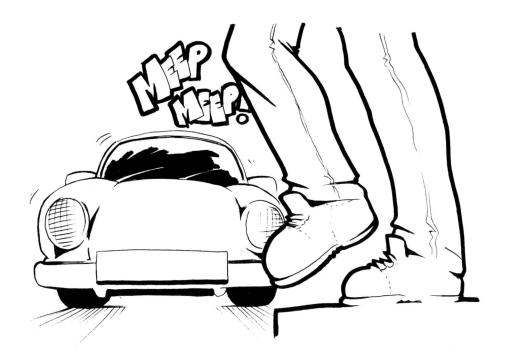

What is hyperventilation?

In hyperventilation, faster breathing with the upper part of the chest occurs so that rapid shallow breaths are taken through the mouth.

It is important to distinguish between the sudden-onset (so-called acute) hyperventilation that occurs during panic, and the problem of longer-term low-key hyperventilation. Low-key hyperventilation reflects 'bad habits' of breathing. In generalised anxiety it is this longer-term so-called chronic hyperventilation that is often more of a problem. Acute hyperventilation can still occur during times of high anxiety or panic.

Important information: Longer-term chronic hyperventilation can cause symptoms such as occasionally blurred vision and a dry mouth. We may notice sensations of tension or tightness in our chest. It can make us feel dizzy or fuzzy-headed. We may feel 'spaced out', distanced, or strangely disconnected from things. There may be a feeling of shortness of breath on occasion when we are anxious, even if we are not exercising. Finally, it can cause sleep problems and lead to longer-term feelings of tiredness. It is important to recognise that although these sensations are unpleasant, **they are not harmful**.

If you would like to find out more about hyperventilation, please read the Worksheet *Overcoming hyperventilation/overbreathing* (p. 11.1).

Depersonalisation: feeling cut-off and disconnected from things

An important difficulty caused by anxiety is that from time to time we can feel mentally disconnected and cut-off from things. The technical term for this is *depersonalisation*. It can sometimes be quite difficult to describe exactly what this feels like. Many people feel a *fuzzy-headed, spaced-out* sort of sensation. We may know that we are fully awake and also exactly where we are, yet in spite of this we feel distanced from things. It can seem as if we are a robot functioning on automatic. Sometimes we feel like an observer looking at everything from a distance as if we are watching television. We may feel not really connected – as if we or the things around us are not completely real. This feeling can be disturbing and often has a clear 'start'. It then just as suddenly stops.

   If you would like to find out more about depersonalisation, please read the worksheet *Understanding depersonalisation* (p. 12.1).

My altered physical symptoms in anxiety

Q. Do I notice a dry mouth when I feel anxious? — Yes ☐ No ☐

Q. Do I sometimes over-breathe with rapid, shallow gasping breaths? — Yes ☐ No ☐

Q. Do I notice my heart racing at times when I am anxious? — Yes ☐ No ☐

Q. Am I restless and unable to relax? — Yes ☐ No ☐

Q. Do I notice a fuzzy-headed/disconnected feeling when I am anxious? — Yes ☐ No ☐

Q. Am I noticing physical tension in my muscles? — Yes ☐ No ☐

Q. Do I feel shaky, hot, cold, sweaty or clammy when I feel anxious? — Yes ☐ No ☐

Q. Am I feeling physically drained and easily tired? — Yes ☐ No ☐

Q. Am I finding it difficult getting off to, or staying, asleep? — Yes ☐ No ☐

Q. Am I feeling off my food? — Yes ☐ No ☐

Q. Do I notice feelings of sickness or butterflies in my stomach? — Yes ☐ No ☐

Summary for Area 4: Altered physical symptoms

Having answered these questions:

Q. Overall, do I have any problems in this area? — Yes ☐ No ☐

These difficulties are potential targets for change. You will find out more about what steps to take to tackle these in Section 4 of the workbook.

You have now completed thinking about how anxiety may be affecting you in four of the five key areas. The next section will help you to consider the final area – how anxiety can affect your behaviour.

Section 3 Unhelpfully altered behaviour in anxiety

This section moves on to consider the fifth and final area of your Five Areas Assessment – altered behaviour. Behaviour may change unhelpfully in two key ways – avoidance and unhelpful behaviours.

Altered behaviour 1: Avoidance

When somebody develops anxiety, it is normal for him or her to try to avoid difficult situations, people or places. This avoidance can make matters worse by making the person lose even more confidence. The result is often an increasingly restricted lifestyle and additional distress. A *Vicious Circle of Avoidance* may result and this is summarised below:

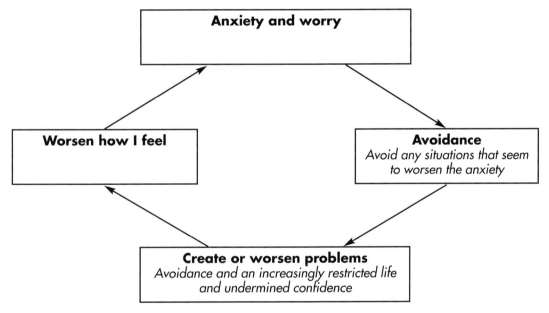

The vicious circle of avoidance

To help you see if this applies to you, ask yourself '*What have I stopped doing because of my anxiety?*'

Question: What have I stopped doing because of my anxiety?

You may find yourself avoiding certain situations, people or places because of how you feel. Try to identify ways in which you might be avoiding things as a result of anxiety. For example, do you avoid going out or mixing with others? Stop for a minute or so and consider what you have avoided doing because of anxiety.

What situations at home, work or in my relationships with others am I avoiding tackling/putting off?

If I didn't have this anxiety, what things would I like to be able to do?

What have I stopped/reduced doing that I used to enjoy because of my anxiety?

Remember, sometimes avoidance can be quite subtle. For example:

- *Putting off dealing with important practical problems* such as paying a bill or replying to an important letter. On a smaller scale this might involve putting off dealing with even everyday tasks which seem too hard/difficult, e.g. going into town shopping, cleaning the house, etc.
- *Not being open and assertive with others*, as in not talking directly and openly with others about important issues that you know really need to be discussed. This problem may also apply to 'smaller' everyday things, such as failing to reply to an invitation to a party rather than directly saying 'no'.
- *Not living life to the full.* You may choose to stay in bed, for example, or in your house/flat brooding.
- *Avoiding sex or physical intimacy* with your partner or spouse either because of tiredness and reduced sex drive (common in anxiety) or because of anxiety about your sexual performance.
- *Asking others to make decisions for you*, rather than deciding yourself.

● *Expecting others to sort things out*, for example to do the shopping, look after the children, wash the dishes, etc.

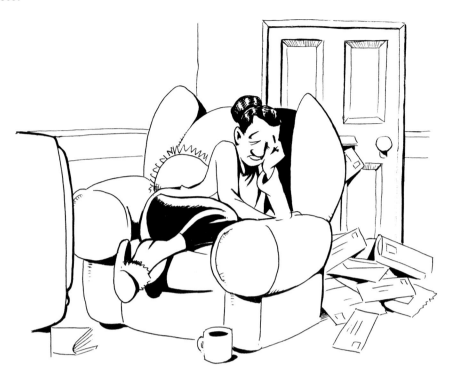

The following checklist will help you consider any areas of avoidance in your life.

Checklist: Identifying the vicious circle of avoidance

As a result of feeling anxious am I:	**Tick here if you have noticed this**
Avoiding dealing with important practical problems (both large and small)?	
Not really being honest with others. For example, saying Yes when I really mean No?	
Trying hard to avoid situations that bring about upsetting thoughts/memories?	
Brooding over things and therefore no longer living life to the full?	
Avoiding opening or replying to letters or bills?	
Sleeping in to avoid doing things or meeting people?	
Avoiding answering the phone, or the door when people visit?	
Avoiding sex?	
Avoiding talking to others face to face?	
Avoiding things in any other way? (Please write in): ✎	

Other areas of avoidance may occur in panic, phobias, obsessive-compulsive disorder and in problems with physical health and are covered in the workbooks addressing those difficulties.

Summary: The vicious circle of avoidance

Having answered these questions, reflect on your responses using the three questions below:

Q. Am I avoiding doing things as a result of anxiety?   Yes ☐   No ☐

Q. Has this reduced my confidence in things and led to an increasingly
restricted life?   Yes ☐   No ☐

Q. Overall, has this worsened how I feel?   Yes ☐   No ☐

If you have replied **Yes** to all three questions, then you are experiencing the vicious circle of avoidance.

Altered behaviour 2: Unhelpful behaviours

When somebody becomes anxious or depressed, it is normal to try to do things to feel better. This altered behaviour may be *helpful* or *unhelpful*. The purpose of both types of activity is to reduce anxiety – at least in the short term.

Helpful activities may include:
- Talking with friends or relatives and receiving helpful support.
- Reading or using self-help materials to find out more about the causes and treatment of the problems.
- Doing activities that provide pleasure or support such as meeting friends, playing sport, attending religious activities and participating in outdoor pursuits.
- Challenging anxious thoughts by stopping, thinking and reflecting rather than accepting them as true.
- Going to see your doctor or health care practitioner or attending a self-help support group.

Write down any *helpful* things you have done here:

You should aim to try to maximise the number of helpful activities you do as part of your recovery plan. Sometimes, however, we may try to block how we feel with a number of **unhelpful behaviours**. For example, when anxiety is at a high level we may choose to act in ways that aim to quickly reduce the level of anxiety – for a while. This is called a *safety behaviour*. These so-called safety behaviours include a range of actions designed to make you feel safer when anxious.

Actions designed to make you feel safer when anxious
- **Quickly leaving anxiety-provoking situations when anxiety is noticed.** Unhelpful behaviours include leaving situations where you feel anxious, or rushing through things as quickly as possible so as to minimise the amount of time spent there.

- **Trying to block how you feel by using drugs/alcohol etc.** Sometimes we may try to block anxiety by:
  - Misusing alcohol or drugs. Alcohol misuse is very common in generalised anxiety. This may start out as just having an extra drink to give you false courage or to help you get off to sleep. The danger is of escalating amounts being taken more and more frequently. The risk is alcohol or drug dependency.
  - Over-using or misusing prescription medication, or taking tablets inappropriately at times when they are not prescribed to try to relax or get off to sleep.
  - Eating too much (*comfort eating*) – particularly sweet foods/carbohydrates. This may result in weight gain.
  - Sleeping with a number of people in an attempt to feel needed/attractive/relaxed.
  - Trying to spend your way out of how you feel by visiting shops and buying things. The purpose is to cheer you up (so-called *retail therapy*).
- **Excessively telling others about your problems and seeking reassurance/advice which doesn't help.** At one extreme, we may choose *not* to talk at all about how we feel. Keeping your problems to yourself may be because of a belief that '*I shouldn't have emotional problems*', or that '*It is a sign of weakness to be upset.*' At the other extreme, we may recurrently seek support and *excessive reassurance* from those around us. This is a good example of an action that in moderation can be *helpful* and a source of support, but which can become *unhelpful* when taken to excess. The result is a feeling of dependency on others and a further loss of confidence in yourself.
- **Overcommitting yourself to work or social activities – or withdrawing from these completely.** At one extreme, sometimes we can withdraw into ourselves and stop going out or even meeting anyone. At the other extreme it can be tempting to throw yourself into excessive activity at home or at work. The intention is to 'work' through the distress. By filling every part of the day with non-stop activity the hope is to avoid noticing how bad you feel.

  This may involve other ways of avoiding emotional distress such as deliberately staying up late watching films, or sleeping in during the day to avoid seeing others. It also could include spending hours on computer games or watching television. Other common activities are listening to music, chatting/surfing on the Internet or texting others all the time. This is not to say that such activities are all unhelpful – more about why they are done. Doing these things because they can help us to avoid life is a very different motivation from doing them because they are fun.

- **Pushing others away.** Another unhelpful reaction is resolving our feelings by turning against those around us. We may become angry, gossipy, and undermine others by spreading rumours or becoming bitter and critical. This particularly can occur towards people who are easy targets and less likely to hit back, such as close relatives and friends. Sometimes this behaviour is a form of testing out the love, friendship and support of others. The consequence may be isolation, rejection and loneliness. Occasionally, the level of frustration can be so high that the result is violence, or the threat of violence.
- **Taking part in risk-taking behaviour.** This might include:
  - Self-harm (by cutting or scratching arms, legs or stomach) is sometimes used as a way of blocking or numbing feelings of tension.
  - Taking part in risk-taking actions. For example crossing the road without looking, or gambling using money you don't really have.

> **Key point:** Remember that the purpose of these unhelpful behaviours is to feel safer/better at least in the short term. They are sometimes therefore called *safety behaviours*. Although each action causes a short-term relief in symptoms, this doesn't last. The anxious worrying returns to the same or an even higher level.

The safety behaviours also teach an unhelpful lesson – *that it is only by leaving the situation/drinking too much/harming yourself/seeking reassurance etc. that you managed to cope.* In the longer term these actions backfire and add to your problems. For example, if we rely on alcohol or sedative drugs to give us false courage, we may find they cause additional problems of their own. A **vicious circle of unhelpful behaviour** can occur. This can further worsen how you feel by increasing self-blame and confirming negative beliefs about yourself or others.

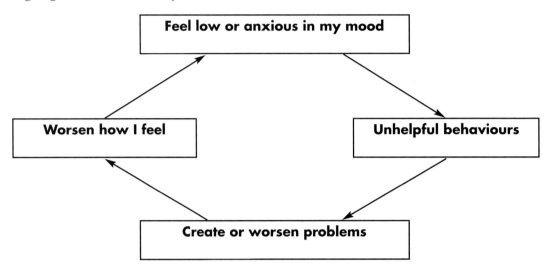

The vicious circle of unhelpful behaviours

Think about how this may apply to you by answering the questions below.

Checklist: Identifying the vicious circle of unhelpful behaviour

	Tick here if you have noticed this
As a result of how I feel, am I:	

Misusing drink/illegal drugs or prescribed medication to block how I feel in general or improve how I sleep etc.?

Eating too much to block how I feel (*'comfort eating'*), or over-eating so much that this becomes a 'binge'?

Trying to spend my way out of how I feel by going shopping (*'retail therapy'*)?

Becoming very demanding or excessively seeking reassurance from others?

Looking to others to make decisions or sort out problems for me?

Throwing myself into doing things so there are no opportunities to stop, think and reflect?

Pushing others away and being verbally or physically threatening/rude to them?

Deliberately harming myself in an attempt to block how I feel?

Taking part in risk-taking actions for example crossing the road without looking, or gambling with money I don't really have?

Checklist: Identifying the vicious circle of unhelpful behaviour

As a result of how I feel, am I:	Tick here if you have noticed this
Compulsively checking, cleaning, or doing things a set number of times or in exactly the 'correct' order so as to make things 'right'?	
Compulsively carrying out mental rituals such as counting or deliberately thinking good thoughts/saying prayers to make things feel 'right'?	
Being overly aware and excessively checking for symptoms of ill health?	
Excessively changing the way I sit or walk to reduce symptoms of physical discomfort? The altered posture then creates or worsens the physical problem.	
Sleeping with a number of people as a means of blocking how I feel or to feel needed, attractive or relaxed?	

Sometimes unhelpful behaviours can lead to quite subtle avoidance during times of anxiety. Do you notice any of the following in your own life?

Unhelpful behaviours leading to subtle avoidance of anxiety-provoking situations.

Am I:

Quickly leaving anxiety-provoking situations?

Rushing though a task as quickly as possible? (e.g. walking or talking faster)

Trying very hard not to think about upsetting thoughts/memories? Trying to distract myself to improve how I feel?

Only going out and doing things when others are there to help?

Taking the easiest option (for example joining the shortest queue in the shop as a result of anxiety, or turning down opportunities that seem scary)?

Deliberately looking away during conversations and avoiding eye contact? Bringing conversations to a close quickly because of not knowing what to say?

Q. Am I avoiding things in other subtle ways?

Write in what you are doing here if this applies to you:

Summary: The vicious circle of unhelpful behaviours

Having answered these questions, reflect on your responses using the three questions below.

Q. Am I doing certain activities or behaviours that are designed to improve
how I feel?   Yes ☐   No ☐

Q. Are some of these activities unhelpful in the short or longer-term either for
me or for others?   Yes ☐   No ☐

Q. Overall has this worsened how I feel?   Yes ☐   No ☐

If you have answered **Yes** to all three questions, you are experiencing the vicious circle of unhelpful
behaviour.

Summary for Area 5: Altered behaviour (avoidance or unhelpful behaviours)

Having answered these questions:

Q. Overall, do I have any problems in this area?   Yes ☐   No ☐

These difficulties are potential targets for change. You will find out more about what steps to take to
tackle these in Section 4 of the workbook.

You have now finished your Five Areas Assessment. Before you move on, please stop for a while and
consider what you have learned. How does what you have read help you to make sense of your
symptoms?

Q. How well does this assessment summarise how you feel?

Poorly ————————————————————— Very well
0   10

The purpose of your assessment

The purpose of the Five Areas Assessment is to help you plan the areas you need to focus on to bring
about change. The workbooks in the *Overcoming Anxiety* course can help you begin to tackle each
of the five problem areas of anxiety.

Section 4   Choosing your targets for change

The main problem areas seen in worry and generalised anxiety are the:
- Current situations, relationship or practical problems
- Altered thinking (with extreme and unhelpful thinking)
- Altered feelings/emotions
- Altered physical symptoms
- Altered behaviour (with avoidance or unhelpful behaviours)

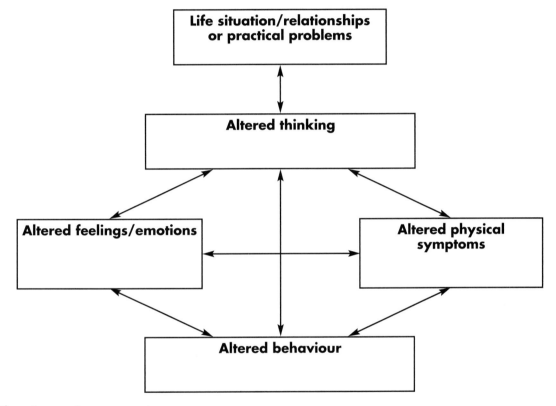

The Five Areas Assessment

You have previously answered questions about each of these five areas. Look again at the answers you gave in your own Five Areas Assessment, in the last two sections of the workbook. Your answers summarise the problems you identified in each area. Since there are links between the areas, it is possible by altering any one of the areas to bring about changes in others, and help improve how you feel.

> **Key point:** By defining your problems, you have now identified possible target areas to focus on. The key is to make sure that you do things **one step at a time**. Slow steady steps are more likely to result in improvement than very enthusiastically starting and then running out of steam.

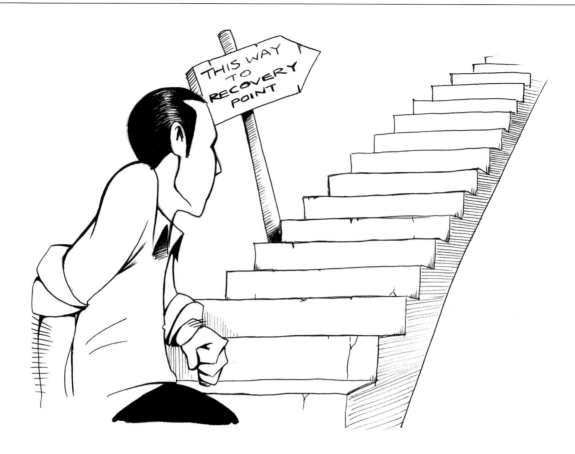

Short-, medium- and longer-term targets

You may have made all sorts of previous attempts to change, but unless you have a clear plan and stick to it, change will be very difficult. Planning and selecting which targets to try and change first is a crucial part of successfully moving forwards. By choosing some specific areas to focus on to start with, this also means that you are actively choosing at first **NOT** to focus on other areas.

Setting yourself targets will help you to focus on how to make the changes needed to get better. To do this you will need to decide:

- Short-term targets: changes you can make today, tomorrow and next week.
- Medium-term targets: changes to be put in place over the next few weeks.
- Long-term targets: where you want to be in six months or a year.

The questions that you have answered in this workbook will have helped you to identify the main problem areas that you currently face. The *Overcoming Anxiety* course (outlined below) can help you to make changes in each of these areas.

The workbooks can be used either alone or as part of a complete course. The Workbooks 1a to 1e in Part 1 are designed to help you to identify your current problem areas. This will help identify which of the Workbooks 2 to 9 in Part 2 you need to read. Finally, you can summarise what you have learned and plan for the future by completing Workbook 10. This will help you keep putting what you have learned into practice.

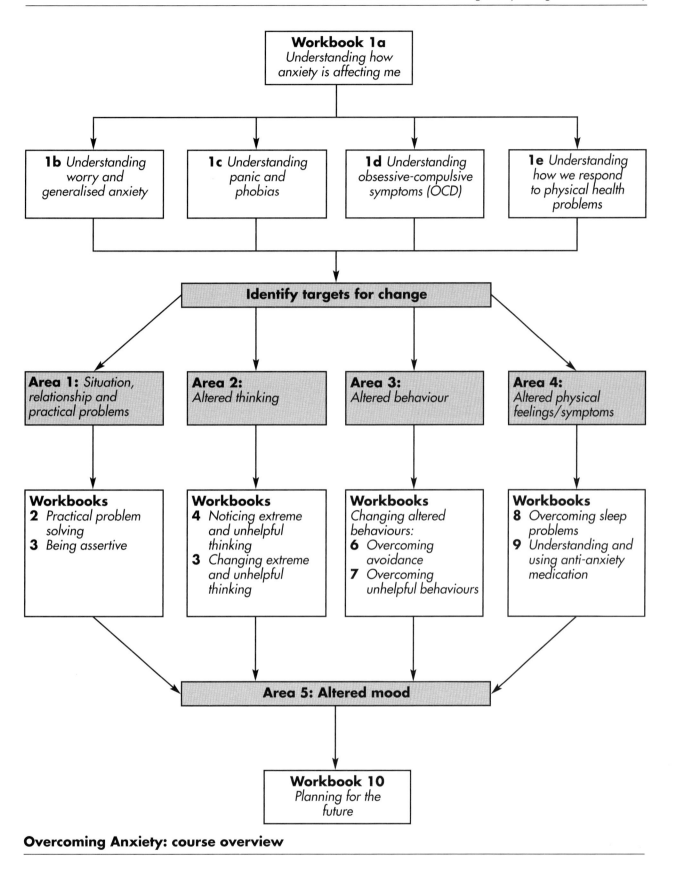

Overcoming Anxiety: course overview

The Overcoming Anxiety course

Understanding anxiety

Workbooks 1a to 1e provide an introduction and overview of anxiety problems. It is recommended that you read these workbooks first to give you an overview of how anxiety can affect you. The five workbooks together cover the common anxiety disorders – worry, panic, phobias, obsessive-compulsive disorder and also how we respond to physical health problems. They will help you identify which of these areas you need to focus on changing and will help you decide which of the remaining workbooks you need to read.

Area 1: Dealing with difficult situations, relationship and practical problems

Workbook 2: *Practical problem solving*

In this workbook you will learn a step-by-step plan that you can use to deal with practical problems. It will provide you with the tools to tackle any practical problems that you face. This will help you to take more control of your life and the decisions that you make. By feeling more in control of your life, you will improve your self-confidence.

Workbook 3: *Being Assertive*

Have you ever thought that no one listens to you, and that other people seem to walk all over you? Have others commented that they think that you always walk over them? You will find out about the difference between passive, aggressive and assertive behaviour and learn how to develop more balanced relationships with others where your opinion is listened to and respected, and you listen to and respect other people.

Area 2: Changing extreme and unhelpful thinking

Workbook 4: *Noticing extreme and unhelpful thinking*

What you think about yourself, others and the situations that occur around you, can alter how you feel and affect what you do. This workbook will help you to learn ways of identifying extreme and unhelpful ways of thinking. You will learn how to notice such thoughts and to understand the impact these have on how you feel and what you do.

Workbook 5: *Changing extreme and unhelpful thinking*

This workbook will teach you the important skill of how to challenge extreme and unhelpful thinking. With practice this will help you change the extreme and unhelpful thinking that is often a major problem in anxiety or depression.

Area 3: Changing altered behaviours

Workbook 6: *Overcoming avoidance*

You will find out more about how avoidance keeps problems going. You will learn ways of changing what you do in order to break the vicious circle of avoidance.

Workbook 7: *Overcoming unhelpful behaviours*

You will learn some effective ways of overcoming unhelpful behaviours such as drinking too much, reassurance seeking and trying to spend your way out of how you feel.

Area 4: Physical symptoms and treatments

Workbook 8: *Overcoming sleep problems*

Often when someone is anxious they not only feel emotionally and mentally low, but they also notice a range of physical changes that are a normal part of anxiety. This workbook will help you find out about these common changes, and in particular will help you to deal with problems of poor sleep.

Workbook 9: *Understanding and using anti-anxiety medication*

When someone is anxious sometimes their doctor suggests they take an anti-anxiety medication. You will find out why doctors suggest this, and also learn about common fears and concerns that people have when first starting to take these tablets so that you can find out for yourself whether this medication may be helpful for you.

Area 5: Altered mood

The fifth and final area, anxious mood, will improve if you work at the other areas where you have problems (the altered thinking, behaviour, physical symptoms and the situations, relationships and practical problems that you face). Once you feel better, the final workbook of the series can be read to help you to summarise what you have learned.

Workbook 10: *Planning for the future*

You will have learned new things about yourself and made changes in how you live your life. This final workbook will help you to identify what you have learned and help you plan for the future. You will devise your own personal plan to cope with future problems in your life so that you can face the future with confidence.

The work you do using the workbooks can supplement the help you receive from your doctor or other health care practitioner or friends. Sometimes more specialist help is needed to help how you feel and your doctor may suggest that you see a trained specialist such as a clinical psychologist, occupational therapist, social worker, psychiatric nurse or a psychiatrist.

Use the following table to help you decide which workbooks are right for you to read now, and over the next few weeks and months. You have already read the current workbook, and it is recommended that you also read Workbook 1a: *Understanding how anxiety is affecting me*. You may find it helpful to discuss this with your health care practitioner or other trusted supporter.

Workbook title	Short-term goals (plan to read in the next week or so)	Medium-term goals (plan to read over the next few weeks)	Long-term goals (plan to read over the next few months)	Tick when completed
Understanding anxiety workbooks				
1a *Understanding how anxiety is affecting me*	✔			
1b *Understanding worry and generalised anxiety*	✔			
1c *Understanding panic and phobias*				
1d *Understanding obsessive-compulsive symptoms (OCD)*				
1e *Understanding how we respond to physical health problems*				
Workbook 2 *Practical problem solving*				
Workbook 3 *Being assertive*				
Workbook 4 *Identifying extreme and unhelpful thinking*				
Workbook 5 *Changing extreme and unhelpful thinking*				
Workbook 6 *Overcoming avoidance*				
Workbook 7 *Overcoming unhelpful behaviours*				
Workbook 8 *Overcoming sleep problems*				
Workbook 9 *Understanding and using anti-anxiety medications*				
Workbook 10 *Staying well*				
Worksheet *Overcoming hyperventilation/ over-breathing*				
Worksheet *Understanding depersonalisation*				

In order to help you to review your progress, it can be useful to record how you feel at different times as you work on your problems. Your health care practitioner may work with you to decide what information it might be helpful to record. Don't expect to feel better all at once. Change can take time, however by working at your problems, most people find that improvement is possible.

> **Key point:** In order to change, you will need to choose to try to apply what you will learn regularly **throughout the week**, and not just when you read the workbook or see your health care practitioner. The workbooks will encourage you to do this by sometimes suggesting certain tasks for you to carry out in the days after reading each workbook.
>
> These tasks will:
> ● help you to put into practice what you have learned in each workbook;
> ● gather information so that you can get the most out of the workbook.
>
> Experience has shown that you are likely to make the most progress if you are able to put into practice what you have learned.

Summary

In this workbook you have learned about:
● the key elements of worry and of generalised anxiety;
● the impact of how what you think can affect how you feel and unhelpfully alter what you do;
● the Five Areas of Anxiety: the *situations, relationship and practical problems* faced, and the *altered thinking, emotional* and *physical feelings* and *behaviour* that occur as part of anxiety;
● the areas you need to tackle in order to overcome your own problems of anxiety.

Putting into practice what you have learned

● Read through the current workbook again. Think in detail about how anxiety is affecting your thinking, emotional and physical feelings, and behaviour. Decide which areas you want to change.
● Choose **two episodes** over the next week when you feel more anxious. Use the blank Five Areas Assessment sheet (p. 1b.34) to record the impact on your thinking, mood, body and behaviour at those times. Try to generate a summary of your own anxiety in each of the five areas (life situation, relationships and practical problems, altered thinking, feelings, physical symptoms and behaviour). Use this workbook to identify whether you showed any of the unhelpful thinking styles during these occasions. What impact did your thoughts have on how you felt and what you did during these two episodes? Can you identify any examples of avoidance or unhelpful behaviours? Please photocopy or draw out additional copies of this diagram as you need it and keep the sheet handy.
● Finally, review your list of which workbooks you will choose to use next and move on to work through these in your own time.

If you have difficulties with these tasks, don't worry. Just do what you can. If you have found any aspects of this workbook unhelpful, upsetting or confusing, please can you discuss this with your health care practitioner or someone else whose opinion you trust.

A request for feedback

An important factor in the development of all the Five Areas Assessment workbooks is that the content is updated on a regular basis based upon feedback from users and practitioners. If there are areas which you find hard to understand, or seem poorly written, please let me know and I will try to improve things in future. I regret that I am unable to provide any specific replies or advice on treatment.

To provide feedback, please contact me via:

Email: Feedback@fiveareas.com

Mail: Dr Chris Williams, Department of Psychological Medicine, Gartnavel Royal Hospital, 1055 Great Western Road, Glasgow, G12 0XH

Acknowledgements

I wish to thank all those who have commented upon this workbook especially Mumtaz Ahmad, Alan Davidson, Julie Hickson, Sandra Johnston, Liz Rafferty, Julie Tiller, Alison Williams and Stephen Williams.

The cartoon illustrations in the workbooks have been produced by Keith Chan (kchan75@hotmail.com) and are copyright of Media Innovations Ltd.

My notes

....

....

....

....

....

....

....

....

....

....

....

....

....

....

....

....

....

....

....

....

....

....

....

....

....

My notes

....

....

Worksheet: A Five Areas Assessment of a specific time when I feel more anxious/worse

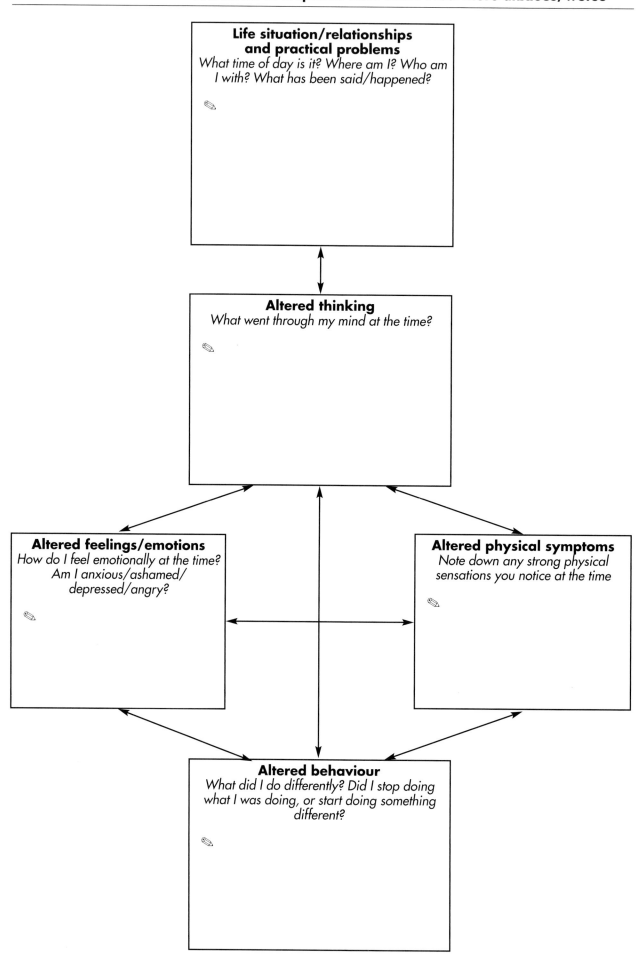

Workbook 1c
Understanding panic and phobias

Dr Chris Williams

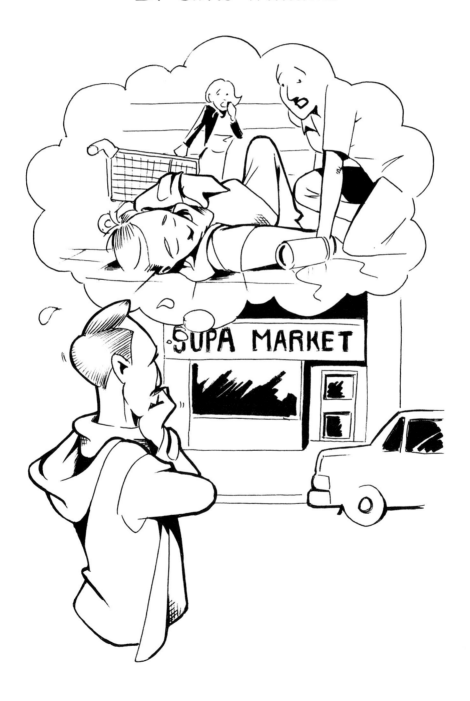

A Five Areas Approach

Section 1   **Introduction**

The workbook will cover:
- how to use the workbook most effectively;
- the key elements of anxiety, panic attacks and phobias so that you will understand how anxiety can affect you;
- the impact of how what you think can affect how you feel and unhelpfully alter what you do;
- the Five Areas of Anxiety: the *situations, relationship and practical problems* faced, and the *altered thinking, emotional* and *physical feelings* and *behaviour* that occur as part of panic and phobias;
- the areas you need to tackle to overcome your own problems of anxiety, panic and phobias.

Don't be concerned if any of these words seem new or difficult to understand. All the terms will be described clearly as you read through the workbook.

How to use this workbook

Take time to read the workbook at your own pace. You don't have to sit down and read it in one go. You might find it most helpful to set yourself the target of reading the workbook one section at a time.
- Try to **answer all the questions** asked. The process of having to *stop, think and reflect* on how the questions might be relevant to you is crucial to getting better.
- **Write down** your own notes in the margins or in the *My notes* area at the back of the workbook to help you remember information that has been helpful. **Plan to review your notes regularly** so that you apply what you have learned.
- Once you have read through the entire workbook once, **put it on one side** and then **re-read it** a few days later. It may be that different parts of it become clearer, or seem more useful on second reading.
- Use the workbook to **build upon the help you receive in other ways,** such as from reading other helpful material, talking to friends, or attending self-help organisations and support groups.
- **Discuss the workbook** with your health care practitioner and those who give you helpful support so that you can work together on overcoming the problems.
- **Remember that although change can seem difficult at first, it is possible.**

Understanding anxiety

Anxiety, tension, stress, and *panic* are all terms that are used to describe what is a widespread problem for many people. Anxiety can affect everyone and anyone. Very high levels of anxiety and fear are described as feelings of panic.

Can anxiety be helpful?

Anxiety is a common and normal emotion, which can be helpful even though it can feel unpleasant. For example, at lower levels it can help motivate us to prepare for events such as interviews or exams. Anxiety is also helpful in situations of sudden danger, where it helps us to respond and get away as rapidly as possible. The problem is when we feel anxious in situations that are not dangerous at all. Another problem is feeling anxious well beyond what is helpful in the circumstances. For example, being so anxious that you cannot cross the road or enter a shop.

What are panic attacks and phobias?

What is a panic attack?

Sometimes anxiety can be so strong, and we feel so mentally and physically tense and unwell that we stop what we are doing and try to leave or escape the situation. Sometimes we may feel paralysed into inactivity like rabbits caught in the headlamps of a car and freeze, expecting disaster to strike at any moment. This feeling of acute fear, dread or terror is called a *panic attack*. Panic attacks rarely last longer than 20–30 minutes.

During panic, there are strong beliefs that something terrible or catastrophic is happening right now. Common fears are '*I'm going to faint*', '*I'm going to suffocate*' '*I'm going to collapse*', '*I'm going to have a stroke*', or '*I'm going to have a heart attack*'. Sometimes the fear is of *going mad* or *losing control*. The key point is that the fear is immediately threatening, scary and catastrophic. We become overly aware of the anxiety and quickly stop what we are doing, and hurry away from the situation.

Sometimes we don't have a specific fear or anxiety. Instead, anxious worries build up and up in our minds. What starts as anxious worrying about difficulties can build up over time until a state of panic develops.

Panic attack checklist

Q. Do I notice anxiety that rises to a peak?   Yes ☐   No ☐

Q. Do I feel mentally very scared and physically unwell during the panic?   Yes ☐   No ☐

Q. Do I fear that something terrible/catastrophic will happen during the panic?   Yes ☐   No ☐

Q. Do I become overly aware of the things that I fear might happen during panic? Yes ☐   No ☐

Q. Am I downplaying my own ability to overcome these problems?   Yes ☐   No ☐

Q. Do I stop what I am doing and try to immediately escape or leave when I feel like this?   Yes ☐   No ☐

If you have answered **Yes** to any of these questions, then panic may be a problem for you.

How common is panic?

Because people often don't want to talk about mental health problems, you may think you are the only person to have these difficulties. This is not true. You may be surprised to learn that about one in twenty people experience problems of panic attacks. Think of the people who live in the same street as you. There are likely to be at least one or two people in your street who currently have problems with panic. There will also be people who have experienced problems of panic in the past.

Panic attacks commonly occur as part of other mental health difficulties:

- *Depression*. This often causes or worsens anxiety. Here, depressing thoughts are linked to low mood, a lack of enjoyment and reduced activity. If you think you may be depressed then you should talk to your health care practitioner to find out more.
- *Generalised anxiety*. Here, worries are anxiously gone over again and again in a way that is unhelpful because it does not actually help to sort out the difficulties that are being worried about. Look at Workbook 1b: *Understanding worry and generalised anxiety* to find out more.
- *Obsessive-compulsive disorder*. Obsessional thoughts seem senseless and unwanted. They go round and round your mind and focus on fears that some harm or damage may result from something you have done or might do. Workbook 1d: *Understanding obsessive-compulsive symptoms (OCD)* addresses this.

What is a phobia?

You may have friends or relatives who are very scared of certain creatures, such as spiders, or of situations, such as heights. You yourself may have such fears. Sometimes even just thinking about the feared situation can cause strong feelings of panic. We may avoid anything to do with that situation as a result. This can lead to an increasingly restricted lifestyle. It also undermines your confidence and causes additional distress. When this occurs, we have a *phobia*. Phobias, worry, obsessive-compulsive disorder, depression and panic attacks can occur together.

Definition: A *phobia* describes high anxiety (often with panic attacks) that regularly occurs in a particular situation. In phobias, we become overly aware of any possible threats relating to our fear and try to avoid or quickly leave any situation, place or person(s) that cause us anxiety. We often know logically that the situation will not harm or kill us, yet we experience the anxiety anyway.

Phobia checklist

Q. Do I notice strong feelings of anxiety or panic when I face particular situations, people or places? Yes ☐ No ☐

Q. Does even thinking about these situations/places/people make me feel nervous? Yes ☐ No ☐

Q. Have I become overly sensitive to anything to do with the phobic fear? Yes ☐ No ☐

Q. Am I downplaying my own ability to overcome these fears? Yes ☐ No ☐

Q. Am I avoiding these situations, places or people? Yes ☐ No ☐

Q. Overall, am I living an increasingly restricted lifestyle as a result? Yes ☐ No ☐

If you have answered **Yes** to any of these questions, then you may have a phobia

---

In the next section of the workbook, you will find out about the different sorts of phobias that can occur.

Section 2   **What are the different types of phobia?**

Remember: A *phobia* describes high anxiety (often with panic attacks) that regularly occurs in a particular situation. We become overly aware of any possible threats relating to our fear and do all we can to escape. We then avoid any situation, place or person(s) that causes us to feel anxious. We know logically that the situation will not harm or kill us, yet we experience the anxiety anyway.

Virtually any situation, place or person/group can become the focus of a phobia. Each phobia has a specific name. This section summarises the most common types.

a) Avoidance of particular situations or objects

Almost any situation or object can become a cause of phobic fear. For example heights and insects (e.g. wasps or spiders). This type of phobia is often called a specific phobia since exposure to this one situation/object results in intense fear, and causes the person to hurry away.

> **Choice point:** If you think that this sort of specific phobia may apply to you, please read the following text. If not, please skip to b) below. The case example here is fear of spiders. If this is a problem for you please note that there are no illustrations of spiders in the following text.

Example: Jane has a strong phobic fear of spiders. One afternoon, a spider scuttles across the carpet in front of her. She immediately screams, and feels great anxiety, panic and fear. Her heart speeds up and races in her chest. She feels very physically tense, shaky and weak. The fear not only affects how she feels, but also affects how she reacts.

Avoidance: Jane leaves the room by jumping onto the settee to get to the door. She then runs out and slams the door behind her.

Unhelpful behaviours: Jane asks her neighbour Helen if she will take the spider well away from the house. She steers well clear as Helen does this. Finally, Jane repeatedly checks that Helen has really removed the spider. She is ashamed she had asked Helen to do this. She can't go back into the room until she knows the spider has gone.

The avoidance is unhelpful because it undermines Jane's confidence in being able to deal with the problem, and it reinforces her belief that she can only cope by leaving the situation.

In extreme form, a fear of spiders prevents the sufferer living their life normally. They think all the time about the possibility of coming across a spider. Any places where spiders might lurk are avoided or approached only gingerly. Even pictures of spiders are avoided.

This example summarises some of the key elements of phobic anxiety. A similar situation exists in the case of any other feared object or situation.

b) Avoidance of specific places from which escape might be difficult

You may have heard of people who have panic attacks on buses or in shops or other crowded situations. This is called *agoraphobia*. This is one of the most common forms of phobia. The term agoraphobia literally means 'fear of the market place' in Greek. The term is now used to describe a focused fear of any specific place from which it is difficult to exit.

It can include situations such as:

- *Being on a bus, train or aeroplane*. This can include being given a lift in a car, or being driven through a place where stopping would be difficult: for example, driving through a long tunnel or across a toll bridge.
- *Sitting in a cinema or theatre* – particularly if you are not sitting near the exit. Sitting in the middle of the row where you have to pass others to leave may also cause problems.
- *Shopping in large shops* (or sometimes smaller ones, too) or *being in long queues* waiting to pay your bill.
- *Eating in restaurants*, particularly if you are some distance from the exit.

The key element is that these are situations where it is either physically difficult to leave (e.g. from a train, when the doors are closed), or it is socially difficult to leave (e.g. from a cinema, pushing past people to get out). The result is that the agoraphobic feels trapped. They experience increasingly catastrophic fears about what might happen if they can't escape from the place or situation.

Choice point: If you think that agoraphobia may apply to you, please read the following text. If not, please skip to c) below.

Example: Harvinder has developed panic attacks whenever he goes shopping. He has had this difficulty for about six months. He starts noticing the anxiety increasing as he plans his weekly shop. On the way to the supermarket he is very aware of his heart thumping. His breathing is faster than usual. As he enters the store his breathing speeds right up and his heart starts racing. He fears that he will pass out and collapse. As he breathes faster and faster he feels even dizzier. Harvinder changes his behaviour to try to make himself feel better.

Avoidance: He stops going to supermarkets as often as in the past and only shops at quieter times.

Unhelpful behaviours: He walks faster than usual as he shops. He also holds tightly to the shopping trolley for support. Previously he has persevered and reached the checkouts, always choosing the till with the shortest queue and having his credit card ready for a quick escape. Today, however, he tries to control his breathing by taking rapid breaths. This makes things worse. After only five minutes he abandons the trolley in the middle of the store and runs outside. He sits on a seat to recover. He decides next time he will bring someone along with him in case he feels like this again. He pledges that he will never go into another supermarket.

Harvinder's panicky fears have affected how he feels emotionally and physically. They have also unhelpfully altered what he does. His altered behaviour succeeds in helping him feel safer in the short term. However in the longer term this action backfires and further undermines his confidence. Leaving the shop has reinforced his underlying belief that he can only cope by *leaving* an anxiety-provoking situation. It has prevented him from staying in the store and testing out if his fear of fainting/collapsing would really result in such an event.

c) Avoidance of conversations with people/being in the spotlight

A degree of shyness affects many people. A *social phobia* occurs where there is an excessive shyness and a very strong fear that others are judging us negatively. This extreme form of shyness affects about one person in thirty-five at some stage in their lives.

Social phobia causes great difficulty in one-to-one situations or whenever the person with this problem thinks that the spotlight is on them. For example, meeting new people or making small talk over coffee can be desperately difficult. In such situations someone suffering from social phobia will mind-read that others don't like them, or that they judge them to be unattractive, boring, inferior or stupid. These thoughts produce great anxiety.

Other situations that social phobics might find difficult include times when others are watching them perform a task, such as giving a talk. Here the fear is focused on public speaking to a group of people. For example, a teacher can become very anxious leading a class. Any other situation where the person is the centre of attention can cause similar anxiety.

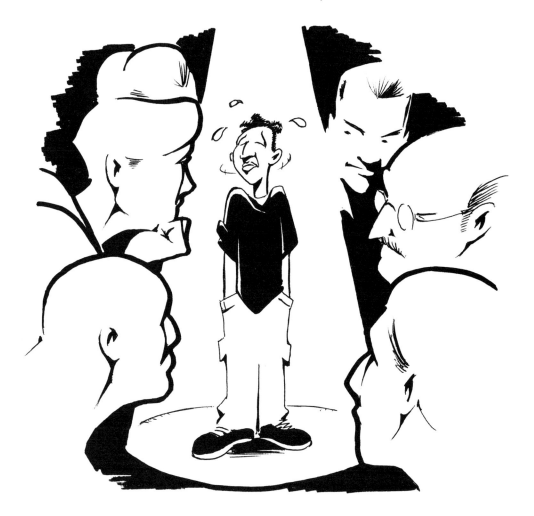

Sometimes, the person with social phobia starts to drink far more than usual to help them cope with the stress of social occasions. This can lead to drink problems and alcohol dependency.

Choice point: If you think that social phobia may apply to you, read the following text. If not, please skip to the next section of the workbook.

Example: Dawn becomes very anxious in social situations. This has worsened since she was a teenager when she had bad acne. Even though the acne has now cleared her anxiety in social situations has become worse and worse. On these occasions she notices strong bodily symptoms of anxiety. She feels hot and flushed, sweaty and slightly shaky. She is very aware of her dry mouth and notices a frog in her throat. She is overly sensitive to these physical symptoms. She constantly predicts that the person she is speaking to will be aware of her discomfort and judge her negatively. Dawn reacts to her fears in two ways.

Avoidance. She chooses to avoid social situations, whenever possible. She tends to say no to invitations to meals out or parties, and tries to keep all social encounters as short as possible. **Unhelpful behaviours.** She tries to avoid eye contact with people. She only makes eye contact briefly and for as short time as possible. She finds herself constantly tempted to cut conversations short and leave abruptly. She is especially aware of feeling hot, flushed and sweaty and uses her handkerchief to repeatedly dab her forehead. She also tries to cool down by fanning herself with her hand and by blowing air from her mouth directed up at her forehead. Finally, she keeps swallowing hard and coughing to try to clear her throat.

What Dawn *thinks* affects how she *feels emotionally and physically*, and has *unhelpfully altered what she does*. The altered behaviour is designed to help Dawn cope with the anxiety of social contact. However, her actions and avoidance can backfire and undermine her confidence even more. Hurrying away will reinforce her underlying belief that she can only cope by leaving a situation. Mopping her brow reinforces her fear that others will judge her negatively because in doing this she is acting differently from the people around her and she is strongly aware of this. Finally, the actions she takes might actually draw *more* attention to her. This is quite the opposite of what she wished.

Section 3 Understanding panic and phobias: my own Five Areas Assessment

A Five Areas Assessment can be helpful in understanding your own symptoms of anxiety, and in choosing targets to change how you feel.

The five areas are:

1 Life situation, relationships, practical problems and difficulties (e.g. problems at home or work)
2 Altered thinking (with extreme and unhelpful thinking)
3 Altered feelings (also called emotions or moods)
4 Altered physical symptoms/feelings in the body
5 Altered behaviour or activity levels (with avoidance, or unhelpful behaviours)

The Five Areas Assessment indicates that what a person thinks about a situation or problem may affect how they feel emotionally and physically, and also alters what they do. Look at the arrows in the diagram. Each of these five areas affects the others and offers possible areas of change to reduce anxiety.

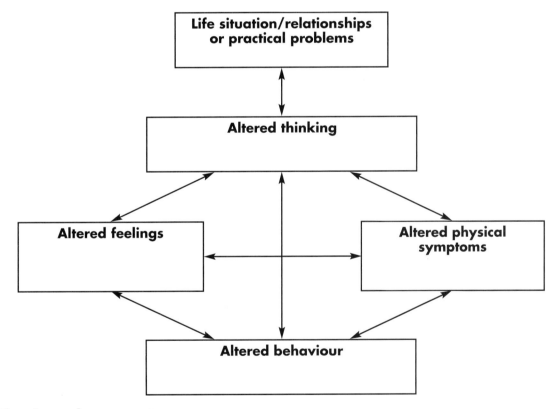

The Five Areas Assessment

Key point: As you go through the Five Areas Assessment, please think about how anxiety has affected you in the last week. Try to answer all the questions and really think about how they apply to you. By doing this you will be able to identify possible target areas for change.

In order to break down the task, areas 1–4 will be covered in this section. Area 5, altered behaviour, will be covered in Section 4.

Area 1: Situation, relationship and practical problems

All of us from time to time face practical problems or difficulties in relationships. When we face a large number of problems we may begin to feel overwhelmed. Difficult situations include everyday events such as comments from family, friends or others that we take personally. Practical problems may include:

- debts, housing or other difficulties;
- problems in relationships with family, friends or colleagues;
- other difficult situations that you face, such as problems at home or work (or lack of work – for example, unemployment).

The following table refers to several common factors that may be associated with anxiety. Are any of these relevant to you?

Situation, relationship and practical problems

I have relationship difficulties (such as arguments).	Yes ☐	No ☐
I can't really talk and receive support from my partner.	Yes ☐	No ☐
There is no one around who I can really talk to.	Yes ☐	No ☐
My children won't do what I tell them.	Yes ☐	No ☐
I have difficulties with money problems or debts.	Yes ☐	No ☐
There are problems with my flat/house.	Yes ☐	No ☐
I am having problems with my neighbours.	Yes ☐	No ☐
I don't have a job.	Yes ☐	No ☐
I have difficulties with colleagues at work.	Yes ☐	No ☐

You may notice that different situations, places or people also seem to worsen your anxiety. Write these here:

You will find out more about these as you complete your own Five Areas Assessment.

Summary for Area 1: Situation, relationship and practical problems

Having answered these questions:

Q. Overall, do I have any problems in this area?   Yes ☐   No ☐

These difficulties are potential targets for change. You will find out more about what steps to take to tackle these in Section 5 of the workbook.

Area 2: Altered thinking in panic and phobias

Thinking can alter in various ways when panic or phobias occur.

The unhelpful thinking styles

During panic, there are strong fears that something terrible or catastrophic is happening right now. You may jump to the very worst conclusion (**catastrophic thinking**). Common fears are '*I'm going to faint*', '*I'm going to suffocate*' '*I'm going to collapse*', '*I'm going to have a stroke*', or '*I'm going to have a heart attack*'. You may fear that you are *going mad* or *are losing control*. You may overlook your own strengths and be very self-critical (**bias against self**). You may be prone to second-guess that others think negatively of you and rarely check out whether these fears are true (**mind-reading**). Overall, your thinking becomes extreme, unhelpful and puts everything out of proportion. By focusing on problems that are taken out of all proportion, your own strengths and ability to cope are overlooked or downplayed. Things are seen as being out of control.

> **Key point:** All these unhelpful thinking styles occur in each of us from time to time. However during times of high anxiety they become more frequent and are harder to dismiss from the mind.

Now, consider your own thinking over the last week:

> **My anxious thinking**
>
> **Q.** Am I being my own worst critic *(bias against myself)*? Yes ☐ No ☐
>
> **Q.** Am I focusing on the bad in situations *(negative mental filter)*? Yes ☐ No ☐
>
> **Q.** Do I have a gloomy view of the future *(make negative predictions)*? Yes ☐ No ☐
>
> **Q.** Am I jumping to the very worst conclusion *(catastrophic thinking)*? Yes ☐ No ☐
>
> **Q.** Am I second-guessing that others think badly of me without actually checking *(mind-reading)*? Yes ☐ No ☐
>
> **Q.** Am I taking responsibility for things that aren't really my fault *(bearing all responsibility/taking all the blame)*? Yes ☐ No ☐
>
> **Q.** Do I have unhelpfully high standards and use the words '*should, must, ought* and *got to*' a lot, or make statements such as '*Just typical*' when something goes wrong *(unhelpfully high standards/rules)*? Yes ☐ No ☐
>
> If you have answered **Yes** to the question about catastrophic thinking, try to identify what sort of thoughts pop into your mind when you feel panicky.

Common catastrophic thoughts during panic

Catastrophic thought	Tick here if you notice this thought
'I'm going to faint or collapse/pass out.'	
'I'm going to suffocate.'	
'I'm going to collapse.'	
'I'm going to have a stroke.'	
'I'm going to have a heart attack.'	
I'm going to go mad.'	
'I'm going to lose control.'	
'I'm going to show myself up/make a fool of myself.'	

Write any other catastrophic fears you have here:

Why are these unhelpful thinking styles so unhelpful?

These extreme thinking styles are called unhelpful because believing them worsens how we feel and unhelpfully alters what we do.

Anxious thoughts ◄————————————► Feel more anxious

Anxious thoughts ◄————————————► Act in ways that worsen how you feel

Think about a recent time when you have felt more anxious or panicky. Were any unhelpful thinking styles present? Did they have an impact on how you felt and what you did at the time?

Read the table below to find more about the links between situations, thoughts, feelings and behaviour.

Situation, relationship or practical problem	Immediate catastrophic thought	Unhelpful thinking style	Emotional and/or physical impact	Behaviour change
Jane is sitting in her main room when suddenly a spider runs across the carpet.	'It's horrible, it will bite me. I can't deal with this.'	Catastrophic thinking and bias against yourself.	Anxiety and feel physically tense.	Runs out of the room (avoidance). Asks neighbour to remove the spider, and repeatedly checks that she has done so (unhelpful behaviour).
Harvinder has had fears of going shopping for over 6 months and these are gradually getting worse. He is now in the middle of a long queue at the supermarket.	'I'm going to collapse and pass out.'	Catastrophic thinking.	Anxiety and physical symptoms, of a faster heart rate and rapid breathing.	Tends to avoid supermarkets, and only shops when it is quieter (avoidance). Walks round the store faster than usual, gripping tightly to the trolley. Abandons the trolley and quickly leaves the store to sit down (unhelpful behaviour).
Dawn is someone with strong social anxiety. She has just been introduced to an attractive stranger.	'He thinks I'm boring and unattractive.'	Mind-reading.	Anxiety and physical symptoms, including going red and feeling hot, sweaty and shaky. Notices a dry mouth and a frog in her throat.	She generally avoids speaking to people and says no to invitations (avoidance). Avoids eye contact as she talks. Brings the conversation to an abrupt end. Clears her throat and swallows to excess (unhelpful behaviour).

The unhelpful thinking styles can thus worsen how you feel emotionally and physically, and unhelpfully alter what you do in both the short and in the longer term.

Other thinking changes also occur in anxiety.

Becoming overly aware of things that seem scary

High anxiety causes us to watch out for anything that is particularly scary to us. This can include difficult situations such as going into shops, seeing a spider, or the reactions of other people.

You may be overly aware of:
- *scary thoughts* (e.g. that you might die). You may try very hard not to think this.
- *Scary physical symptoms.* During times of high anxiety, all sorts of physical changes occur. This is a standard bodily response in times of threat or danger. Your heart rate and breathing both speed up. This allows more blood to get to your muscles to defend yourself or run away. These intense physical reactions can reinforce underlying fears that something terrible is about to happen. You will find out more about this later in this workbook.

Images and mental pictures – an important part of anxiety

Another way that we think is often in mental pictures. Some people (although not all) notice mental pictures or images in their mind when they become anxious. Images are a form of thought and may be 'still' images (like a photograph), or are moving (like a video). Images may be in black and white or in colour. They may include a mental picture of something catastrophic happening to you. You may see yourself collapsing, suffocating, or see an image of your own funeral. As with all extreme and unhelpful fears, the images add to feelings of anxiety.

Summary for Area 2: Altered thinking

Having answered the questions about altered thinking in this workbook:

Q. Overall, do I have any problems in this area?   Yes ☐   No ☐

These difficulties are potential targets for change. You will find out more about what steps to take to tackle these in Section 5 of the workbook.

Area 3: Altered feelings/emotions in anxiety

In times of high anxiety and panic, the following are common altered feelings:

- **Anxiety (also often called 'stress' or 'tension')**

In anxiety, the person feels troubled, unsettled and uneasy in himself or herself. At high levels of anxiety this can reach the level of intense fear seen in panic. Such high levels of anxiety are unpleasant but not dangerous.

- **Anger or irritability**

Little things that normally wouldn't bother you may now seem to really irritate or upset you. Anger tends to happen when you, or someone else, break a rule that you think is important, or acts to threaten or frustrate you in some way.

- **Shame**

Feelings of shame occur when you see yourself as having undesirable qualities which if revealed to others will result in ridicule and humiliation. For example this might be of your:
- *physical appearance (e.g. how your nose, ears, face, bottom, breasts etc. appear to others);*
- *emotions (e.g. shame at being anxious);*
- *personality (e.g. that you are not confident in everything you do);*
- *or actions (e.g. that you lied and avoided going to the party because of anxiety).*
These concerns lead to behaviours to hide these perceived 'faults' from others.

- **Low mood**

Depression may occur at the same time as panic or phobias. It can either start or worsen symptoms of anxiety. Common terms that people use to describe low mood include depression, or feeling low/sad/blue/upset/down/miserable or fed up. Typically in severe depression the person feels excessively down and few, if any, things cheer them up. If you feel like this, speak to your health care practitioner.

My altered feelings

Q. Do I feel very anxious or fearful/panicky at times?   Yes ☐   No ☐

Q. Do I get easily angry, frustrated or more irritable than previously?   Yes ☐   No ☐

Q. Do I feel shame about aspects of my actions or myself?   Yes ☐   No ☐

Q. Am I feeling depressed, upset or low in mood and no longer enjoy things
as before?   Yes ☐   No ☐

Summary for Area 3: Altered feelings/emotions

Having answered these questions:

Q. Overall, do I have any problems in this area?   Yes ☐   No ☐

These difficulties are potential targets for change. You will find out more about what steps to take to tackle these in Section 5 of the workbook.

Area 4: Altered physical sensations in high anxiety and panic

When a person becomes anxious, they may notice altered physical sensations such as feeling restless and unable to relax. Feelings of **mental tension** can also cause **physical tension** in your muscles and joints. This may cause feelings of shakiness, pain, weakness or tiredness. It can be surprising how tiring anxiety can be and some people may feel completely exhausted when they have felt anxious for a time. This muscle tension can cause symptoms such as tension headaches, stomach or chest pains. Sensations of being hot or cold, sweaty or clammy are common. Your heart may seem to be racing, and you may feel fuzzy-headed or disconnected from things.

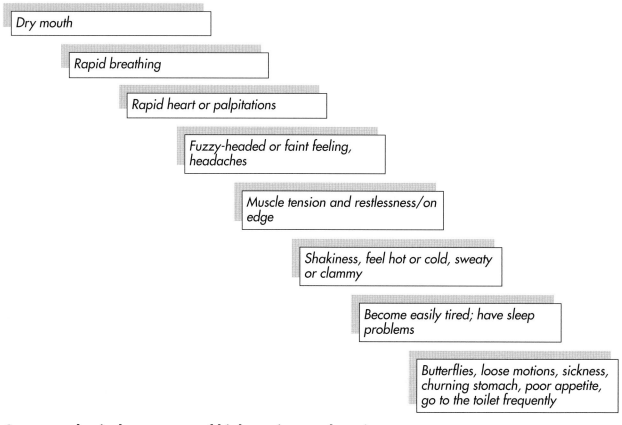

Dry mouth

Rapid breathing

Rapid heart or palpitations

Fuzzy-headed or faint feeling, headaches

Muscle tension and restlessness/on edge

Shakiness, feel hot or cold, sweaty or clammy

Become easily tired; have sleep problems

Butterflies, loose motions, sickness, churning stomach, poor appetite, go to the toilet frequently

Common physical symptoms of high anxiety and panic

What causes these physical symptoms?

Your body reacts to extreme and unhelpful frightening thoughts just as it would to a physical danger. The **fight or flight adrenaline response** creates all of the symptoms described above. Your heart rate and breathing both speed up so that your muscles are ready to react to defend yourself or run away. This is very useful when the danger is real. Think about a time when you have had a sudden shock – perhaps you have stepped into the road when a car was coming and didn't realise till you heard the car horn. Your body releases adrenaline which makes your heart beat faster. The fight or flight adrenaline response causes the person to pay particular attention to any potential threats around them. There may be other physical responses such as feeling sweaty or restless and tense. Blood is pumped faster round the body so that the muscles are ready to react. Breathing may speed up to allow more oxygen to get to the muscles. Sometimes rapid breathing continues long enough to cause a state of anxious over-breathing – also known as *hyperventilation*.

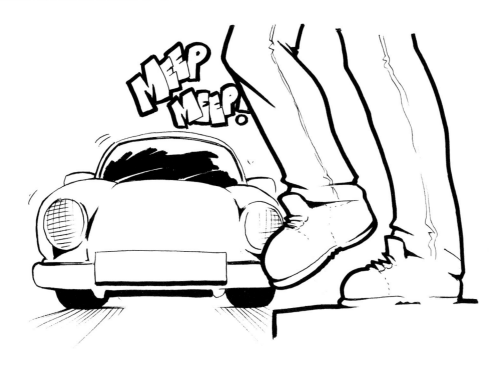

How do these physical changes and our catastrophic fears relate to each other?

The fight or flight adrenaline response causes us to pay particular attention to any potential threats around us. Each of us will focus on threats that are especially scary for us. For example, the experience of a very rapid heart or chest pain in panic may reinforce the fear that '*I'm having a heart attack*'. Feelings of dizziness and blurred vision caused by overbreathing can reinforce fears that '*I am about to faint/collapse*' or that '*I'm having a stroke*'.

It is important to recognise that although these sensations are unpleasant, **they are not harmful**.

What is hyperventilation?

In hyperventilation, fast breathing with the upper part of the chest occurs so that rapid shallow breaths are taken through the mouth.

It is important to distinguish between the sudden-onset (so-called acute) hyperventilation that occurs during panic, and the problem of longer-term low-key hyperventilation. Low-key hyperventilation reflects 'bad habits' of breathing. In acute hyperventilation the person begins to over-breathe very quickly with rapid shallow breaths. It is this sort of breathing that tends to occur in times of high anxiety and panic. Even though the person is getting more than enough oxygen into the blood supply, they begin to notice a range of unpleasant physical symptoms.

> **Important information:** When somebody develops sudden-onset hyperventilation, this makes him or her feel even more breathless. It causes other symptoms such as blurred vision, a dry mouth, and also sensations of tension or tightness in the chest. This may create a 'choking' sensation. There may be tingling in the tips of the nose, feet, fingers or hands and this can occasionally lead to muscle spasms in the hands or face. Finally, hyperventilation can cause the person to feel dizzy or fuzzy-headed so that he/she feels 'spaced out', distanced, or strangely disconnected from things.
>
> These symptoms occur because of breathing out too much carbon dioxide. You may have heard that people who are hyperventilating are sometimes given paper bags to place over their mouths for a few minutes. This helps them to slow their breathing and to re-capture some of the carbon dioxide so that they quickly begin to feel better again.

If you would like to find out more about hyperventilation, please read the worksheet *Overcoming hyperventilation/overbreathing* (p. 11.1). This includes tips for dealing with hyperventilation, though the use of a paper bag is not recommended.

Depersonalisation: feeling cut-off and disconnected from things

An important difficulty caused by anxiety is that from time to time we can feel mentally disconnected and cut-off from things. The technical term for this is *depersonalisation*. It can sometimes be quite difficult to describe exactly what this feels like. Many people feel a *fuzzy-headed, spaced-out* sort of sensation. We may know that we are fully awake and also exactly where we are, yet in spite of this we feel distanced from things. It can seem as if we are a robot functioning on automatic. Sometimes we feel like an observer looking at everything from a distance as if we are watching television. We may feel not really connected – as if we or the things around us are not completely real. This feeling can be disturbing and often has a clear 'start'. It then just as suddenly stops.

If you would like to find out more about depersonalisation, please read the worksheet *Understanding depersonalisation* (p. 12.1).

My altered physical symptoms in times of high anxiety

Q. Do I notice a dry mouth when I feel very anxious? Yes ☐ No ☐

Q. Do I sometimes over-breathe with rapid, shallow gasping breaths? Yes ☐ No ☐

Q. Do I notice my heart racing at times when I am anxious? Yes ☐ No ☐

Q. Am I restless and unable to relax? Yes ☐ No ☐

Q. Do I notice a fuzzy-headed/disconnected feeling when I am anxious? Yes ☐ No ☐

Q. Am I noticing physical tension or pain in my chest or head when I feel anxious? Yes ☐ No ☐

Q. Do I feel shaky, hot, cold, sweaty or clammy when I feel anxious? Yes ☐ No ☐

Q. Do I feel physically drained and weak after a period of high anxiety? Yes ☐ No ☐

If you over-breathe, which symptoms do you notice at that time?

A sensation of not getting enough air into my body?	Yes ☐	No ☐
A dry mouth?	Yes ☐	No ☐
Blurred vision?	Yes ☐	No ☐
Sensations of increased chest tension?	Yes ☐	No ☐
Tingling in the nose, mouth, fingers or hands?	Yes ☐	No ☐
Feeling jelly-legged or faint/dizzy?	Yes ☐	No ☐
A strange fuzzy-headed/disconnected feeling where everything seems to go quite distant?	Yes ☐	No ☐

Summary for Area 4: Altered physical symptoms

Having answered these questions:

Q. Overall, do I have any problems in this area? Yes ☐ No ☐

These difficulties are potential targets for change. You will find out more about what steps to take to tackle these in Section 5 of the workbook.

You have now completed thinking about how anxiety may be affecting you in four of the five key areas. The next section will help you to consider the final area – how anxiety can affect your behaviour.

Section 4 Unhelpfully altered behaviour in panic and phobias

This section moves on to consider the fifth and final area of your Five Areas Assessment – altered behaviour. Behaviour may change unhelpfully in two key ways – avoidance and unhelpful behaviours.

Altered behaviour 1: Avoidance

When somebody develops anxiety, it is normal for him or her to try to avoid difficult situations, people or places. This avoidance can make matters worse by making the person lose even more confidence. The result is often an increasingly restricted lifestyle and additional distress. A **vicious circle of avoidance** may result. This is summarised in the diagram below.

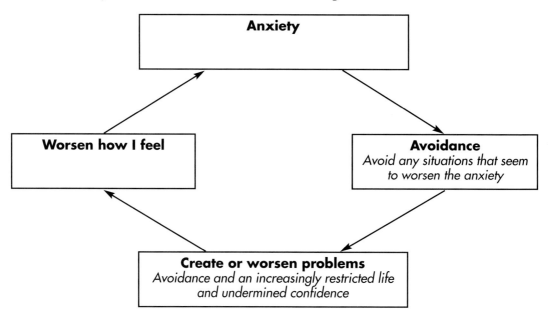

The vicious circle of avoidance

For example, someone who has panic attacks in shops may begin to avoid going there, or will only go into smaller shops when they are likely to be empty. To help you see if this applies to you, ask yourself '*What have I stopped doing because of my anxiety?*'

Question: What have I stopped doing because of my anxiety?

You may find yourself avoiding certain situations, people or places because of how you feel. Try to identify ways in which you might be avoiding things as a result of anxiety. For example, do you avoid going out or mixing with others? Consider what you are avoiding because of anxiety.

What situations at home, work or in my relationships with others am I avoiding tackling/putting off?

If I didn't have this anxiety, what things would I like to be able to do?

What have I stopped/reduced doing that I used to enjoy because of my anxiety?

Remember, sometimes avoidance can be quite subtle. For example, choosing a time or place when you think the anxiety-provoking situation will be easier to deal with, or choosing the easiest option when making decisions.

The following checklist will help you consider any areas of avoidance in your life.

Checklist: Identifying the vicious circle of avoidance

As a result of feeling anxious am I:

Tick here if you have noticed this

Avoiding dealing with important practical problems (both large and small)?

Not really being honest with others. For example, saying Yes when I really mean No?

Trying hard to avoid situations that bring about upsetting thoughts/memories?

Brooding over things and therefore not longer living life to the full?

Avoiding opening or replying to letters or bills?

Sleeping in to avoid doing things or meeting people?

Avoiding answering the phone, or the door when people visit?

Avoiding sex?

Avoiding talking to others face to face?

Avoiding being with others in crowded or hot places?

Avoiding busy or large shops, or finding that I have to think about where and when I go shopping etc.?

Avoiding going on buses, in cars, taxis etc., or any places where it is difficult to escape?

Avoiding walking alone far from home?

Avoiding situations, objects, places or people because of fears about what harm might result?

Avoiding physical activity or exercise as a result of concerns about my physical health?

Q. Am I avoiding things in other ways?

Write in here how you are doing this if this is applicable to you.

Summary: the vicious circle of avoidance

Having answered these questions, reflect on your responses using the three questions below:

Q. Am I avoiding doing things as a result of anxiety?   Yes ☐   No ☐

Q. Has this reduced my confidence in things and led to an increasingly
restricted life?   Yes ☐   No ☐

Q. Overall, has this worsened how I feel?   Yes ☐   No ☐

If you have answered **Yes** to all three questions, you are experiencing the vicious circle of avoidance.

Before moving on, think back on what you have learned and think about how avoidance may be affecting your life. Take time to think this through and take a break now if you wish to.

Altered behaviour 2: Unhelpful behaviours

When somebody becomes anxious or depressed, it is normal to try to do things that make them feel better. This altered behaviour may be *helpful* or *unhelpful*. The purpose of both types of activity is to reduce anxiety – at least in the short term.

Helpful activities may include:
Talking with friends or relatives and receiving helpful support.

- Reading or using self-help materials to find out more about the causes and treatment of the problems.
- Doing activities that provide pleasure or support such as meeting friends, playing sport, and attending religious activities.
- Challenging anxious thoughts by stopping, thinking and reflecting rather than accepting them as true.
- Going to see your doctor or health care practitioner or attending a self-help support group.

Write down any *helpful* things you have done here.

You should aim to try to maximise the number of helpful activities you do as part of your recovery plan. Sometimes, however, we may try to block how we feel with a number of **unhelpful behaviours**. These are designed to make us feel safer.

Unhelpful actions designed to make you feel safer
Unhelpful behaviours include *leaving situations where you feel anxious*, or *rushing through things as quickly as possible* so as to minimise the amount of time spent in the uncomfortable situation.

Sometimes a person may carry out a *mental task* such as counting things a set number of times, repeating positive statements such as '*I won't panic*', or saying a prayer again and again. These are sometimes called *distraction techniques* – because the person is trying to distract from how they feel. They may also try to do this by clenching their muscles tightly, digging their nails hard into their hands, or gripping onto things such as a shopping trolley as tightly as they possibly can to distract from how they feel.

Other ways that we block how we feel may include *over-eating*, *using illegal drugs* or *misusing prescription medication* by taking tablets at times when they are not prescribed to try to relax. *Alcohol misuse* is very common in anxiety. This may start out as just having an extra drink to help us get off to sleep. The danger is of escalating amounts being taken more and more frequently. The risk is alcohol or drug dependency.

Reassurance-seeking and *asking others to accompany you* whenever you do anything that causes anxiety also commonly occurs. This is a good example of an action that in moderation can be helpful and a source of support, but which can become unhelpful when taken to excess. The result is a feeling of dependency on others and a further loss of confidence in yourself.

It can sometimes be tempting to throw yourself into *excessive activity at home or at work*. The intention is to 'work' through the distress. By filling every part of the day with non-stop activity the hope is to avoid noticing how bad you feel. This may involve other ways of avoiding emotional distress, such as deliberately staying up late watching films, or sleeping in during the day to avoid seeing others. It also could include spending hours on computer games or watching television. Other common activities are listening to music, chatting/surfing on the Internet or texting others all the time. This is not to say that such activities are all unhelpful – but we need to ask *why* they are done. Doing these things because they can help us to avoid life has a very different motivation from doing them because they are fun.

> **Keypoint:** The purpose of all the unhelpful behaviours is to feel safer/better at least in the short term. They are sometimes therefore called *safety behaviours* as a result. Although they lead to a short-term relief in symptoms, this doesn't last. **The anxiety returns to the same or even higher level**.

The safety behaviours also teach an unhelpful lesson – *that it is only by relying on these unhelpful behaviours that you managed to cope*. In the longer term these actions can backfire and add to your problems.

For example, if we rely on alcohol or sedative drugs to give us false courage, we may find they cause us additional problems of their own. A **vicious circle of unhelpful behaviour** can occur. This can further worsen how you feel by increasing self-blame and confirming negative beliefs about yourself or others.

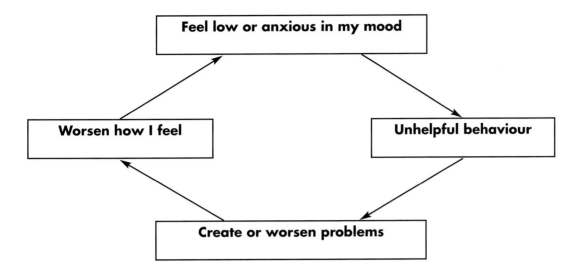

The vicious circle of unhelpful behaviour

A useful question to identify unhelpful behaviours is to ask yourself 'What am I doing differently to cope with how I feel?'

The following checklists will help you to identify any unhelpful behaviour in your life. At times these actions can be quite subtle and often revolve around avoidance of people, places or events.

Unhelpful behaviours leading to avoidance of anxiety-provoking situations.

Am I:

Quickly leaving anxiety-provoking situations?

Rushing through a task as quickly as possible? (e.g. walking or talking faster).

Trying very hard not to think about upsetting thoughts/memories? Trying to distract myself to improve how I feel?

Only going out and doing things when others are there to help?

Taking the easiest option (for example joining the shortest queue in the shop as a result of anxiety, or turning down opportunities that seem scary)?

Deliberately looking away during conversations and avoiding eye contact? Bringing conversations to a close quickly because of not knowing what to say?

Q. Am I avoiding things in other subtle ways?

Write in what you are doing here if this applies to you.

In addition, a number of other unhelpful behaviours may occur as a means of blocking or improving how you feel.

Checklist: Identifying the vicious circle of unhelpful behaviour

As a result of how I feel, am I:	Tick here if you have noticed this
Misusing drink/illegal drugs or prescribed medication to block how I feel in general or improve how I sleep?	
Eating too much to block how I feel (*comfort eating*), or over-eating so much that this becomes a 'binge'?	
Trying to spend my way out of how I feel by going shopping (*retail therapy*)?	
Becoming very demanding or excessively seeking reassurance from others?	
Looking to others to make decisions or sort out problems for me?	
Throwing myself into doing things so there are no opportunities to stop, think and reflect?	
Pushing others away and being verbally or physically threatening/rude to them?	
Deliberately harming myself in an attempt to block how I feel?	

Checklist: Identifying the vicious circle of unhelpful behaviour

As a result of how I feel, am I:

Tick here if you have noticed this

Taking part in risk-taking actions for example crossing the road without looking, or gambling with money I don't really have?

Compulsively checking, cleaning, or doing things a set number of times or in exactly the 'correct' order so as to make things 'right'?

Carrying out mental rituals such as counting or deliberately thinking 'good' thoughts/saying prayers to make things feel 'right'?

Being overly aware and excessive checking for symptoms of ill health?

Excessively changing the way I sit or walk to reduce symptoms of physical discomfort? The altered posture then creates or worsens the physical problem.

Sleeping with a number of people as a means of blocking how I feel or to feel needed, attractive or relaxed?

Summary: the vicious circle of unhelpful behaviours

Having answered these questions, reflect on your responses using the three questions below:

Q. Am I doing certain activities or behaviours that are designed to improve how I feel?   Yes ☐   No ☐

Q. Are some of these activities unhelpful in the short or longer-term either for me or for others?   Yes ☐   No ☐

Q. Overall has this worsened how I feel?   Yes ☐   No ☐

If you have answered **Yes** to all three questions, you are experiencing the vicious circle of unhelpful behaviour.

Summary for Area 5: Altered behaviour (avoidance or unhelpful behaviours)

Having answered these questions:

Q. Overall, do I have any problems in this area?   Yes ☐   No ☐

These difficulties are potential targets for change. You will find out more about what steps to take to tackle these in Section 5 of the workbook.

You have now finished your Five Areas Assessment. Before you move on, please stop for a while and consider what you have learned. How does what you have read help you to make sense of your symptoms?

Q. How well does this assessment summarise how you feel?

Poorly   Very well
0 ———————————————————————— 10

The purpose of your assessment

The purpose of the Five Areas Assessment is to help you plan the areas you need to focus on to bring about change. The workbooks in the *Overcoming Anxiety* course can help you begin to tackle each of the five problem areas of anxiety.

Section 5 Choosing your targets for change

The main problem areas seen in high levels of anxiety, panic and phobias are the:
- Current situations, relationship or practical problems
- Altered thinking (with extreme and unhelpful thinking)
- Altered feelings /emotions
- Altered physical symptoms
- Altered behaviour (with avoidance or unhelpful behaviours)

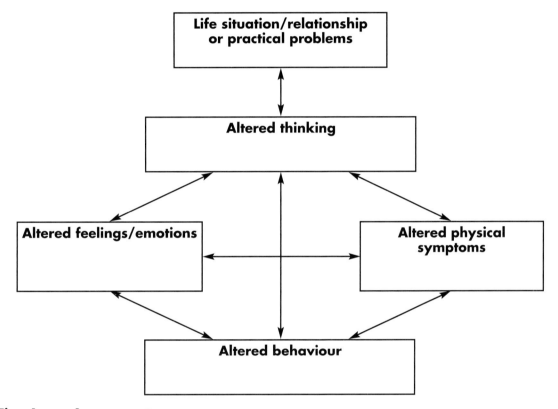

The Five Areas Assessment

You have previously answered questions about each of these five areas. Look again at the answers you gave in your own Five Areas Assessment, in the last two sections of the workbook. Your answers summarise the problems you identified in each area. Since there are links between the areas, it is possible by altering any one of the areas to bring about changes in others, and help improve how you feel.

Key point: By defining your problems, you have now identified possible target areas to focus on. The key is to make sure that you do things **one step at a time**. Slow steady steps are more likely to result in improvement than very enthusiastically starting and then running out of steam.

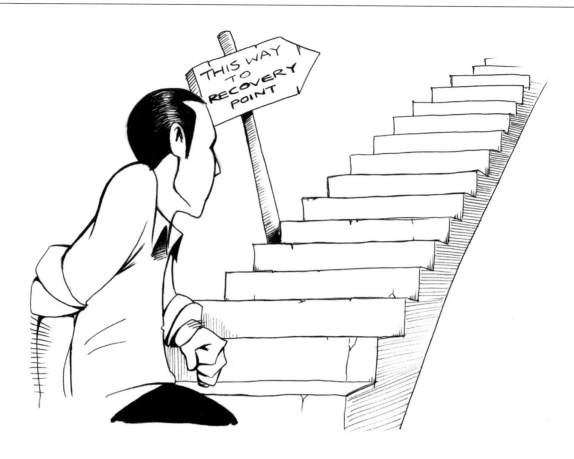

Short-, medium- and longer-term goals

You may have made all sorts of previous attempts to change, but unless you have a clear plan and stick to it, change will be very difficult. Planning and selecting which targets to try and change first is a crucial part of successfully moving forwards. By choosing some specific areas to focus on to start with, this also means that you are actively choosing at first **NOT** to focus on other areas.

Setting yourself targets will help you to focus on how to make the changes needed to get better. To do this you will need to decide:

- Short-term targets: changes you can make today, tomorrow and next week.
- Medium-term targets: changes to be put in place over the next few weeks.
- Long-term targets: where you want to be in six months or a year.

The questions that you have answered in this workbook will have helped you to identify the main problem areas that you currently face. The *Overcoming Anxiety* course (outlined below) can help you to make changes in each of these areas.

The workbooks can be used either alone or as part of a complete course. The workbooks 1a to 1e in Part 1 are designed to help you to identify your current problem areas. This will help identify which of the workbooks 2 to 9 in Part 2 you need to read. Finally, you can summarise what you have learned and plan for the future by completing Workbook 10. This will help you keep putting what you have learned into practice.

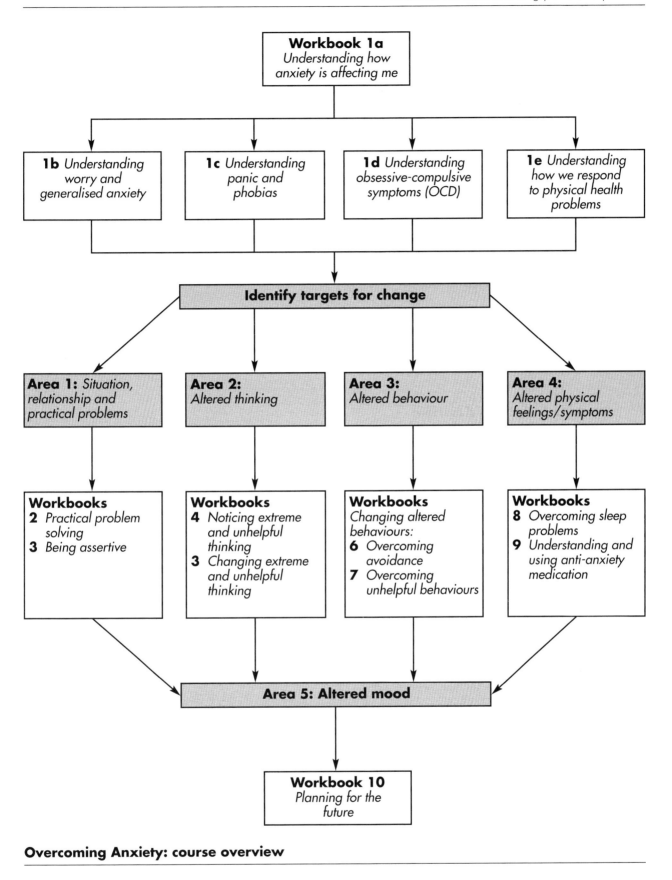

Overcoming Anxiety: course overview

The Overcoming Anxiety course

Understanding anxiety

Workbooks 1a to 1e provide an introduction and overview of anxiety problems. It is recommended that you read these workbooks first to give you an overview of how anxiety can affect you. The five workbooks together cover the common anxiety disorders – worry, panic, phobias, obsessive-compulsive disorder and also how we respond to physical health problems. They will help you identify which of these areas you need to focus on changing and will help you decide which of the remaining workbooks you need to read.

Area 1: Dealing with difficult situations, relationship and practical problems

Workbook 2: *Practical problem solving*

In this workbook you will learn a step-by-step plan that you can use to deal with practical problems. It will provide you with the tools to tackle any practical problems that you face. This will help you to take more control of your life and the decisions that you make. By feeling more in control of your life, you will improve your self-confidence.

Workbook 3: *Being Assertive*

Have you ever thought that no one listens to you, and that other people seem to walk all over you? Have others commented that they think that you always walk over them? You will find out about the difference between passive, aggressive and assertive behaviour and learn how to develop more balanced relationships with others where your opinion is listened to and respected, and you listen to and respect other people.

Area 2: Changing extreme and unhelpful thinking

Workbook 4: *Noticing extreme and unhelpful thinking*

What you think about yourself, others and the situations that occur around you, can alter how you feel and affect what you do. This workbook will help you to learn ways of identifying extreme and unhelpful ways of thinking. You will learn how to notice such thoughts and to understand the impact these have on how you feel and what you do.

Workbook 5: *Changing extreme and unhelpful thinking*

This workbook will teach you the important skill of how to challenge extreme and unhelpful thinking. With practice this will help you change the extreme and unhelpful thinking that is often a major problem in anxiety or depression.

Area 3: Changing altered behaviours

Workbook 6: *Overcoming avoidance*

You will find out more about how avoidance keeps problems going. You will learn ways of changing what you do in order to break the vicious circle of avoidance.

Workbook 7: *Overcoming unhelpful behaviours*

You will learn some effective ways of overcoming unhelpful behaviours such as drinking too much, reassurance seeking and trying to spend your way out of how you feel.

Area 4: Physical symptoms and treatments

Workbook 8: *Overcoming sleep problems*

Often when someone is anxious they not only feel emotionally and mentally low, but they also notice a range of physical changes that are a normal part of anxiety. This workbook will help you find out about these common changes, and in particular will help you to deal with problems of poor sleep.

Workbook 9: *Understanding and using anti-anxiety medication*

When someone is anxious sometimes their doctor suggests they take an anti-anxiety medication. You will find out why doctors suggest this, and also learn about common fears and concerns that people have when first starting to take these tablets so that you can find out for yourself whether this medication may be helpful for you.

Area 5: Altered mood

The fifth and final area, anxious mood, will improve if you work at the other areas where you have problems (the altered thinking, behaviour, physical symptoms and the situations, relationships and practical problems that you face). Once you feel better, the final workbook of the series can be read to help you to summarise what you have learned.

Workbook 10: *Planning for the future*

You will have learned new things about yourself and made changes in how you live your life. This final workbook will help you to identify what you have learned and help you plan for the future. You will devise your own personal plan to cope with future problems in your life so that you can face the future with confidence.

The work you do using the workbooks can supplement the help you receive from your doctor or other health care practitioner or friends. Sometimes more specialist help is needed to help how you feel and your doctor may suggest that you see a trained specialist such as a clinical psychologist, occupational therapist, social worker, psychiatric nurse or a psychiatrist.

Use the following table to help you decide which workbooks are right for you to read now, and over the next few weeks and months. You have already read the current workbook, and it is recommended that you also read Workbook 1a: *Understanding how anxiety is affecting me*. You may find it helpful to discuss this with your health care practitioner or other trusted supporter.

Workbook title	Short-term goals (plan to read in the next week or so)	Medium-term goals (plan to read over the next few weeks)	Long-term goals (plan to read over the next few months)	Tick when completed
Understanding anxiety workbooks				
1a *Understanding how anxiety is affecting me*	✔			
1b *Understanding worry and generalised anxiety*				
1c *Understanding panic and phobias*	✔			
1d *Understanding obsessive-compulsive symptoms (OCD)*				
1e *Understanding how we respond to physical health problems*				
Workbook 2 *Practical problem solving*				
Workbook 3 *Being assertive*				
Workbook 4 *Identifying extreme and unhelpful thinking*				
Workbook 5 *Changing extreme and unhelpful thinking*				
Workbook 6 *Overcoming avoidance*				
Workbook 7 *Overcoming unhelpful behaviours*				
Workbook 8 *Overcoming sleep problems*				
Workbook 9 *Understanding and using anti-anxiety medications*				
Workbook 10 *Staying well*				
Worksheet *Overcoming hyperventilation/ over-breathing*				
Worksheet *Understanding depersonalisation*				

In order to help you to review your progress, it can be useful to record how you feel at different times as you work on your problems. Your health care practitioner may work with you to decide what information it might be helpful to record. Don't expect to feel better all at once. Change can take time, however by working at your problems, most people find that improvement is possible.

> **Key point:** In order to change, you will need to choose to try to apply what you will learn regularly **throughout the week**, and not just when you read the workbook or see your health care practitioner. The workbooks will encourage you to do this by sometimes suggesting certain tasks for you to carry out in the days after reading each workbook.
>
> These tasks will:
> ● help you to put into practice what you have learned in each workbook;
> ● gather information so that you can get the most out of the workbook.
>
> Experience has shown that you are likely to make the most progress if you are able to put into practice what you have learned.

Summary

In this workbook you have learned about:
● the key elements of anxiety, panic and phobias;
● how what you think can affect how you feel and unhelpfully alter what you do;
● the Five Areas of Anxiety: the *situations, relationship and practical problems* faced, and the *altered thinking, emotional* and *physical feelings* and *behaviour* that occur as part of panic and phobias;
● the areas you need to tackle in order to overcome your own problems of anxiety. You should now be able to identify the workbooks you will read next in the short-, medium- and longer-term.

Putting into practice what you have learned

● Read through the current workbook again. Think in detail about how anxiety is affecting your thinking, emotional and physical feelings, and behaviour. Decide which areas you want to change.
● Choose **two episodes** over the next week when you feel more anxious. Use the blank Five Areas Assessment sheet (p. 1c.38) to record the impact on your thinking, mood, body and behaviour at those times. Try to generate a summary of your own anxiety in each of the five areas (life situation, relationships and practical problems, altered thinking, feelings, physical symptoms and behaviour). Use this workbook to identify whether you showed any of the unhelpful thinking styles during these occasions. What impact did your thoughts have on how you felt and what you did during these two episodes? Can you identify any examples of avoidance or unhelpful behaviours? Please photocopy or draw out additional copies of this diagram as you need it and keep the sheet handy.
● Finally, review your list of which workbooks you will choose to use next and move on to work through these in your own time.

If you have difficulties with these tasks, don't worry. Just do what you can. If you have found any aspects of this workbook unhelpful, upsetting or confusing, please can you discuss this with your health care practitioner or someone else whose opinion you trust.

A request for feedback

An important factor in the development of all the Five Areas Assessment workbooks is that the content is updated on a regular basis based upon feedback from users and practitioners. If there are areas which you find hard to understand, or which seem poorly written, please let me know and I will try to improve things in future. I regret that I am unable to provide any specific replies or advice on treatment.

To provide feedback, please contact me via:

Email: Feedback@fiveareas.com

Mail: Dr Chris Williams, Department of Psychological Medicine, Gartnavel Royal Hospital, 1055 Great Western Road, Glasgow, G12 0XH

Acknowledgements

I wish to thank all those who have commented upon this workbook especially Nick Bell, Joan Bond, Frances Cole, Anne Joice, Catriona Kent, Willie Munro, Celia Scott-Warren and Susan Shaw.

The cartoon illustrations in the workbooks have been produced by Keith Chan (kchan75@hotmail.com) and are copyright of Media Innovations Ltd.

My notes

....

....

....

....

....

....

....

....

....

....

....

....

....

....

....

....

....

....

....

....

....

....

....

....

....

....

....

....

....

....

Worksheet: A Five Areas Assessment of a specific time when I feel more anxious/worse

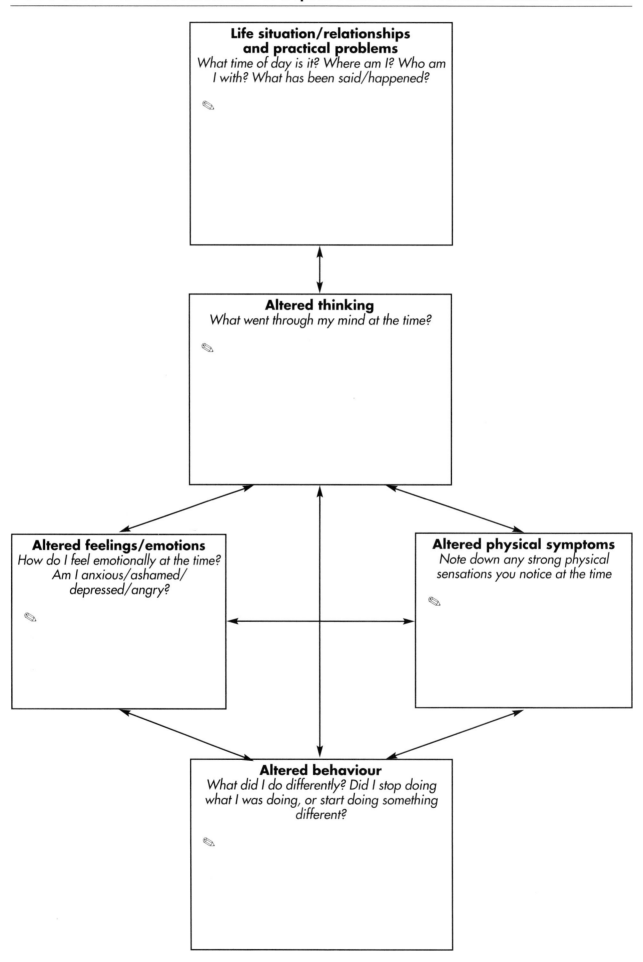

Workbook 1d

Understanding obsessive-compulsive symptoms

Dr Chris Williams

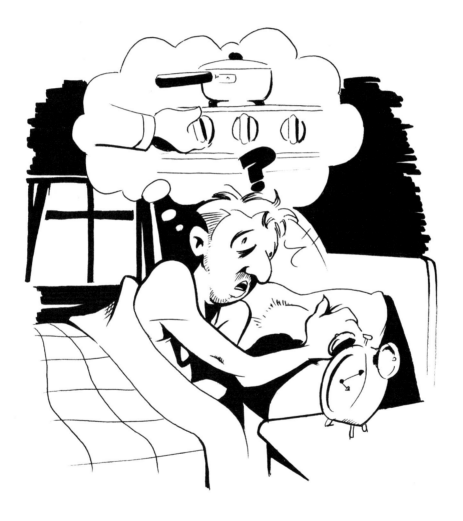

A Five Areas Approach

Section 1   **Introduction**

This workbook will cover:
- how to use the workbook most effectively;
- the key elements of obsessions and compulsions so that you will understand how they can affect you;
- the impact of how what you think can affect how you feel and unhelpfully alter what you do;
- the Five Areas of Anxiety: the *situations, relationship and practical problems* faced, and the *altered thinking, emotional* and *physical feelings* and *behaviour* that occur as part of obsessive-compulsive problems;
- the areas you need to tackle in order to overcome your own problems of obsessive-compulsive symptoms.

Don't be concerned if any of these words seem new or difficult to understand. All the terms will be described clearly as you read through the workbook.

How to use this workbook

Take time to read the workbook at your own pace. You don't have to sit down and read it in one go. You might find it most helpful to set yourself the target of reading the workbook one section at a time.
- Try to **answer all the questions** asked. The process of having to *stop, think and reflect* on how the questions might be relevant to you is crucial to getting better.
- **Write down** your own notes in the margins or in the *My notes* area at the back of the workbook to help you remember information that has been helpful. **Plan to review your notes regularly** so that you apply what you have learned.
- Once you have read through the entire workbook once, **put it on one side** and then **re-read it** a few days later. It may be that different parts of it become clearer, or seem more useful on second reading.
- Use the workbooks to **build upon the help you receive in other ways**, such as from reading other helpful material, talking to friends, or attending self-help organisations and support groups.
- Discuss the workbook with your health care practitioner and those who give you helpful support so that you can work together on overcoming the problems.

- **Remember that although change can seem difficult at first, it is possible.**

What is anxiety?

Anxiety, tension, stress, and *panic* are all terms that are used to describe what is a widespread problem for many people. Anxiety can affect everyone and anyone. At any one time, over one in ten people experience high levels of anxiety.

Can anxiety be helpful?

Anxiety is a common and normal emotion that at times can be helpful even though it can feel unpleasant. For example, at lower levels it can help motivate us to prepare for events such as interviews or exams. Anxiety is also helpful in situations of sudden danger, where it helps us to respond and get away as rapidly as possible. The problem is when we feel anxious in situations that are not dangerous at all. Another problem is feeling anxious well beyond what is helpful in the circumstances. For example, becoming very anxious about whether a light switch is turned off or not.

What are obsessions and compulsions?

In obsessive-compulsive disorder (OCD), the anxiety focuses upon two main areas:
- Obsessional thoughts
- Compulsive actions

Obsessional thoughts

Many people occasionally have the experience of noticing that a tune or piece of music seems to get 'stuck' and goes round and round in their mind for a time before eventually disappearing. In most cases this is seen as 'okay' (the person just hums along); at worst it is annoying, and eventually it stops. The term *obsessional thoughts* describes a similar situation, but the anxious or upsetting thoughts come more persistently to mind even though the person concerned does not wish this. The thoughts are unwanted and distressing. They are distressing because they focus on the threat that something the person has or might do will result in terrible harm for themselves or others.

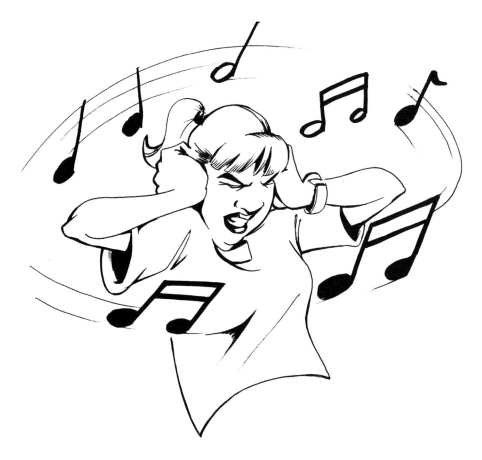

Compulsive actions

What people think affects how they feel and what they do. If we believe that the upsetting thoughts or images which pop into mind are important and might predict future events, we are likely to become scared by them. Then certain actions are completed to try to prevent or reverse harm. It is these actions that can become compulsive and make up the other feature of obsessive-compulsive disorder. The actions aim to try to avoid the chance of harm occurring, however slim this chance might be. The problem in obsessive-compulsive disorder is that doing the compulsive actions just once is never enough. The person becomes trapped in a cycle of doubt and resulting actions that goes on and on. For example, a person who has obsessional doubts that *unless* they check that the oven is off then there will be an explosion will check that the cooker is switched off again and again. You will find out later that these actions may in fact keep the problems going.

Who is affected by obsessive-compulsive symptoms?

Although the full symptoms of obsessive-compulsive disorder affect between one and two in every hundred people, it is quite common for people to occasionally experience some obsessive-compulsive symptoms. Many people live their lives with some degree of obsession – so that they need to always have things perfectly controlled, neat, ordered or tidy. It is also quite common for people to experience a wide range of obsessional thoughts.

Mild obsessive-compulsive symptoms

These occur in almost everybody. Think about some practical situations that you or your friends may have come across to illustrate this:

Q. Do you know anyone (particularly in childhood) who has avoided walking
on cracks or walking under ladders?   Yes ☐   No ☐

Q. Have you met anyone who 'touches wood' or will look for another magpie
if they see just one?   Yes ☐   No ☐

Q. Do you know anyone who will avoid sitting on public toilets and hover
above the toilet seat 'just in case' they get an infection?   Yes ☐   No ☐

If you consider most of the symptoms of OCD, they are usually extreme versions of quite commonly held and at times helpful beliefs. What is different in OCD is that the extent of anxiety and guilt associated with these thoughts and actions becomes enormously increased so that they come to dominate our life. **We have become afraid of the thoughts themselves.** This is one of the things that keeps obsessive-compulsive disorder going. You will find out more about this in the next section of the workbook.

What is the impact of the OCD on me?

The first step towards change is to try and work out the impact on you of your OCD at the moment. Start by thinking about how the OCD has affected you, your friends and relatives. Has it actually enhanced your life and made you feel more in control, or has it worsened how you feel? The following questions will help you think about this further.

The impact of obsessive-compulsive symptoms on me

Q. How long have I had the obsessive-compulsive symptoms? _____ months/years (please delete)

Q. On average, how much of my waking time do I spend thinking my obsessional thoughts each day? _____ hours (approximately)

Q. How intense does my anxiety seem at its worst?   Low ☐   Moderate ☐   High ☐

Q. On average, how much of my waking time do I spend each day carrying out compulsive actions? _____ hours (approximately)

Q. Despite my compulsive actions, have my obsessional thoughts continued
to take over my life?   Yes ☐   No ☐

Obsessive-compulsive symptoms can also be mixed in with other problems:

● **Depression:** This can cause or worsen obsessive-compulsive symptoms. People with depression have low mood, a lack of enjoyment and reduced activity. If you think you may be depressed then you should talk to your health care practitioner about this.

● **Generalised anxiety:** Worrying thoughts are anxiously brooded over in a way that is unhelpful because it does not actually help to sort out the difficulties that are being worried about. Look at Workbook 1b: *Understanding worry and generalised anxiety* to find out more about this.

● **Panic attacks:** These occur when high levels of anxiety and fear occur. If you think this might apply to you, Workbook 1c: *Understanding panic and phobias* will help you find out more.

The next section of the workbook will help you to identify exactly how anxiety linked to obsessive-compulsive disorder is affecting you.

Section 2 Understanding obsessive-compulsive disorder: my own Five Areas Assessment

A Five Areas Assessment can be helpful in understanding your own symptoms of anxiety and obsessive-compulsive symptoms, and in choosing targets to change how you feel.

The five areas are:

1 Life situation, relationships, practical problems and difficulties (e.g. problems at home or work)
2 Altered thinking (with extreme and unhelpful thinking)
3 Altered feelings (also called emotions or moods)
4 Altered physical symptoms/feelings in the body
5 Altered behaviour or activity levels (with avoidance, or unhelpful behaviours)

The Five Areas Assessment indicates that what we think about a situation or problem may affect how we feel emotionally and physically, and also alters what we do. Look at the arrows in the diagram. Each of these five areas affects the others and offers possible areas of change to reduce anxiety.

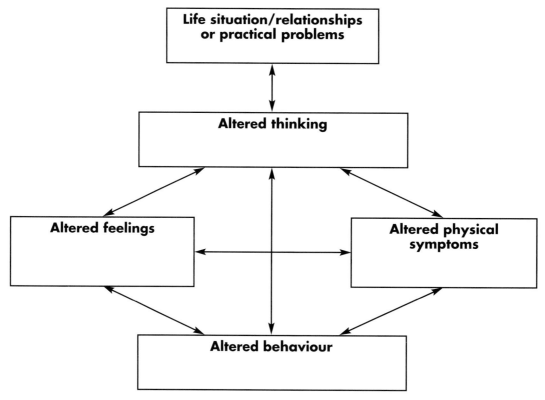

The Five Areas Assessment

Key point: As you go through the Five Areas Assessment, please think about how obsessive-compulsive symptoms have affected you in the last week. Try to answer all the questions and really think about how they apply to you. By doing this you will be able to identify possible target areas for change.

In order to break down the task, areas 1–4 will be covered in this section. Area 5, altered behaviour, is covered in Section 3.

Area 1: Situation, relationship and practical problems

All of us from time to time face practical problems or difficulties in relationships. When we face a large number of problems we may begin to feel overwhelmed. Difficult situations include everyday events such as comments from family, friends or others that we take personally. Practical problems may include:

- debts, housing or other difficulties;
- problems in relationships with family, friends or colleagues;
- other difficult situations that you face, such as problems at home or work (or lack of work – for example, unemployment).

The following table refers to several common situation, relationship and practical problems. Are any of these relevant to you?

Situation, relationship and practical problems

I have relationship difficulties (such as arguments).	Yes ☐	No ☐
I can't really talk and receive support from my partner.	Yes ☐	No ☐
There is no one around who I can really talk to.	Yes ☐	No ☐
My children won't do what I tell them.	Yes ☐	No ☐
I have difficulties with money problems or debts.	Yes ☐	No ☐
There are problems with my flat/house.	Yes ☐	No ☐
I am having problems with my neighbours.	Yes ☐	No ☐
I don't have a job.	Yes ☐	No ☐
I have difficulties with colleagues at work.	Yes ☐	No ☐

In obsessive-compulsive disorder the practical problems faced by the person can affect them in two ways:

1 As a source of **additional pressure and stress**. Many people who experience obsessive-compulsive disorder notice that the obsessional thoughts and compulsive actions seem worse when other life pressures have built up at the same time. Think about a pressure cooker in a kitchen. If the heat is turned up the pressure in the cooker rises and rises. Steam then begins to increasingly blow off to reduce the pressure. Compulsive actions can be seen a little like this. When life's pressures build up, the pressure leading to compulsive actions also can increase. The problem is that these actions end up turning up the pressure even more.

2 We may **avoid places, objects, people or situations**, which we fear might result in harm to ourselves or others. For example, if we have a fear that we might hit out, stab or hurt others, we may avoid getting near to others, or being close to any knives, 'just in case'.

There may therefore be a number of different situations, places or people that seem to worsen your obsessive-compulsive symptoms.

Write any such situations here:

> ✎

You will find out more about this as you complete your own Five Areas Assessment.

Summary for Area 1: Situation, relationship and practical problems

Having answered these questions:

Q. Overall, do I have any problems in this area?   Yes ☐   No ☐

These difficulties are potential targets for change. You will find out more about what steps to take to tackle these in Section 4 of the workbook.

Area 2: Altered thinking in obsessive-compulsive disorder

Anxious thinking is central to obsessive-compulsive disorder and the problems it causes. The first step in understanding obsessional thinking is therefore to understand the sorts of thinking that usually occur in anxiety.

The unhelpful thinking styles

Anxious thinking shows certain common themes and often becomes extreme, unhelpful and puts things out of all proportion. By focusing on problems that are taken out of all proportion, the person's own strengths and ability to cope are overlooked or played down. Things are seen as being out of control.

Consider your own thinking over the last week:

The unhelpful thinking styles in obsessive-compulsive disorder

Q. Am I being my own worst critic (bias against myself)?   Yes ☐   No ☐

Q. Am I focusing on the bad in situations (negative mental filter)?   Yes ☐   No ☐

Q. Do I have a gloomy view of the future (make negative predictions)?   Yes ☐   No ☐

Q. Am I jumping to the very worst conclusion (catastrophic thinking)?   Yes ☐   No ☐

Q. Am I second-guessing that others think badly of me without actually checking (mind-reading)?   Yes ☐   No ☐

Q. Am I taking unfair responsibility for things that aren't really my fault (bearing all responsibility/taking all the blame)?   Yes ☐   No ☐

Q. Do I have unhelpfully high standards and use the words 'should, must, ought and got to' a lot, or make statements such as 'Just typical' when something goes wrong (unhelpfully high standards/rules)?   Yes ☐   No ☐

If you have answered **Yes** to any of the questions it is likely that extreme anxious thoughts are adding to you problems.

The unhelpful thinking styles occur in each of us from time to time. However, during times of anxiety (including obsessive-compulsive disorder) they become more frequent and are harder to dismiss. By focusing on and unhelpfully exaggerating your problems, you let them build up and up in your mind without actually tackling them effectively.

Now think about how this may apply to the situation in obsessive-compulsive disorder.

Why are the unhelpful thinking styles so unhelpful?

In both anxiety and obsessive-compulsive disorder, the *unhelpful* thinking styles are called unhelpful because believing them worsens how we feel and pushes you into behaving in ways you do not wish to.

Obsessional thoughts ⟷ Feel more anxious

Obsessional thoughts ⟷ Act in ways that worsen how you feel

The obsessional thoughts can therefore worsen how you feel emotionally and physically, and unhelpfully alter what you do in both the short and the longer term. Think about a recent time when you have felt more anxious or noticed any obsessional thoughts. Were any unhelpful thinking styles present? Did they have an impact on how you felt and what you did at the time?

Thinking in obsessive-compulsive disorder

You have already read that in obsessive-compulsive disorder the key problem is that upsetting thoughts come into mind again and again. These thoughts may be memories from the past, ideas, doubts, fears, or images/mental pictures. The thoughts commonly include a fear of **harm arising because of something you have done or might have done.** Sometimes, the fear is of causing harm as a result of not having done something. In both situations we are constantly worried that a really bad consequence may happen to us or to others. Although we know that no harm is really *likely* to occur, the obsessional fears continue to dominate our thoughts. This even occurs when we recognise that the thoughts are silly or senseless. Sometimes obsessive thinking results in us becoming crippled by doubt about a particular issue. We go round and round trying to answer a particular question to the very last detail. An example is where we think again and again about the evidence of our own sexual orientation.

Obsessive fears and compulsive behaviours actions always revolve around themes that are deeply disturbing to us. Obsessional fears latch on to our Achilles heel – the last thing in the world we wish to have happen. Common examples of obsessional thoughts include fears that terrible harm may arise:

- *by an action you have (or might have) done*: for example, thoughts that someone may have been hurt when you brushed past them on the way home;
- *by an action you fear you might do*: for example, a loving mother of a newborn baby might have the obsessional fear that she will harm or kill her child; a quiet, shy person might fear shouting or swearing out loud in public; a person who hates the idea of violence fears they will stab or hit others.
- *by an action you haven't done*: for example, doubts about whether the cooker has really been switched off, or whether the door has been locked properly, or whether things have been cleaned well enough to prevent others getting infected.

The feared consequences might include a fire, death, separation or destruction. In each case, the results are always seen as *horrible* and cause deep upset. As with any threatening situation, the thoughts lead to anxiety.

Obsessive thinking checklist

Q. Do I have thoughts, memories, impulses, images or ideas that seem to go round and round in my mind?	Yes ☐	No ☐
Q. Are these thoughts unpleasant and/or upsetting to me?	Yes ☐	No ☐
Q. Have I become overly sensitive to these thoughts/fears?	Yes ☐	No ☐
Q. Am I downplaying my own ability to overcome these problems?	Yes ☐	No ☐
Q. Do I dwell on things I have (or could have) done that *might* result in harm to others?	Yes ☐	No ☐
Q. Do I fear I *might* lose control and do something that will harm or upset others?	Yes ☐	No ☐
Q. Do I worry that things I haven't done properly *might* result in harm to others?	Yes ☐	No ☐
Q. Do I have doubts and go over the same questions again and again with no chance of ever finding a solution?	Yes ☐	No ☐

This checklist illustrates an important point. Obsessional thoughts focus on a fear of harm arising. The harm might be very unlikely, but it doesn't *feel* this way. There is often an overestimation of the probability of the feared event occurring. In life many things *might* occur; however, the chances of them occurring are usually judged as being very unlikely. Dirtiness *can* spread infection, ovens *can* be left on by mistake and cause fires, doors *can* be left unlocked and result in a burglary. It makes perfect sense to check things or keep things clean *to a reasonable extent*. The problem in obsessive-compulsive disorder is that the fears and actions get out of all proportion. It is important to remember that the intrusive thoughts are only seen as distressing depending on how we interpret them.

> **Key point:** The fear is that something terrible *might* occur, and the chances of this occurring are over-estimated.

Obsessional thoughts – the big bully[1]

Imagine a child who is bullied at school. We can all understand how scared they may become and how they may hand over whatever the bully demands because they are terrified of being hurt or humiliated. In fact, this is quite a good short-term way of solving the problem. They hand over their pocket money and the bully goes away. However, giving in to the bully makes it more likely they will come back. In fact, the more you give the more they return. What would happen if every time the bully returned the child did not hand over what they wanted? It is easy to imagine the initial anxiety the child would feel, but bullies usually make empty threats. They also stop coming back if it is no longer worthwhile for them to do so. We can see the same pattern with obsessive-compulsive disorder. Letting ourselves be pushed around by unwanted intrusive thoughts reduces anxiety in the short-term but they just keep them coming back. We can also get the same increase in self-confidence through resisting them that the child in the story would feel.

---

1 Thank you to Dale Huey for this example.

Example:
- *'The light switch may be on. If it is it could short out and burn the house down.'*
- *'If I don't do the compulsive action (check the switch is off again)* **then** *the house will burn down.'*

The person who has such a fear becomes increasingly distressed, and often will then check the light switch is off. They feel compelled to do this even if they know they have checked it and made sure it was off just 20 minutes ago. We can let such intrusive doubts push us into behaving in ways we don't want to. It is easy to believe that if we give in the doubts will go away.

Images and mental pictures – an important part of obsessional thinking

Another way that we think is often in mental pictures. Some people (although not all) notice mental pictures or images in their mind when they become anxious and fearful. Images are a form of thought and may be 'still' images (like a photograph), or moving (like a video). Images may be in black and white or in colour. They may include a mental picture of some bad event occurring. For example, an image of a fire starting if the cooker is left unchecked. This then leads to someone being trapped in the fire. As with all fears, the images add to feelings of anxiety.

Q. Am I prone to noticing intrusive upsetting images or mental pictures?　　　　Yes ☐　　No ☐

The three key elements of obsessive-compulsive disorder

The three key unhelpful thinking styles present in obsessive-compulsive disorder are:

1　A **prediction** that something terrible will occur and an over-estimation of the probability of this happening (*making negative predictions* and *catastrophic thinking*).

2　A feeling of **personal responsibility** for the harm (*bearing all responsibility/taking all the blame*).

3　Having **very high standards and rules.** The unrealistically high standards do not allow you to rest if there is any chance of harm occurring. It is the very high standards that drive the compulsive actions. These aim to prevent or reverse any possible harm. Unfortunately, the compulsive actions can backfire and actually worsen the situation. This is described in the next section of the workbook.

The next task will help you to identify whether these three key unhelpful thinking styles are affecting you.

Write in your own obsessional thought(s) or images here:

Consider the thought(s):

Q. Am I predicting that some terrible harm will/might occur?   Yes ☐   No ☐

If yes:

Q. Am I possibly over-estimating the probability that this will occur?   Yes ☐   No ☐

Q. Would I feel personally responsible if it occurred?   Yes ☐   No ☐

Q. Can I allow myself to rest if there is any chance of it occurring?   Yes ☐   No ☐

Summary for Area 2: Altered thinking

Having answered these questions:

Q. Overall, do I have any problems in this area?   Yes ☐   No ☐

These difficulties are potential targets for change. You will find out more about what steps to take to tackle these in Section 4 of the workbook.

Area 3: Altered feelings/emotions

In obsessive-compulsive disorder, the following are common altered emotional feelings.

- **Anxiety (also often called 'stress' or 'tension')**

In anxiety, you feel troubled, unsettled and uneasy in yourself. This may be present for large parts of the day as you desperately struggle not to think the upsetting obsessional thoughts or try to resist the compulsive actions.

- **Anger or irritability**

Little things that normally wouldn't bother you may now seem to really irritate or upset you. Anger tends to happen when you, or someone else, break a rule that you think is important, or acts to threaten or frustrate you in some way.

- **Guilt**

Feelings of guilt arise when you judge that you have done wrong, and failed against some external or internal standard or code. You think that you have let yourself or others down by your actions, or lack of action.

- **Shame**

Feelings of shame occur when you see yourself as having undesirable qualities which if revealed to others will result in ridicule and humiliation. For example, this might be shame at experiencing obsessional thoughts which are seen as bad or wrong, or that you carry out actions that you recognise are excessive and senseless. These concerns lead to actions to hide these perceived 'faults' from others.

- **Low mood**

Depression may occur at the same time as obsessive-compulsive disorder. It can both start or worsen obsessive-compulsive symptoms. Common terms that people use to describe depression include feeling low/sad/blue/upset/down/miserable or fed up. You may find that you are more easily moved to tears and that things you would normally cope with really seem to strike home. Typically in severe depression the person feels excessively down and few if any things can cheer them up. If you feel like this, speak to your doctor or health care practitioner.

My altered feelings

Q. Do I feel anxious/very tense when I notice obsessional thoughts or when I resist the compulsive actions?   Yes ☐   No ☐

Q. Do I get more easily angry, frustrated or irritable than previously?   Yes ☐   No ☐

Q. Do I feel guilty and overly responsible for bad things that happen?   Yes ☐   No ☐

Q. Do I feel shame about aspects of my actions or myself?   Yes ☐   No ☐

Q. Am I feeling depressed, upset or low in mood and no longer enjoy things as before?   Yes ☐   No ☐

Summary for Area 3: Altered feelings/emotions

Having answered these questions:

Q. Overall, do I have any problems in this area?   Yes ☐   No ☐

These difficulties are potential targets for change. You will find out more about what steps to take to tackle these in Section 4 of the workbook.

Area 4: Altered physical sensations in obsessive-compulsive disorder

When a person becomes anxious, they may notice altered physical sensations such as feeling restless and unable to relax. Feelings of **mental tension** can also cause **physical tension** in your muscles and joints. This may cause feelings of shakiness, pain, weakness or tiredness. It can be surprising how tiring anxiety can be and some people may feel completely exhausted when they have felt anxious for a time. This muscle tension can cause symptoms such as tension headaches, stomach or chest pains. Anxiety can also cause other physical symptoms. Sensations of being hot or cold, sweaty or clammy are common. Your heart may seem to be racing, and you may feel fuzzy-headed or disconnected from things.

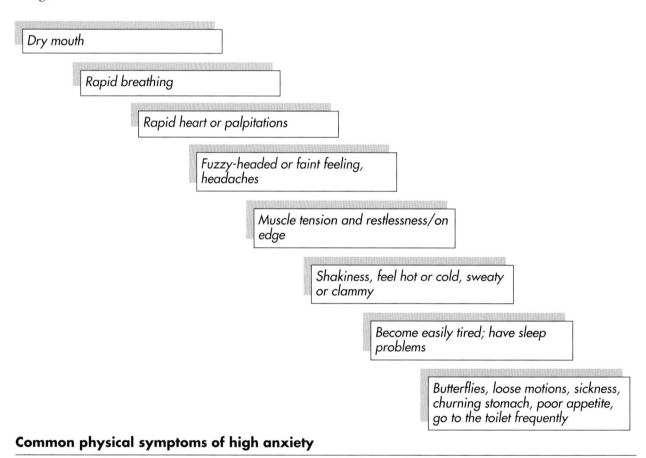

Dry mouth

Rapid breathing

Rapid heart or palpitations

Fuzzy-headed or faint feeling, headaches

Muscle tension and restlessness/on edge

Shakiness, feel hot or cold, sweaty or clammy

Become easily tired; have sleep problems

Butterflies, loose motions, sickness, churning stomach, poor appetite, go to the toilet frequently

Common physical symptoms of high anxiety

What causes these physical symptoms?

When intrusive thoughts seem believable your body reacts to them as it would to a physical danger. The **fight or flight adrenaline response** creates all of the symptoms described above. This is very useful when the danger is real. Think about a time when you have had a sudden shock – perhaps you have stepped into the road when a car was coming and didn't realise till you heard the car horn.

Your body releases adrenaline which makes your heart beat faster. The purpose is to prepare the body to defend yourself or to run away. Blood is pumped faster round the body so that the muscles are ready to react and breathing may speed up to allow more oxygen to get to the muscles. Sometimes rapid breathing continues long enough to cause a state of anxious over-breathing. This is also known as *hyperventilation.*

What is hyperventilation?

In hyperventilation, faster breathing with the upper part of the chest occurs so that rapid shallow breaths are taken through the mouth.

If you would like to find out more about hyperventilation, please read the worksheet *Overcoming hyperventilation/overbreathing* (p. 11.1).

Depersonalisation: feeling cut-off and disconnected from things

An important difficulty caused by anxiety is that from time to time we can feel mentally disconnected and cut-off from things. The technical term for this is *depersonalisation.* It can sometimes be quite difficult to describe exactly what this feels like. Many people feel a *fuzzy-headed, spaced-out* sort of sensation. We may know that we are fully awake and also exactly where we are, yet in spite of this we feel distanced from things. It can seem as if we are a robot functioning on automatic. Sometimes we feel like an observer looking at everything from a distance as if we are watching television. We may feel not really connected – as if we or the things around us are not completely real. This feeling can be disturbing and often has a clear 'start'. It then just as suddenly stops.

If you would like to find out more about depersonalisation, please read the worksheet *Understanding depersonalisation* (p. 12.1).

My altered physical symptoms in anxiety		
Q. Do I notice a dry mouth when I feel anxious?	Yes ☐	No ☐
Q. Do I sometimes over-breathe with rapid, shallow gasping breaths?	Yes ☐	No ☐
Q. Do I notice my heart racing at times when I am anxious?	Yes ☐	No ☐
Q. Am I restless and unable to relax?	Yes ☐	No ☐
Q. Do I notice a fuzzy-headed/disconnected feeling when I am anxious?	Yes ☐	No ☐
Q. Am I noticing physical tension in my muscles?	Yes ☐	No ☐
Q. Do I feel shaky, hot, cold, sweaty or clammy when I feel anxious?	Yes ☐	No ☐
Q. Am I feeling physically drained and easily tired?	Yes ☐	No ☐
Q. Am I finding it difficult getting off to, or staying, asleep?	Yes ☐	No ☐
Q. Am I feeling off my food?	Yes ☐	No ☐
Q. Do I notice feelings of sickness or butterflies in my stomach?	Yes ☐	No ☐

Summary for Area 4: Altered physical symptoms.

Having answered these questions:

Q. Overall, do I have any problems in this area?　　　Yes ☐　　　No ☐

These difficulties are potential targets for change. You will find out more about what steps to take to tackle these in Section 4 of the workbook.

You have now completed thinking about how anxiety caused by obsessive-compulsive disorder is affecting you in four of the five key areas. We have yet to look in detail at the actions that we do to try to neutralise or reverse the impact of intrusive thoughts. Section 3 will help you to consider the final area – how anxiety has affected your behaviour.

Section 3 Unhelpfully altered behaviour in obsessive-compulsive disorder

This section moves on to consider the fifth and final area of your Five Areas Assessment – altered behaviour. Behaviour may change unhelpfully in two key ways – unhelpful behaviours and avoidance.

Altered behaviour 1: Unhelpful behaviours

When somebody is anxious or depressed about anything, it is normal to try to do things to feel better. This altered behaviour may be *helpful* or *unhelpful*. The purpose of both types of activity is to reduce anxiety – at least in the short term.

Helpful activities may include:
- Talking with friends or relatives and receiving helpful support.
- Reading or using self-help materials to find out more about the causes and treatment of the problems.
- Doing activities that provide pleasure or support such as meeting friends, playing sport, attending religious activities and participating in outdoor pursuits.
- Challenging anxious thoughts by stopping, thinking and reflecting rather than accepting them as true.
- Going to see your doctor or health care practitioner or attending a self-help support group.

Write down any *helpful* things you have done here:

```
✎
```

You should aim to try to maximise the number of helpful activities you do as part of your recovery plan. Sometimes, however, we may try to block how we feel with a number of **unhelpful behaviours**. For example, when anxiety is at a high level we may choose to act in ways that reduce the level of anxiety – for a while. This is called a *safety behaviour*. These so-called safety behaviours include a range of actions designed to make you feel safer when anxious.

Unhelpful actions designed to make you feel safer

> **Key point:** The unhelpful actions that aim to neutralise or reverse the chance of harm arising are part of the problem rather than part of the solution. These actions worsen the problem of obsessive-compulsive disorder and are therefore a key target for change.

Unhelpful thinking

Trying to resist the thoughts by trying hard not to think them

Because obsessional thoughts focus on a fear that something terrible will happen, it can be frightening just to have the thoughts themselves – just in case the worst happens. In response you may desperately try **not** to think the thoughts. Is this an effective strategy?

Experiment: A hallmark of obsessive-compulsive thinking is that you may try to cope with the upsetting thoughts by trying not to think them. In order to see if this works, try this practical experiment. Please try as hard as you can **not** to think about the following object. Please try very hard for the next 30 seconds not to think about a white polar bear.

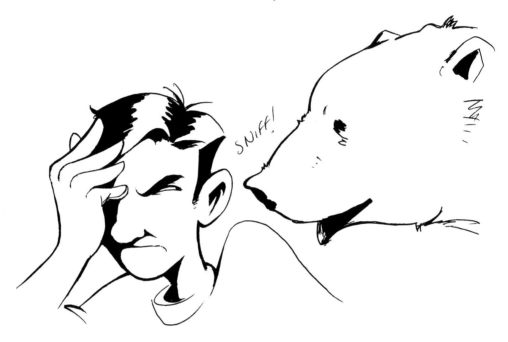

After you have done this, think about what happened. Was it easy not to think about the bear, or did it take a lot of effort? You may have noticed that trying hard not to think about it actually made it worse. Alternatively, you may have spent a lot of mental effort trying hard to think about something else such as a *black polar bear* instead. For many people, trying hard to ignore their obsessional thoughts doesn't work and may actually worsen the problem. Sometimes people who experience obsessive-compulsive disorder have tried very hard not to think about their distressing thoughts for many months and years. This can be mentally exhausting.

Q. Do I end up putting a lot of mental effort into trying hard not to think the
upsetting thoughts?   Yes ☐   No ☐

Q. If I try not to think the thoughts, does it work?   Yes ☐   No ☐

Recurrent mental rituals

Sometimes the person will use various mental rituals to try to prevent or reverse the impact of the obsessional thoughts. These are often largely hidden from others. It might involve carrying out a mental task such as counting things a set number of times (such as an even number of times), or deliberately thinking a 'good' thought or mentally repeating a prayer in order to prevent harm being done. The aim is to make things 'right'.

Unhelpful actions (compulsive actions)

Recurrent compulsive actions

As a result of the obsessional fears, the person tries to carry out actions in order to prevent or reverse the harm from occurring. These flow from the underlying obsessional fears the person has. Because the person feels personally responsible if harm were to occur, and because they have very high standards, they feel compelled to act. The word 'compelled' is important. In many cases the person knows that logically there is very little chance that harm will occur, yet feels rising distress and anxiety until the action is done. In other words a compulsion is when we feel compelled to act even if we don't want to. We feel pushed into the action – just as if we are being bullied into it.

These *compulsive actions* include:

- **Checking.** This might include going back over a recent journey to check if anyone has been hit by the car, or picking up all objects in the gutter as you walk along just in case they may hit someone. You may check that light switches are off or a door is locked. Even though logically you may know you have checked things many times already, you feel very uncomfortable until you go and check it again '*just one more time*'. This can be very disruptive and cause you to have to go back into work or get out of bed repeatedly at night to check things again and again.

- **Cleaning.** If you fear contamination by germs or that you might infect others, you may end up excessively cleaning yourself or your surroundings far beyond a reasonable or normal extent. This may include scrubbing your hands with soap or disinfectant or showering or bathing for hours on end. The result is that your hands may become red and raw. You may also be unable to go out or mix with others properly as a result.

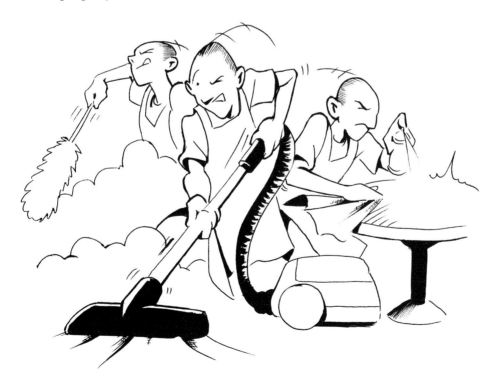

- **Carrying out tasks in the 'right' order or a set number of times.** Many children will avoid walking on the cracks in the pavement. This action is like a superstitious behaviour with fears that that unless it is done something bad will happen. In obsessive-compulsive disorder a similar compulsion to do things in the 'right' way may occur. For example, the person may feel compelled to put on their clothes in *exactly* the right order. If things are not done 'right' it has to be repeated again and again until it is done right. Just getting dressed might take up to two or three hours as a result. A variation of this is where the person has an uncomfortable feeling unless they do things a **set number of times** (e.g. to look round three times before setting off). This sort of superstitious thinking is sometimes called 'magical' thinking. The thinking only makes sense if we believe the initial bullying thought.

Excessively checking with others in order to seek reassurance

At one extreme we may choose not to talk at all about how we feel. Keeping your problems to yourself may be because of a belief that '*I shouldn't have emotional problems*', or that '*It is a sign of weakness to be upset.*'

At the other extreme, we may recurrently seek support and *excessive reassurance* from those around us. This is a good example of an action that in moderation can be *helpful* and a source of support, but which can become *unhelpful* when taken to excess. The result is a feeling of dependency on others and a further loss of confidence in yourself. With reassurance the more you get the more you seek.

Quickly leaving anxiety-provoking situations as soon as any anxiety is noticed

For example, leaving places where obsessional thoughts seem to worsen. If your obsessional thoughts are focused on a fear of stabbing others this place could be the kitchen, where there are knives.

Trying to block how you feel

Sometimes people try to block anxiety by:
- **Misusing alcohol or drugs.** Alcohol misuse is very common in obsessive-compulsive disorder. This may start out as just having an extra drink to help you try to block the intrusive thoughts or to get off to sleep. The danger is of escalating amounts being taken more and more frequently. The risk is alcohol dependency. The same misuse can be made of drugs.
- **Over-using or misusing prescription medication,** or taking tablets inappropriately at times when they are not prescribed to try to relax, block the thoughts or overcome your compulsion to act.
- **Eating too much** (*comfort eating*) – particularly sweet foods/carbohydrates. This may result in weight gain. Compulsive over-eating may sometimes result in binge eating and lead to an eating disorder.
- **Trying to spend your way out of how you feel** by visiting the shops and buying new clothes/goods. The purpose is to cheer you up (so-called *retail therapy*). This may overlap with compulsive shopping – buying things to make you feel better – in the short-term.
- **Sleeping with a number of people** in an attempt to feel needed, attractive or relaxed.

Over-committing yourself to work or social activities

Sometimes we may throw ourselves into excessive activity at home or at work. The intention is to 'work' through the distress. By filling every part of our day with non-stop activity the hope is to avoid noticing how we feel. This may involve other ways of avoiding emotional distress such as deliberately staying up late watching films, or sleeping in during the day to avoid seeing others. It also could include spending hours on computer games or watching television. Other common activities are listening to music, chatting/surfing on the Internet or texting others all the time. This is not to say that such activities are all unhelpful, but we need to look at why they are done. Doing these things because they can help us to avoid life is a very different matter from doing them because they are fun.

Pushing others away

Another unhelpful reaction is resolving our feelings by turning against those around us. We may become angry, gossipy, and undermine others by spreading rumours or becoming bitter and critical. This particularly can occur towards people who are easy targets and less likely to hit back, such as close relatives and friends. Sometimes this behaviour is a form of testing out the love, friendship and support of others. The consequence may be isolation, rejection and loneliness.

Taking part in risk-taking behaviour

This might include:

- Self-harm (for example, by cutting or scratching arms, legs or stomach) to block or numb feelings of tension.
- Taking part in risk-taking actions (for example, crossing the road without looking, or gambling using money you don't really have).

> **Key point:** Remember that the purpose of these unhelpful behaviours is to feel safer/better at least in the short term. They are sometimes therefore called *safety behaviours*. **Although each action causes a short-term relief in symptoms, this doesn't last and the tension always returns.**

A second problem with all these behaviours is that acting on the obsessional thoughts tends to confirm and strengthen the underlying fears. As in the case of the child giving into the bully, this can make the problem even worse. In the long term instead of helping reduce them the compulsive activities only reinforce your fears, causing them to take over more and more of your life. This can worsen the problems for yourself, your family and your friends.

A **vicious circle of unhelpful behaviour** can occur. This can further worsen how you feel by increasing self-blame and confirming negative beliefs about yourself or others as a result.

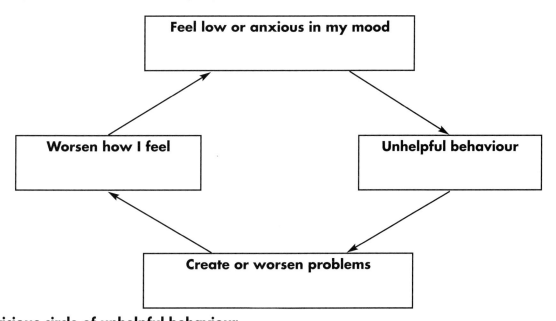

The vicious circle of unhelpful behaviour

A useful question in order to identify unhelpful behaviours is to ask yourself '*What am I doing differently to cope with how I feel?*'

The following checklists will help you to identify any unhelpful behaviour in your life. At times these actions can be quite subtle.

Core unhelpful behaviours in obsessive-compulsive disorder:	**Tick here if you have noticed this**
Compulsively checking, cleaning, or doing things a set number of times or in exactly the 'correct' order so as to make things 'right'?	
Compulsively carrying out mental rituals such as counting or deliberately thinking 'good' thoughts/saying prayers to make things feel 'right'?	

In addition, a number of other unhelpful behaviours may occur as a means of blocking or improving how you feel.

Checklist: Identifying the vicious circle of unhelpful behaviour

As a result of how I feel, am I:	**Tick here if you have noticed this**
Misusing drink/illegal drugs or prescribed medication to block how I feel in general or improve how I sleep?	
Eating too much to block how I feel (*comfort eating*), or over-eating so much that this becomes a 'binge'?	
Trying to spend my way out of how I feel by going shopping (*retail therapy*)?	
Becoming very demanding or excessively seeking reassurance from others?	
Looking to others to make decisions or sort out problems for me?	
Throwing myself into doing things so there are no opportunities to stop, think and reflect?	
Pushing others away and being verbally or physically threatening/rude to them?	
Deliberately harming myself in an attempt to block how I feel?	
Taking part in risk-taking actions for example crossing the road without looking, or gambling with money I don't really have?	
Being overly aware and excessively checking for symptoms of ill health?	
Excessively changing the way I sit or walk to reduce symptoms of physical discomfort? The altered posture then creates or worsens the physical problem.	
Sleeping with a number of people as a means of blocking how I feel or to feel needed, attractive or relaxed?	

Sometimes unhelpful behaviours can lead to quite subtle avoidance. Do you notice any of the following in your own life?

Unhelpful behaviours leading to subtle avoidance of anxiety-provoking situations.

Am I:

Quickly leaving anxiety-provoking situations?

Rushing through a task as quickly as possible? (e.g. walking or talking faster).

Trying very hard not to think about upsetting thoughts/memories? Trying to distract myself to improve how I feel?

Only going out and doing things when others are there to help?

Taking the easiest option (for example joining the shortest queue in the shop as a result of anxiety, or turning down opportunities that seem scary)?

Deliberately looking away during conversations and avoiding eye contact? Bringing conversations to a close quickly because of not knowing what to say?

Q. Am I avoiding things in other subtle ways?

Write in what you are doing here if this applies to you.

> **Summary: Altered behaviour 1: the vicious circle of unhelpful behaviours**
>
> Having answered these questions, reflect on your responses using the three questions below:
>
> **Q.** Am I doing certain activities or behaviours that are designed to improve how I feel?   Yes ☐   No ☐
>
> **Q.** Are some of these activities unhelpful in the short or longer term either for me or for others?   Yes ☐   No ☐
>
> **Q.** Overall has this worsened how I feel?   Yes ☐   No ☐
>
> If you have answered **Yes** to all three questions, you are experiencing the vicious circle of unhelpful behaviour. Before moving on, think back on what you have learned and think about how unhelpful behaviour may be affecting your life. Take time to think this through and take a break now if you wish to.

Altered behaviour 2: Avoidance

When somebody develops anxiety of any sort, it is normal for him or her to try to avoid any threatening situations. In obsessive-compulsive disorder, the person tries to avoid situations that seem to make the obsessive-compulsive symptoms worse and which they believe may result in distress or harm to themselves or to others.

Example: Someone with obsessional fears about germs and infection will avoid any circumstances where there is such a risk. This could mean not cleaning the toilet, shaking hands or touching anything that might be a source of contamination. This might include avoiding touching or moving letters and/or free weekly newspapers that are delivered, so that these pile up behind the front door.

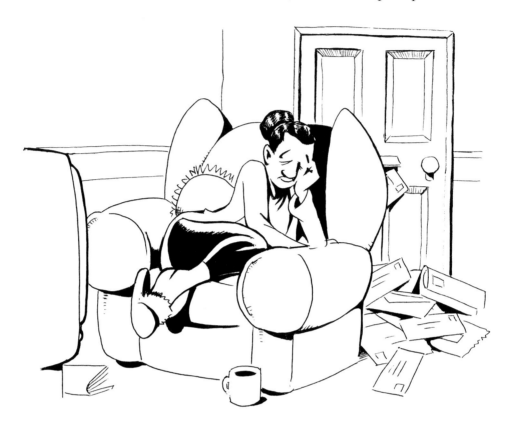

Try to identify ways in which you might be avoiding things as a result of anxiety. For example, do you avoid going out, mixing or touching others? Are you avoiding certain objects, such as knives, because of a fear that you might use them to kill or harm others? Are other forms of avoidance present, such as avoiding dealing with bills? Stop for a minute or so and consider what you might be avoiding because of your problems.

What have I stopped doing/avoided because of my fears about what harm might result?

What other things am I avoiding in life. For example any situations at home, work or in my relationships with others?

The result is often an increasingly restricted lifestyle and additional distress. A *vicious circle of avoidance* may result and this is summarised below:

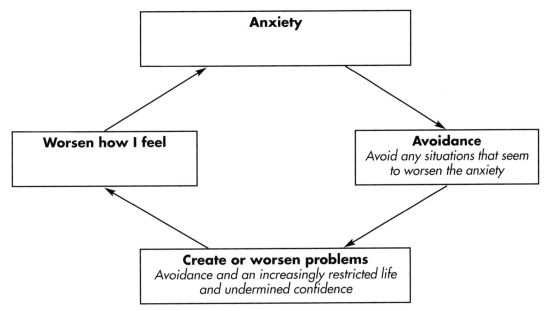

The vicious circle of avoidance

To help you see if this applies to you, ask yourself '*What have I stopped doing because of my obsessions and compulsions?*'

Remember, sometimes avoidance can be quite subtle. The following checklist will help you consider any areas of avoidance in your life.

Checklist: Identifying the vicious circle of avoidance

As a result of feeling anxious am I:	**Tick here if you have noticed this**
Avoiding dealing with important practical problems (both large and small)?	
Not really being honest with others. For example saying yes when I really mean no?	
Trying hard to avoid situations that bring about upsetting thoughts/memories?	
Brooding over things and therefore no longer living life to the full?	
Avoiding opening or replying to letters or bills?	
Sleeping in to avoid doing things or meeting people?	
Avoiding answering the phone, or the door when people visit?	
Avoiding sex?	
Avoiding talking to others face to face?	
Avoiding being with others in crowded or hot places?	
Avoiding busy or large shops, or finding that I have to think about where and when I go shopping etc.?	
Avoiding going on buses, in cars, taxis etc., or any places where it is difficult to escape?	

Checklist: Identifying the vicious circle of avoidance

As a result of feeling anxious am I:	**Tick here if you have noticed this**
Avoiding walking alone far from home?	
Avoiding situations, objects, places or people because of fears about what harm might result?	
Avoiding physical activity or exercise as a result of concerns about my physical health?	

Q. Am I avoiding things in other ways?

Write in here how you are doing this if this is applicable to you.

Summary: Altered behaviour 2: the vicious circle of avoidance

Having answered these questions, reflect on your reponses using the three questions below:

Q. Am I avoiding doing things as a result of anxiety?   Yes ☐   No ☐

Q. Has this reduced my confidence in things and led to an increasingly restricted life?   Yes ☐   No ☐

Q. Overall, has this worsened how I feel?   Yes ☐   No ☐

If you have replied **Yes** to all three questions, then you are experiencing the vicious circle of avoidance.

Experiment: The purpose behind the compulsive actions, avoidance and other unhelpful behaviours is to help relieve your anxiety. Answer the following questions to see how well it achieves this.

Q. Does carrying out the mental ritual or compulsive action(s) make me feel better **in the short term?**   Yes ☐   No ☐

If so, how long do I feel better for?
Less than 30 mins ☐   30–60 mins ☐   1–3 hours ☐   All day ☐   All week ☐   All month ☐
It lasts forever ☐

Q. Overall, does carrying out the compulsive actions, avoidance and other unhelpful behaviours make me feel better **in the long term?**   Yes ☐   No ☐

Q. What impact do they have on my confidence and ability to live my life as I would want?

If you have ticked Yes to the first question, this could be one of the factors that is keeping your OCD going. Feeling better (even if for only a short time) can be a powerful reinforcer of your compulsive actions and act to keep your problems going. The good news is that you have now identified an important area you can focus on changing.

Having completed these questions, think back on what you have learned about unhelpful behaviours in this section of the workbook, then answer the questions below.

Summary for Area 5: Altered behaviour

Having answered the questions about avoidance and unhelpful behaviours:

Q. Overall, do I have any problems in this area?   Yes ☐   No ☐

These difficulties are potential targets for change. You will find out more about what steps to take to tackle these in Section 4 of the workbook.

You have now finished your five areas assessment. Before you move on, please stop for a while and consider what you have learned. How does what you have read help you to make sense of your symptoms?

Q. How well does this assessment summarise how you feel?

Poorly ——————————————————— Very well
0   10

The purpose of the Five Areas Assessment is to help you plan the areas you need to focus on to bring about change. The workbooks in the *Overcoming Anxiety* course can help you begin to tackle each of the five problem areas of anxiety.

Section 4 **Choosing your targets for change**

The main problem areas seen in obsessive-compulsive disorder are the:

- Current situations, relationship or practical problems
- Altered thinking (with extreme and unhelpful thinking)
- Altered feelings/emotions
- Altered physical symptoms
- Altered behaviour (with avoidance or unhelpful behaviours)

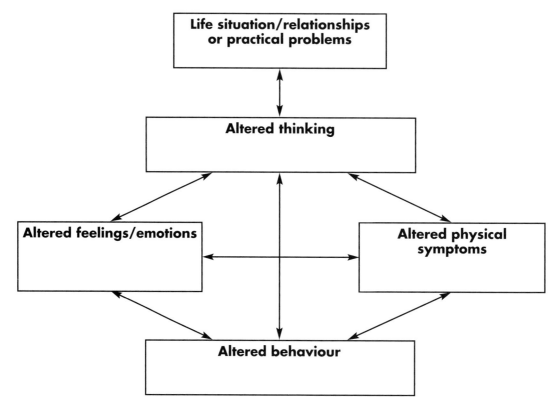

The Five Areas Assessment

You have previously answered questions about each of these five areas. Look again at the answers you gave in your own Five Areas Assessment, in the last two sections of the workbook. Your answers summarise the problems you identified in each area. Since there are links between the areas, it is possible by altering any one of the areas to bring about changes in others, and help improve how you feel.

> **Key point:** By defining your problems, you have now identified possible target areas to focus on. The key is to make sure that you do things **one step at a time**. Slow steady steps are more likely to result in improvement than very enthusiastically starting and then running out of steam.

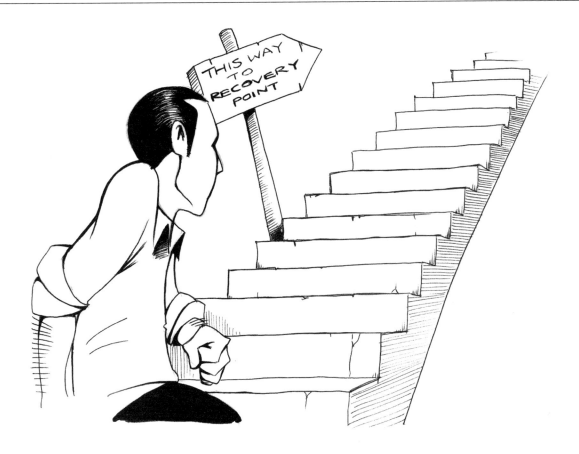

Short-, medium- and longer-term goals

You may have made all sorts of previous attempts to change, but unless you have a clear plan and stick to it, change will be very difficult. Planning and selecting which targets to try and change first is a crucial part of successfully moving forwards. By choosing some specific areas to focus on to start with, this also means that you are actively choosing at first **NOT** to focus on other areas.

Setting yourself targets will help you to focus on how to make the changes needed to get better. To do this you will need to decide:

- Short-term targets: changes you can make today, tomorrow and next week.
- Medium-term targets: changes to be put in place over the next few weeks.
- Long-term targets: where you want to be in six months or a year.

The questions that you have answered in this workbook will have helped you to identify the main problem areas that you currently face. The *Overcoming Anxiety* course (outlined below) can help you to make changes in each of these areas.

The workbooks can be used either alone or as part of a complete course. The Workbooks 1a to 1e in Part 1 are designed to help you to identify your current problem areas. This will help identify which of the Workbooks 2 to 9 in Part 2 you need to read. Finally, you can summarise what you have learned and plan for the future by completing Workbook 10. This will help you keep putting what you have learned into practice.

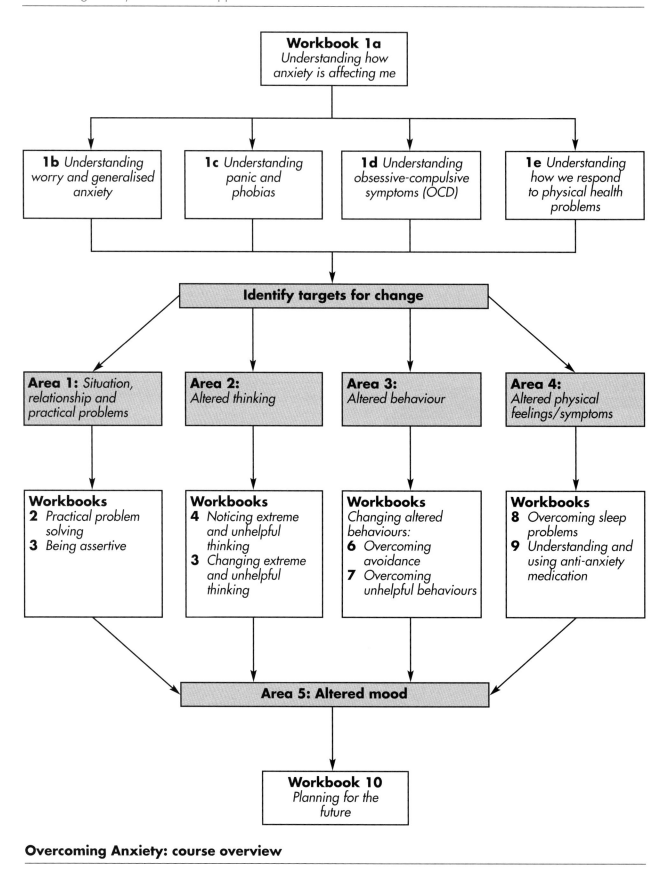

Workbook 1a
Understanding how anxiety is affecting me

1b *Understanding worry and generalised anxiety*

1c *Understanding panic and phobias*

1d *Understanding obsessive-compulsive symptoms (OCD)*

1e *Understanding how we respond to physical health problems*

Identify targets for change

Area 1: *Situation, relationship and practical problems*

Area 2: *Altered thinking*

Area 3: *Altered behaviour*

Area 4: *Altered physical feelings/symptoms*

Workbooks
2 *Practical problem solving*
3 *Being assertive*

Workbooks
4 *Noticing extreme and unhelpful thinking*
3 *Changing extreme and unhelpful thinking*

Workbooks
Changing altered behaviours:
6 *Overcoming avoidance*
7 *Overcoming unhelpful behaviours*

Workbooks
8 *Overcoming sleep problems*
9 *Understanding and using anti-anxiety medication*

Area 5: Altered mood

Workbook 10
Planning for the future

Overcoming Anxiety: course overview

The Overcoming Anxiety course

Understanding anxiety

Workbooks 1a to 1e provide an introduction and overview of anxiety problems. It is recommended that you read these workbooks first to give you an overview of how anxiety can affect you. The five workbooks together cover the common anxiety disorders – worry, panic, phobias, obsessive-compulsive disorder and also how we respond to physical health problems. They will help you identify which of these areas you need to focus on changing and will help you decide which of the remaining workbooks you need to read.

Area 1: Dealing with difficult situations, relationship and practical problems

Workbook 2: *Practical problem solving*

In this workbook you will learn a step-by-step plan that you can use to deal with practical problems. It will provide you with the tools to tackle any practical problems that you face. This will help you to take more control of your life and the decisions that you make. By feeling more in control of your life, you will improve your self-confidence.

Workbook 3: *Being Assertive*

Have you ever thought that no one listens to you, and that other people seem to walk all over you? Have others commented that they think that you always walk over them? You will find out about the difference between passive, aggressive and assertive behaviour and learn how to develop more balanced relationships with others where your opinion is listened to and respected, and you listen to and respect other people.

Area 2: Changing extreme and unhelpful thinking

Workbook 4: *Noticing extreme and unhelpful thinking*

What you think about yourself, others and the situations that occur around you, can alter how you feel and affect what you do. This workbook will help you to learn ways of identifying extreme and unhelpful ways of thinking. You will learn how to notice such thoughts and to understand the impact these have on how you feel and what you do.

Workbook 5: *Changing extreme and unhelpful thinking*

This workbook will teach you the important skill of how to challenge extreme and unhelpful thinking. With practice this will help you change the extreme and unhelpful thinking that is often a major problem in anxiety or depression.

Area 3: Changing altered behaviours

Workbook 6: Overcoming avoidance

You will find out more about how avoidance keeps problems going. You will learn ways of changing what you do in order to break the vicious circle of avoidance.

Workbook 7: Overcoming unhelpful behaviours

You will learn some effective ways of overcoming unhelpful behaviours such as drinking too much, reassurance seeking and trying to spend your way out of how you feel.

Area 4: Physical symptoms and treatments

Workbook 8: Overcoming sleep problems

Often when someone is anxious they not only feel emotionally and mentally low, but they also notice a range of physical changes that are a normal part of anxiety. This workbook will help you find out about these common changes, and in particular will help you to deal with problems of poor sleep.

Workbook 9: Understanding and using anti-anxiety medication

When someone is anxious sometimes their doctor suggests they take an anti-anxiety medication. You will find out why doctors suggest this, and also learn about common fears and concerns that people have when first starting to take these tablets so that you can find out for yourself whether this medication may be helpful for you.

Area 5: Altered mood

The fifth and final area, anxious mood, will improve if you work at the other areas where you have problems (the altered thinking, behaviour, physical symptoms and the situations, relationships and practical problems that you face). Once you feel better, the final workbook of the series can be read to help you to summarise what you have learned.

Workbook 10: Planning for the future

You will have learned new things about yourself and made changes in how you live your life. This final workbook will help you to identify what you have learned and help you plan for the future. You will devise your own personal plan to cope with future problems in your life so that you can face the future with confidence.

The work you do using the workbooks can supplement the help you receive from your doctor or other health care practitioner or friends. Sometimes more specialist help is needed to help how you feel and your doctor may suggest that you see a trained specialist such as a clinical psychologist, occupational therapist, social worker, psychiatric nurse or a psychiatrist.

Use the following table to help you decide which workbooks are right for you to read now, and over the next few weeks and months. You have already read the current workbook, and it is recommended that you also read Workbook 1a: Understanding how anxiety is affecting me. You may find it helpful to discuss this with your health care practitioner or other trusted supporter.

Workbook title	Short-term goals (plan to read in the next week or so)	Medium-term goals (plan to read over the next few weeks)	Long-term goals (plan to read over the next few months)	Tick when completed
Understanding anxiety workbooks				
1a *Understanding how anxiety is affecting me*	✔			
1b *Understanding worry and generalised anxiety*				
1c *Understanding panic and phobias*				
1d *Understanding obsessive-compulsive symptoms (OCD)*	✔			
1e *Understanding how we respond to physical health problems*				
Workbook 2 *Practical problem solving*				
Workbook 3 *Being assertive*				
Workbook 4 *Identifying extreme and unhelpful thinking*				
Workbook 5 *Changing extreme and unhelpful thinking*				
Workbook 6 *Overcoming avoidance*				
Workbook 7 *Overcoming unhelpful behaviours*				
Workbook 8 *Overcoming sleep problems*				
Workbook 9 *Understanding and using anti-anxiety medications*				
Workbook 10 *Staying well*				
Worksheet *Overcoming hyperventilation/ over-breathing*				
Worksheet *Understanding depersonalisation*				

In order to help you to review your progress, it can be useful to record how you feel at different times as you work on your problems. Your health care practitioner may work with you to decide what information it might be helpful to record. Don't expect to feel better all at once. Change can take time, however by working at your problems, most people find that improvement is possible.

Key point: In order to change, you will need to choose to try to apply what you will learn regularly **throughout the week**, and not just when you read the workbook or see your health care practitioner. The workbooks will encourage you to do this by sometimes suggesting certain tasks for you to carry out in the days after reading each workbook.

These tasks will:
● Help you to put into practice what you have learned in each workbook.
● Gather information so that you can get the most out of the workbook.

Experience has shown that you are likely to make the most progress if you are able to put into practice what you have learned.

Summary

In this workbook you have learned about:
● the key elements of obsessions and compulsions and the key ways that they affect you;
● the impact of how what you think can affect how you feel and unhelpfully alter what you do;
● the Five Areas of Anxiety: the *situations, relationship and practical problems* faced, and the *altered thinking, emotional* and *physical feelings* and *behaviour* that occur as part of obsessive-compulsive problems;
● the areas you need to tackle in order to overcome your own problems of anxiety.

Putting into practice what you have learned

● Read through the current workbook again. Think in detail about how anxiety is affecting your thinking, emotional and physical feelings, and behaviour. Decide which areas you want to change.
● Choose **two episodes** over the next week when you feel more anxious or notice the obsessive-compulsive symptoms. Use the blank Five Areas Assessment sheet (p. 1d.37) to record the impact on your thinking, mood, body and behaviour at those times. Try to generate a summary of your own anxiety in each of the five areas (life situation, relationships and practical problems, altered thinking, feelings, physical symptoms and behaviour). Use this workbook to identify whether you showed any of the unhelpful thinking styles during these occasions. What impact did your thoughts have on how you felt and what you did during these two episodes? Can you identify any examples of avoidance or unhelpful behaviours? Please photocopy or draw out additional copies of this diagram as you need it and keep the sheet handy.
● Finally, review your list of which workbooks you will choose to use next and move on to work through these in your own time.

If you have difficulties with these tasks, don't worry. Just do what you can. If you have found any aspects of this workbook unhelpful, upsetting or confusing, please can you discuss this with your health care practitioner or someone else whose opinion you trust.

A request for feedback

An important factor in the development of all the Five Areas Assessment workbooks is that the content is updated on a regular basis based upon feedback from users and practitioners. Please let me know if you have found the content helpful or unhelpful. If there are areas which you find hard to understand, or which seem poorly written, please let me know and I will try to improve things in future. I regret that I am unable to provide any specific replies or advice on treatment.

> **To provide feedback, please contact me via:**
>
> **Email:** Feedback@fiveareas.com
>
> **Mail:** Dr Chris Williams, Department of Psychological Medicine, Gartnavel Royal Hospital, 1055 Great Western Road, Glasgow, G12 0XH

Acknowledgements

I wish to thank all those who have commented upon this workbook especially Mark Freeston, Judith Halford, Dale Huey and Eileen Riddoch.

The cartoon illustrations in the workbooks have been produced by Keith Chan (kchan75@hotmail.com) and are copyright of Media Innovations Ltd.

My notes

....

....

....

....

....

....

....

....

....

....

....

....

....

....

....

....

....

....

....

....

....

....

....

....

....

My notes

....

Worksheet: A Five Areas Assessment of a specific time when I feel more anxious/worse

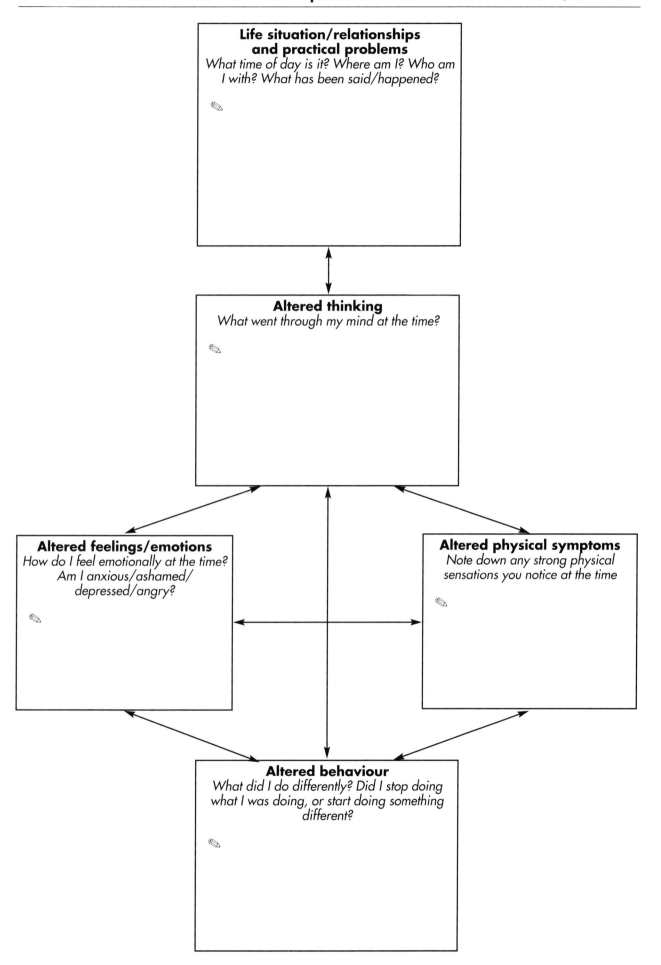

Workbook 1e

Understanding how we respond to physical health problems

Dr Chris Williams

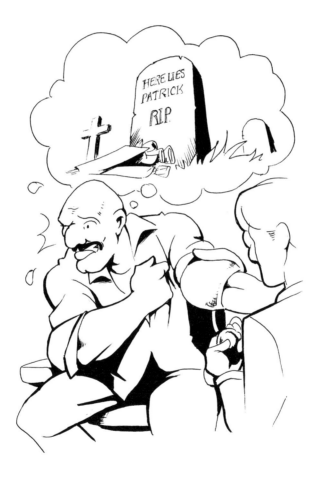

A Five Areas Approach

Section 1   **Introduction**

This workbook will cover:
- how to use the workbook most effectively;
- how we respond to physical health problems;
- the key ways that physical health problems can affect your life;
- the Five Areas Assessment: the *situations, relationship and practical problems* we face, and the *altered thinking*, *emotional* and *physical feelings* and *behaviour* that make up our response to the challenge of illness;
- how our thoughts and concerns about illness can worsen how we feel;
- the areas you need to tackle in order to overcome your own problems.

The workbook addresses two main areas:

1 How we cope with long-term illness. This includes problems like heart or lung disease, cancer and arthritis and any longer-term illness. It will help you understand your response to illness, and help you reflect on the impact of illness on how you feel. You will learn to identify effective ways of responding to physical symptoms such as tiredness, stiffness, breathlessness and pain etc.

2 The situation of health anxiety, where medical investigation has ruled out physical disease, yet we continue to worry about illness and feel unwell in spite of this. This is addressed in Section 4 of the workbook.

In both situations, a psychological approach can help how we cope with illness. Don't be concerned if any of these words seem new or difficult to understand. All the terms will be described clearly as you read through the workbook.

How to use this workbook

Take time to read the workbook at your own pace. You don't have to sit down and read it in one go. You might find it most helpful to set yourself the target of reading the workbook one section at a time.

- Try to **answer all the questions** asked. The process of having to *stop, think and reflect* on how the questions might be relevant to you is crucial to getting better.
- **Write down** your own notes in the margins or in the *My notes* area at the back of the workbook to help you remember information that has been helpful. **Plan to review your notes regularly** so that you apply what you have learned.
- Once you have read through the entire workbook once, **put it on one side** and then **re-read it** a few days later. It may be that different parts of it become clearer, or seem more useful on second reading.
- Use the workbooks to **build upon the help you receive in other ways,** such as from reading other helpful material, talking to friends, or attending self-help organisations and support groups.
- Discuss the workbook with your health care practitioner and those who give you helpful support so that you can work together on overcoming the problems.
- **Remember that although change can seem difficult at first, it is possible.**

How do we respond when we feel ill?

Think about the way that people react when they are ill or off colour. There is a range of different things we normally do. As well as going to the doctor, we may:

- Reduce or stop what we are doing and stay at home. We also may stop doing core tasks around the house such as cleaning or cooking for a time.
- Wear different clothes such as pyjamas, loose fitting clothes or dressing gowns.
- Eat and drink different foods. This might include 'bland' foods, such as toast. We may drink 'energy-filled' drinks. Depending on our cultural background, we may choose to eat 'hot' or 'cold' foods.
- Expect others to help us out – perhaps by making us food and bringing us drinks.

All sorts of things affect our response to illness. This includes the severity of the illness and also our own expectations about how we 'should' respond to illness. Our gender and social background also affect how we react. Think about the people you know – your own friends, relatives and others you know. Each will have very different ways of reacting to illness. You will probably know people who 'soldier on' in the face of illness and also others who are in bed with 'flu' at the first sign of a blocked nose. Each of these reactions is quite normal, and part of the usual range of reaction to illness.

Another important aspect of the illness is that others also have expectations of us. Friends, relatives, work colleagues and others expect us to take things easy. They also expect us to go to see our doctor or health care practitioner and take their advice and treatment. They have an expectation that such treatment will lead to recovery. When we recover we are then expected to return to our previous activities, jobs and roles.

The expectations of others can also affect how we communicate our illness. Think about a time in the past when you have been in bed with a bad cold. Someone phones up – perhaps a colleague from work or a friend. Do you ever make sure that you cough, or clear your throat during the conversation just to make sure they know you are under the weather? Many people – including the author – do. This reflects the importance that we place on making sure that others realise that we are not putting on symptoms or 'hamming things up'.

My reaction to illness: do I usually notice any of the following changes when I am ill?

Q. Do I reduce or stop what I do or take things easy?   Yes ☐   No ☐

Q. Do I wear different clothes?   Yes ☐   No ☐

If so – which ones:

> ✎

Q. Do I eat different foods?

If so – which ones:

> ✎

Others' reactions to illness

Q. Do others make food for me?   Yes ☐   No ☐

Q. Do others support me more than usual?   Yes ☐   No ☐

These are common and normal reactions in the face of illness.

Write in here any other actions that you or others do when you are ill:

> ✎

Our expectations of how we 'should/must/ought' to react when we are ill

One problem is that we have a number expectations of how we 'should', 'must', 'ought' to react when we are ill. We should stop doing things. We should seek treatment and take this. We should get better and move on from our illness to recovery. We should act differently when ill – wear different clothes, eat different foods, rest and cough! These 'rules' often work well for short-term illnesses such as colds, flu, a broken ankle or problems such as appendicitis that resolve over a number of days and weeks. It can be very difficult though either when we find that illness does not get better quickly, or when the illness is not 'obvious' to others.

When our illness is long-term

If our illness lasts for a number of weeks, months or years, you may find that the initial support offered by others can slowly drop off. Some may not know how to respond or offer support beyond short-term flowers and 'Get well' cards. They may still want to help, but are uncertain how to best do this. They may struggle to know what to say when they visit. They may avoid visiting as a result.

Sometimes, similar difficulties may occur with those we see in the health service. Most health care practitioners are able to offer helpful support to people with longer-term (sometimes called chronic) illness. However, from time to time even those working in the caring professions may not be as good at offering the kind of support that you need.

Where our illness isn't 'obvious' to others

When illness leads to a broken leg, there is a large plaster cast on the leg to see. Similarly with a chest infection we have lots of green phlegm to cough into little pots by our bedside. In cancer or heart disease there is a clearly diagnosed disease. However, some illnesses are not so visible: for example, mental illness such as depression or anxiety. Sometimes physical symptoms are also not 'visible' – such as problems of tiredness and pain. The problems are equally real, but because they are less obvious sometimes the reaction of others is less supportive. Part of this reflects difficulties they may have in understanding illness. For example, there is often a stigma surrounding mental health problems.

Identifying problems with longer-term physical illness

Q. Is anyone I know unsure about how to best support me?   Yes ☐   No ☐

Q. Has anyone begun to drop away from offering me support?   Yes ☐   No ☐

Q. Is my own health care practitioner able to offer me the kind of supportive
care I need?   Yes ☐   No ☐

Q. Do I have an illness that isn't 'visible' and obvious to others?   Yes ☐   No ☐

If **Yes**: Does this seem to affect how others react towards me?   Yes ☐   No ☐

Write in what you have noticed here:

The Five Areas approach to understanding illness

You can already see that the problems faced in long-term illness are very complex. A Five Areas Assessment provides a clear summary of the difficulties faced in each of the following areas:
1 Life situation, relationships, practical problems and difficulties
2 Altered thinking
3 Altered feelings (also called emotions or moods)
4 Altered physical symptoms/feelings in the body
5 Altered behaviour or activity levels (with reduced activity, avoidance or unhelpful behaviours)

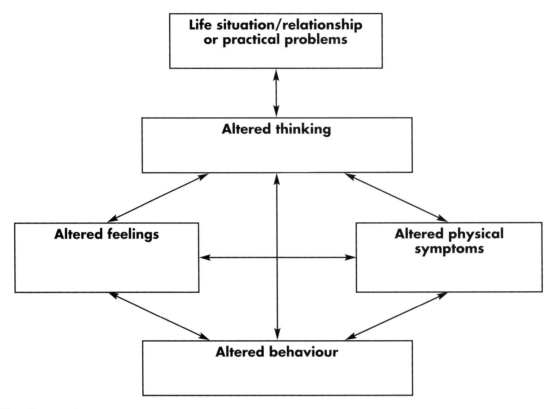

The Five Areas Assessment

Look at the arrows in the diagram. Each of the five areas affects the others and offers possible areas of change to improve how you feel. Because of the links between each of the areas, the physical impact of illness has an impact on other aspects of your life. For example, being ill can be frustrating or emotionally demoralising. This is especially the case when illness lasts for many months or years, or where symptoms stop you living your life as you would wish. Long-term illness can grind us down. We may begin to think that nothing can be done and that nothing we do can make a difference to how we feel. The Five Areas Assessment also indicates that what a person thinks about a situation or problem may affect how they feel emotionally and physically, and also alters what they do. The good news is that the Five Areas Assessment can help you to identify clear target areas that you can change so as to make a difference to how you feel. You will learn more about this as you read this workbook.

Don't be concerned if this approach seems difficult to understand at first. You will find out more later. In the next section of the workbook you have the chance to complete your own Five Areas Assessment.

Section 2   **Carrying out your own Five Areas Assessment**

A Five Areas Assessment can be helpful in understanding how illness is affecting you.
The five areas are:

- Situation, relationship or practical problems
- Altered thinking
- Altered feelings/emotions/mood
- Altered physical symptoms
- Altered behaviour or activity levels in the face of illness

---

Key point: As you go through the five areas assessment, please think about how illness has affected you in the last week. Try to answer all the questions and really think about how they apply to you. By doing this you will be able to identify possible target areas for change.

In order to break down the task, areas 1 to 4 will be covered in this section. Area 5, altered behaviour, is covered in Section 3.

Area 1: Situation, relationship and practical problems

All of us from time to time face practical problems or difficulties in relationships. When we face a large number of problems we may begin to feel overwhelmed. This may be particularly the case at times when we feel ill. Illness reduces our ability to respond well to other problems in life. Opening letters, paying bills or keeping up with the house may just not seem as important when we are in pain, feel ill or have difficulties coping. These everyday difficulties are just one more source of unwanted pressure. Symptoms often seem worse when several life pressures occur at the same time.
These practical problems and life difficulties may include:

- debts, housing or other difficulties;
- problems in relationships with family, friends or colleagues;
- other difficult situations that you face such as problems at home or work (or lack of work – for example, unemployment or problems with benefits).

The following table refers to several common situation, relationship and practical problems. Are any of these relevant to you?

Situation, relationship and practical problems

I have relationship difficulties (such as arguments).	Yes ☐	No ☐
I can't really talk and receive support from my partner.	Yes ☐	No ☐
There is no one around who I can really talk to.	Yes ☐	No ☐
My children won't do what I tell them.	Yes ☐	No ☐
I have difficulties with money problems or debts.	Yes ☐	No ☐
I have difficulties with benefits.	Yes ☐	No ☐
There are problems with my flat/house.	Yes ☐	No ☐
I am having problems with my neighbours.	Yes ☐	No ☐
I don't have a job.	Yes ☐	No ☐
I have difficulties with colleagues at work.	Yes ☐	No ☐

Write down any other difficult situations, relationship or practical problems here:

Ideally we would want to be able to count on others to support us when ill. Sometimes family, friends or others don't know how best to help. In Section 1 of the workbook you found that sometimes those around us can withdraw at least to some extent. Sometimes the opposite occurs and others offer us too much input. They may offer 'helpful advice' all the time and want to do *everything* for us. There can be many motivations for this. Often the cause is concern, friendship and love for us. Sometimes it may be the result of anxiety, or occasionally guilt. Whatever the cause, when others offer too much help and want to do everything for us, their actions can backfire in several ways:

- Their special attention may feel **suffocating and frustrating**. We can end up feeling we are treated like a child. Arguments and little irritations build up and are upsetting to us both.
- Although they mean well, their actions can actually **undermine how we feel**. When trying to cope with long-term illness it is important to continue to do as many things as you are able within the confines of how you feel. If others take responsibility for doing everything for us, the danger is that we are not as active as we could be. You will find out later that this can play a role in worsening how we feel. This is covered in Section 3 of this workbook.
- Those who help us also need to pace themselves and allow time and space for their own needs. **Depression is very common amongst carers.** The danger is that our carer is so busy supporting us that they may end up becoming stressed or depressed.

Problems of unhelpful support from others

Q. Do you find that anyone who offers you support has started to drift away from you?   Yes ☐   No ☐

Q. Do you think that anyone is overly supporting you in a suffocating way?   Yes ☐   No ☐

Q. Do you find that any family, friends or others seem over-committed and need some space for themselves?   Yes ☐   No ☐

If the answer is **Yes** to any of these questions, you may need to try to rebalance how you relate to some key people. There may be a need for open and honest communication. You should aim for a level of support that is helpful for you both rather than undermining.

Workbooks 2 (*Practical problem solving*) and 3 (*Being Assertive*) may be helpful if you need to alter or rebalance your relationships in some way.

Summary for Area 1: Situation, relationship and practical problems

Having answered these questions:

Q. Overall, do I have any problems in this area?   Yes ☐   No ☐

These difficulties are potential targets for change. You will find out more about what steps to take to tackle these in Section 5 of the workbook.

Area 2: Altered thinking in physical health problems

What we think can have a large impact on how we feel and on what we do. There are various ways that our thinking can affect how we feel during illness. As you read through the list, try to think whether they apply to you. The purpose is to try to identify any areas that might act to worsen how you feel.

Our view of our illness

When illness lasts for a number of weeks or months, we can feel very uncertain about the future. This uncertainty includes:

Uncertainty about the causes of the illness

Sometimes the causes of illness are clear – for example infection, trauma or cancer. However, sometimes, in spite of medical investigation, they are not. The cause may be so long in the past that it is not now going to be confirmed. This situation can be very upsetting. It is important to understand why we feel as we do. However, the danger of becoming overly focused on the past is that this can prevent us from focusing our attention on how to overcome the symptoms now.

Uncertainty about the diagnosis

It can be very important to know what illness we have. For example, in the area of mental health sometimes it can be a big relief for someone with depression to find that they have a depressive illness. Before this 'diagnosis' they might find themselves in the situation where they feel really down, cry a lot of the time, and experience very low energy and poor concentration. They may be off their food and lose weight as well as having problems sleeping. To discover that these symptoms are all recognised features of depression can help make sense of these very different problems and provide a clear target for treatment.

We often may have a clear diagnosis such as '*heart disease*', '*asthma*', '*arthritis*' etc. Sometimes, however, there are symptoms such as fever, a rash, pain, swelling or fatigue and no clear diagnosis. A danger is that we can become '*stuck*' until we receive a diagnosis. This uncertainty can be very frustrating. Although diagnostic labels matter, what matters more is using any effective ways to overcome the impact of illness.

Uncertainty about the future

Long-term illness brings with it many threats and uncertainties. We may have all sorts of concerns about the future and can doubt that improvement can occur. We may be anxious about a possible loss of independence and the challenge of symptoms such as pain. We may fear that we will not be able to cope or that we will not receive the level of support we need.

Uncertainty about the extent you can do anything to improve things

Our ability to change things for the better and take control over symptoms is challenged when illness becomes long-term. The result may be a reduction in our belief that we can change things or make any difference in how we feel.

Uncertainty and illness: what areas of uncertainty do I notice?

Q. Am I preoccupied with finding out the cause of why I became ill in the first place?   Yes ☐   No ☐

Q. Am I feeling 'stuck' until a clear diagnosis is made?   Yes ☐   No ☐

Q. Am I concerned about what the future holds and how the illness will affect me?   Yes ☐   No ☐

Q. Am I worried that nothing I do will lead to any benefit?   Yes ☐   No ☐

Write any other concerns you have about your illness here:

Our view of doctors and others around us

How we react to illness is partially affected by the illness itself. It will also be affected by other central attitudes we have. This includes how we judge ourselves and others, and how we make sense of the world around us. These sorts of rules often have their origin very early on in our lives. For example, if throughout our lives we have held views that '*others let me down*', then we are likely to also believe this of our friends, practitioners and even our closest loved ones. Trust can take time to develop as a result. These beliefs can affect our ability to work collaboratively with others such as health care practitioners.

Long-term belief: do I hold any of these beliefs?

Hospitals let you down.   Yes ☐   No ☐

Doctors always make mistakes.   Yes ☐   No ☐

No one understands me.   Yes ☐   No ☐

I don't deserve help.   Yes ☐   No ☐

Others let you down.   Yes ☐   No ☐

Write down any other thoughts you have that might affect how you react to others around you.

✎

In long-term illness by definition there is no quick cure. This can lead to frustration all round. If you hold any of the above beliefs, it is more likely that you will find it difficult working with others if there isn't a rapid improvement in how you feel. You may be prone to doubt the competency of those trying to help, or believe that you or they are wasting scarce time. It is perhaps better to have an open discussion about the frustration of little perceived progress than voting with your feet.

Images and mental pictures – an important part of how we think

We often think in mental pictures. Some people (although not all) notice mental pictures or images in their mind when they think about their illness. Images are a form of thought and may be 'still' images (like a photograph), or moving (like a video). Images may be in black and white or in colour. They may include mental pictures of painful parts of our bodies such as joints, or pictures of a stomach ulcer or cancer. As with all thoughts, mental images can be helpful and accurate; however, sometimes they can be very inaccurate or **portray the very worst** outcome. For example, there may be anxious pictures of severe suffering or our eventual death. They may sometimes focus on fearful themes and cause feelings of anxiety or upset.

Q. Am I prone to noticing intrusive upsetting images or
mental pictures?   Yes ☐   No ☐

The spotlight of the mind

Our minds and bodies are not in separate 'boxes'. Each can affect each other to a very great extent. One of the ways that our minds can influence how we react to physical injury and illness depends upon the extent to which our mind is focused on that injury. This is described as the *spotlight of the mind*. Where this spotlight is focused affects the things we are most aware of.

Illustration: In the past have you ever been engrossed in a sport or an activity? You may have fallen over and scuffed a knee but continued playing. After the game you suddenly realise that you have been bleeding. It is only then that you notice the pain. In this example, the spotlight of the mind was originally focused on the excitement of the game. Although the knee has been injured all this time, the pain is only noticed when the game ends.

> **Key point:** The spotlight of the mind can have a large impact on how we are affected by the physical symptoms of illness. If our focus is mainly on our symptoms, they will preoccupy our thoughts and this will worsen how we feel. Paying attention to symptoms can sometimes cause them to build up and up. Finding other things that we can become interested, occupied or active in can be a big help in coping with long-term symptoms.

Experiment: To see if this process might affect your own experience, try the following experiment.

i) On the scale below, rate how much you notice your symptoms **now**.

Not present at all   **The worst it's ever been**
0   1   2   3   4   5   6   7   8   9   10

ii) Now, focus on your symptoms. Consider how you feel, and how they are affecting you. Do this for a short time and then again record how much you notice them.

Not present at all   **The worst it's ever been**
0   1   2   3   4   5   6   7   8   9   10

iii) At a later time, repeat the rating when you are engrossed in something – for example, watching your favourite soap, talking to someone, or reading a book.

Not present at all   **The worst it's ever been**
0   1   2   3   4   5   6   7   8   9   10

Review: Having done this, what impact does paying attention to your symptoms (ii), and being engrossed in other things (iii) have on you?

Write your conclusions here:

You may find that that there is no impact, in which case the spotlight of the mind may not be relevent to you.

If you found that the rating worsened at all when you paid attention to it, or reduced at all when you were engrossed, then this is very useful information. It means that your focus on the symptoms may play a part in how you feel. This gives you a possible area to work on as you consider ways of moving forwards.

Paying attention to physical symptoms/bodily processes alters how they feel

A second aspect of the spotlight of the mind is that when we pay attention to something it can begin to feel different/strange. To illustrate this, have you ever talked to someone who you know has nits in their hair, or a skin problem such as scabies? As you talk to them, do you notice any difference in how your own scalp feels? You may have begun to notice a sensation of itching. If you then scratch that area, the itching often then spreads around your scalp. You may notice that other parts of your body also start to feel itchy and uncomfortable.

To find out whether this same process affects you at all, try the following experiments.

Experiment 1 At rest, pay attention to your breathing for several minutes.[1] Think in detail about the whole process of breathing – especially how much you breathe in and out. Think about how this process seems to work.

Experiment 2 As you walk around, pay great attention to the process of walking.[2] Think about how you keep balanced and stable as you do this.

Write what you notice here:

✎

Q. Does paying attention to your body alter how it feels?   Yes ☐   No ☐

If **Yes**: does it feel normal or begin to feel abnormal/odd in
any way?   Normal ☐   Abnormal/odd ☐

Review: Sometimes paying attention to quite normal everyday bodily functions makes them seem a little odd or different from usual. You will find out more about this in the next section of the workbook.

What about the impact of activity and relaxation on how you feel?

Although it can sometimes seem that '*Nothing I do makes any difference*', this may well not be the case. How we feel can be affected by all sorts of different things we do throughout the day. These changes may be so subtle that at first we are not even aware of them. To find out what life factors seem to link with an improvement or worsening in how you feel, try this experiment.

---

1 Do not do this experiment if you have lung disease or you are anxious about your breathing.
2 Do not do this experiment if you have a walking or balance disorder.

> **Experiment:** Create a diary containing three columns. Every hour throughout your waking day record what you are doing and the severity of your symptoms on a regular basis, under the following headings:
>
> i) The *time of day*.
>
> ii) *What you are doing*. This might include things like lying in bed listening to the radio; washing the dishes; talking to the boss; sitting in the chair talking to someone on the phone, having a bath, etc.
>
> iii) *The intensity of your main symptom*. You may have a number of different symptoms depending upon your own illness. Choose to monitor just **one** main symptom (e.g. breathlessness, pain, tiredness, stiffness etc.) and record the intensity of this key symptom at this time. Use a scale where 0 means not present at all, and 10 means the worst it has ever been. A score of 5/10 records a moderately severe level.

Example: Patrick's diary. Patrick is in his late forties and has had a heart attack some months ago. He is now noticing chest pain throughout the day. He records his symptoms of chest pain on an hourly basis. He uses a watch with an hourly bleep on it as a reminder to fill in the diary. The following is part of his diary where he records his symptoms of chest pain.

Time	What am I doing at the moment?	Intensity of the main symptom (0–10)
9 am	Getting up and having a shower.	0/10
10 am	Opening the gas bill, which is higher than expected.	7/10
11 am	Talking to personnel on the phone about returning to work.	9/10
12 pm	Talking to my wife about our holiday plans for next year.	3/10
1 pm	Going to see my doctor about the investigations.	5/6 before going in to see her, rising to 7/8 as we talked about the results and she took my blood pressure.
2 pm	Listening to the match on the radio.	2/10. It was a good match. We won!
3 pm	Going for a walk with my wife.	2/10 to start with, increasing to 6/10 when we walked faster than I felt comfortable with.

You can see from his diary that Patrick has discovered something important. His chest pain is not unchanging throughout the day. Instead he feels better when he is taking a shower, talking to his wife about nice things such as holidays, and engrossed in following his favourite team. In contrast, it worsens when he is talking about the symptoms to his doctor, dealing with stressful events such as the gas bill and personnel, and when he walks faster than he feels comfortable with.

The implication of this is:

- Learning to relax and planning in times to wind down may help the pain.
- Anxiety may worsen the symptoms.
- Physical exercise may worsen the symptoms. For example, angina may cause chest pain when he exercises. Specific investigations and advice from his doctor would be needed to find out if this is the case.

The diary therefore provides Patrick with some clear ideas on what he could try out. For example, he could build in some time to relax each day during a bath or shower. He could also learn ways to challenge his worries that arise when he thinks about bills and returning to work. He should arrange to see his doctor to see if his chest pain is caused by a physical problem such as angina. In the mean time he should continue to walk at a pace he can cope with and not stop exercising completely.

You will find a blank copy of this diary for you to use at the end of the workbook. Use this to find out what factors might have a similar impact in your own life. Discuss what you find with your health care practitioner or a trusted friend.

How we interpret things: a crucial factor

Have you ever watched the Oxford and Cambridge boat race or any similar sporting event where there are two fiercely competitive teams? In this race there are two super-fit crews. Each crew puts all their efforts into propelling their boat to victory. Imagine it is one of those years where the boats are neck and neck as they approach the finishing line. As they cross it, one boat just inches ahead and wins. The cameras focus in on the winning team, who are jubilant. They wave their arms in the air and slap each other on the back.

In contrast, the losing crew looks very different. They are silent and dejected, breathing heavily and slumped into their boat. They feel the agony in their arms and legs caused by their exertions. Yet, if it were suddenly announced that the first boat was being disqualified, there would be a rapid change in the second boat. Smiles would break out. There would be loud shouts, and jubilation. Members of the crew would be thrown into the water. Their focus on their tired and strained bodies would quickly disappear.

This short description illustrates an important point. How we interpret things – as victory or defeat – can have a marked impact on how we feel. The difference can be dramatic as shown above. Of course, this is an extreme example. However there is something useful to be learned. In times of illness we are sometimes very aware of symptoms such as pain, or tiredness or sickness. How we interpret and make sense of these will affect how we feel. It will affect if we feel calm and peaceful or depressed, angry, worried or ground down.

The unhelpful thinking styles

It is very common in long-term illness to feel anxious, demoralised, frustrated and fed up from time to time. At times like this, thinking becomes altered. The way we interpret things – including our health – can become quite extreme and unhelpful. These ways of seeing things are sometimes called *unhelpful thinking styles*. They show certain common themes. Our problems may be taken out of all proportion and our strengths and ability to cope overlooked or played down. Things can seem to be out of our control.

Consider your own thinking over the last week:

The unhelpful thinking styles

Q. Am I being my own worst critic *(bias against myself)*? Yes ☐ No ☐

Q. Am I focusing on the bad in situations *(negative mental filter)*? Yes ☐ No ☐

Q. Do I have a gloomy view of the future *(make negative predictions)*? Yes ☐ No ☐

Q. Am I jumping to the very worst conclusion *(catastrophic thinking)*? Yes ☐ No ☐

Q. Am I second-guessing that others think badly of me without actually checking *(mind-reading)*? Yes ☐ No ☐

Q. Am I taking unfair responsibility for things that aren't really my fault *(bearing all responsibility/taking all the blame)*? Yes ☐ No ☐

Q. Do I have unhelpfully high standards and use the words '*should, must, ought* and *got to*' a lot, or make statements such as '*Just typical*' when something goes wrong *(unhelpfully high standards/rules)*? Yes ☐ No ☐

If you have answered **Yes** to any of the questions it is likely that unhelpfully altered thinking is adding to you problems.

The unhelpful thinking styles occur in each of us from time to time. However, during times of distress (including times when we are struggling hard against physical illness) they become more frequent and are harder to dismiss. By focusing on and unhelpfully exaggerating your problems, you may allow them to build up and up in your mind, without their actually being tackled. In illness particularly, we may be prone to seeing our illness in catastrophic ways and predict that the worst will occur. Of course, in physical illness sometimes the future is difficult or bleak. However, the unhelpful thinking styles refer to unrealistic, extreme and unhelpful ways of seeing things. Such thoughts dominate our thinking and worsen how we feel.

Why are the unhelpful thinking styles so unhelpful?

The *unhelpful* thinking styles are so called because believing them worsens how we feel and causes us to act in ways that are unhelpful.

Unhelpful thoughts ←——————————→ Feel more anxious
Unhelpful thoughts ←——————————→ Act in ways that worsen how you feel

The unhelpful thoughts can thus worsen how you feel emotionally and physically, and unhelpfully alter what you do in both the short and the longer term.

Experiment: To see if these extreme and unhelpful ways of seeing things may occur in your own life, think about a recent time when you have felt more distressed.

Q. Were any unhelpful thinking styles present? Yes ☐ No ☐

Q. Did they have an impact on how you felt and what you did at the time? Yes ☐ No ☐

If **Yes**, was this helpful or unhelpful? Helpful ☐ Unhelpful ☐

How do we respond when we notice worrying thoughts about illness?

A common response from friends and relatives and some health care practitioners when we try to cope with long-term illness is to say 'Try not to think about it'.

Experiment: In order to see if trying not to think about worrying thoughts about illness is effective, try this practical experiment. Please try as hard as you can **not** to think about the following object. Please try very hard for the next 30 seconds not to think about a white polar bear.

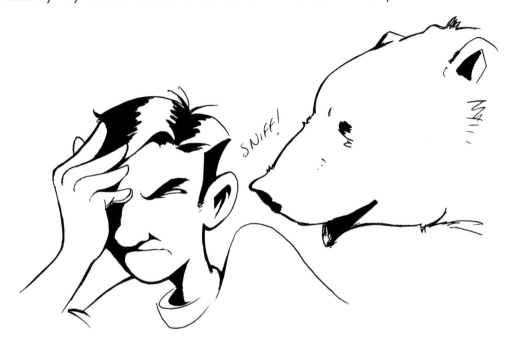

After you have done this, think about what happened. Was it easy not to think about the polar bear, or did it take a lot of effort? You may have noticed that trying hard not to think about it actually made it worse. Alternatively, you may have spent a lot of mental effort trying hard to think about something else such as a *black polar bear* instead. For many people, trying hard to ignore their worrying thoughts and not think about them doesn't work and may actually worsen the problem.

Q. Do I end up putting a lot of mental effort into trying hard not to think worrying thoughts?   Yes ☐   No ☐

Q. If I try not to think the thoughts, does it work?   Yes ☐   No ☐

Summary for Area 2: Altered thinking

Having answered these questions:

Q. Overall, do I have any problems in this area?   Yes ☐   No ☐

These difficulties are potential targets for change. You will find out more about what steps to take to tackle these in Section 5 of the workbook.

Area 3: Altered feelings

Illness can result in a range of possible emotions. These include:

- **Anxiety (also often called 'stress' or 'tension')**

In anxiety, people feel troubled, unsettled and uneasy in themselves.

- **Anger or irritability**

Little things that normally wouldn't bother you may now seem to really irritate or upset you. Anger tends to happen when you, or someone else, break a rule that you think is important, or acts to threaten or frustrate you in some way.

- **Shame**

Feelings of shame occur when you see yourself as having undesirable qualities which if revealed to others will result in ridicule and humiliation. For example, this might be shame at being ill or seeing yourself as not coping. These concerns lead to actions to hide these perceived 'faults' from others.

- **Low mood**

Common terms that people use to describe depression include feeling low/sad/blue/upset/ down/miserable or fed up. You may find that you are more easily moved to tears and that things you would normally cope with really seem to strike home. Typically in severe depression the person feels excessively down and few if any things can cheer them up. During times of depression it becomes harder to cope with physical ill health. Depression can also cause or worsen specific symptoms such as pain, low energy, poor appetite and disrupted sleep patterns. If you feel like this, speak to your doctor or health care practitioner.

My altered feelings

Q. Do I feel anxious or very tense about my physical health or about other life worries?   Yes ☐   No ☐

Q. Do I get more easily angry, frustrated or irritable than previously?   Yes ☐   No ☐

Q. Do I feel shame about aspects of my actions or myself?   Yes ☐   No ☐

Q. Am I feeling depressed, upset or low in mood and no longer enjoy things as before?   Yes ☐   No ☐

Summary for Area 3: Altered feelings/emotions

Having answered these questions:

Q. Overall, do I have any problems in this area?   Yes ☐   No ☐

These difficulties are potential targets for change. You will find out more about what steps to take to tackle these in Section 5 of the workbook.

Area 4: Altered physical reactions in physical ill health

Disease directly causes a range of physical symptoms. These physical symptoms can sometimes be made worse by symptoms of anxiety or depression that occur at the same time. For example, when a person becomes anxious, they may notice altered physical sensations, such as feeling restless and unable to relax. Feelings of mental tension can also cause physical tension in your muscles and joints. This may cause feelings of shakiness, pain, weakness or tiredness. It can be surprising how tiring anxiety can be. Some people may feel completely exhausted when they have felt anxious for a time. Their muscles are so tense it can seem as if they have run a marathon all day. This muscle tension can cause other problems, such as tension headaches, stomach or chest pains. Anxiety can also cause other physical symptoms. Sensations of being hot or cold, sweaty or clammy are common. Your heart may seem to be racing, and you may feel fuzzy-headed or disconnected from things.

Depression can also lead to a number of well-recognised symptoms. These are summarised in the table below.

Physical symptoms common during anxiety	Tick here if you notice this symptom	Physical symptoms common during depression	Tick here if you notice this symptom
Loss of appetite.		Reduced or increased appetite (comfort eating). Weight loss or gain (as a result of comfort eating and underactivity).	
Reduced concentration.		Reduced concentration.	
Tiredness and low energy.		Tiredness and low energy, especially in the morning.	
Problems going off or staying asleep.		Sleep problems are common in depression. You may waken earlier than normal feeling unrested and not be able to get off to sleep again.	
Pain – with tension headaches, stomach pain, eyestrain or chest pain. Muscle tension/shakiness.		Pain is common in depression – especially pain that is worse in the mornings, and which is unaffected by painkillers.	
Feel dizzy/fuzzy-headed or cut-off from things.		Feel dizzy/fuzzy-headed or cut-off from things.	
There may be anxiety about sex and avoidance of sex as a result.		There may be a reduced libido/sex drive.	
Butterflies, loose bowels, sickness, churning stomach, going to the toilet frequently.		Constipation may occur.	
Restless and tense. Rapid heart/palpitations. Sweaty, clammy, shaky. Dry mouth. Shallow rapid breathing.		You may feel physically tense, with restlessness and tension. You feel physically and mentally at your worst first thing in the morning.	
Key symptoms: Going over problems again and again in your mind without resolving them. Feel physically tense and on edge and want to escape. Start to avoid doing things, or to avoid situations, people or places that worsen anxiety.		**Key symptoms:** Low mood and no enjoyment/pleasure or sense of achievement in things. Reduced levels of activity.	

You will have the opportunity to think more about whether anxiety or depression are worsening how you feel physically at the end of this section of the workbook.

Depersonalisation: feeling cut-off and disconnected from things

An important difficulty caused by anxiety is that from time to time we can feel mentally disconnected and cut-off from things. The technical term for this is *depersonalisation*. It can sometimes be quite difficult to describe exactly what this feels like. Many people feel a *fuzzy-headed, spaced-out* sort of sensation. We may know that we are fully awake and also exactly where we are, yet in spite of this we feel distanced from things. It can seem as if we are a robot functioning on automatic. Sometimes we feel like an observer looking at everything from a distance as if we are watching television. We may feel not really connected – as if we or things around us are not completely real. This feeling can be disturbing and often has a clear 'start'. It then just as suddenly stops.

If you would like to find out more about depersonalisation, please read the worksheet *Understanding depersonalisation* (p. 12.1).

Summary for Area 4: Altered physical symptoms

Having answered the questions about physical symptoms:

Q. Overall, do I have any problems in this area?   Yes ☐   No ☐

These difficulties are potential targets for change. You will find out more about what steps to take to tackle these in Section 5 of the workbook.

Anxiety, depression and physical ill health

Physical symptoms can have various causes. These include:
- Physical disease, such as infection, trauma, cancer, hormone problems, etc.
- Anxiety and depression and some other types of mental disorder.

We can feel ill as a result of either of these types of problem. Both types can occur at the same time. Physical illness can also sometimes cause some of the physical symptoms seen in anxiety and depression. For example, painful arthritis can disrupt sleep. A stomach ulcer can cause you to have a reduced appetite and lead to weight loss. Because of this it can sometimes be difficult to be sure whether anxiety or depression are playing a part in worsening how you feel. The Five Areas Assessment can help you identify if anxiety or depression are present. If you have a number of symptoms of anxiety or depression across the whole of the Five Areas Assessment, this makes it more likely that anxiety or depression are present.

Five Areas anxiety checklist	Tick here if you notice this symptom
Situation, relationship and practical problems	
Q. Am I facing various threats or life difficulties?	Yes ☐ No ☐
Altered thinking	
Q. Am I worried about things on most days and finding it difficult to stop worrying?	Yes ☐ No ☐
Q. Am I anxiously going over things again and again in my mind in a way that hasn't actually helped me sort out my problems?	Yes ☐ No ☐
Q. Have I become over-sensitive to possible difficulties and potential threats?	Yes ☐ No ☐
Q. Am I downplaying my own ability to overcome these problems?	Yes ☐ No ☐
Altered feelings	
Q. Do I feel anxious and unsettled about things?	Yes ☐ No ☐
Altered physical symptoms	
Q. Do anxious worries cause me to feel physically on edge and tense?	Yes ☐ No ☐
Q. Do I feel physically tired as a result of anxiety?	Yes ☐ No ☐
Q. Do I have problems sleeping because of worry?	Yes ☐ No ☐
Altered behaviour	
Q. Have anxious thoughts caused me to reduce or stop what I do?	Yes ☐ No ☐
Q. Have worrying thoughts caused me to avoid dealing with difficult situations or people?	Yes ☐ No ☐

If you have answered **Yes** to questions in most of the five areas then anxiety is a problem for you.

Next step: Make sure you finish reading the current workbook. You should then also read Workbook 1b: *Understanding worry and generalised anxiety.*

The following checklist will help you to identify whether you have any of the common symptoms of depression.

Five Areas depression checklist

	Tick here if you notice this symptom
Situation, relationship and practical problems	
Q. Have I had any recent significant life losses or life difficulties?	Yes ☐ No ☐
Altered thinking	
Q. Have I become very much more critical of myself?	Yes ☐ No ☐
Q. Am I very negative about things in general?	Yes ☐ No ☐
Q. Am I sometimes hopeless about the future and the possibility of recovery?	Yes ☐ No ☐
Q. Am I finding it more difficult to keep my mind focused on things?	Yes ☐ No ☐
Altered feelings	
Q. Do I feel depressed or weepy?	Yes ☐ No ☐
Q. Is my ability to enjoy things lower than normal?	Yes ☐ No ☐
Altered physical symptoms	
Q. Has there been a change in my appetite, energy levels, or sleep?	Yes ☐ No ☐
Altered behaviour	
Q. Have I begun to reduce or stop doing things that previously gave me a sense of pleasure or achievement?	Yes ☐ No ☐
Q. Have I begun to be less socially active/staying in more?	Yes ☐ No ☐

If you have answered **Yes** to questions in most of the five areas, you are probably experiencing a depressive illness, and it is depression that is affecting your thinking, feelings, body, behaviour and social activities to a significant extent. Talk to your health care practitioner to find out more about this. They will be able to offer you important information that will help you to work out together whether you are experiencing a depressive disorder.

Misinterpretation of non-threatening symptoms as evidence of serious disease

Sometimes we can become overly sensitive to illness and misinterpret everyday symptoms as being evidence of serious disease. For example, someone like Patrick who has heart disease may pay especial attention to quite normal variations in his heart rate. He becomes scared of doing things that raise his heart rate just in case it is dangerous. This is not to say that someone in that situation should exercise excessively. However, it raises the possibility that we can sometimes be overly protective of ourselves. To make a decision about the *right balance* of activity we need to seek clear advice from doctors and health care practitioners that is based on their professional assessment of our current physical state. Problems arise when we either ignore this and overdo things, or become overly aware of illness and avoid doing anything at all.

How does this situation arise?

Have you changed where you live recently or do you know of anyone who has? Think about that experience. As someone looks to buy or rent a flat or house, they suddenly begin to notice that there are a lot of houses advertised wherever they go. Similarly when someone changes their car they find that everyone is now driving the same model! The key point is that we become very aware of things that are relevant to us at the time. This applies to flats, houses and cars. It also applies to physical health symptoms and health-related information. When we are worried about illness and its consequences, we tend to watch out for information or symptoms that are relevant to us. This especially applies to anything that might be threatening or scary to us.

For example, if you have rheumatoid arthritis, you are more likely to pay attention to newspaper or television reports about new treatments of this disease. The same principle applies to how we scan and pay especial attention to scary physical symptoms that seem particularly threatening. Patrick has had a previous heart attack. He is therefore more likely to pay especial attention to the speed of his pulse, and to any twinges of pain in his chest – whatever the cause. Of course in moderation this is sensible. However, it can backfire if it leads him to become so anxious about his pulse that he is taking it all the time. When going to such extremes, Patrick may find that he is unable to do any exercise at all, even though physically it might be completely safe (and actually recommended as part of his heart recovery programme).

These responses occur in us all. For example:

- Large screening programmes by occupational health departments often pick up possible problems such as high blood pressure (hypertension) or abnormal ECG heart tracing results. Those people are then referred on for a specialist assessment 'just to be sure'. Most of those people are then given a clean bill of health. However, in spite of this they are more likely to feel unwell than before the tests were done in the first place. The health 'scare' has upset them. Even though they are not ill, they feel worse than before.
- Medical students often visit the doctor with health concerns about the area of health that they are studying at the time. For example, they are more prone to present with bowel symptoms shortly after learning about all the different diseases that affect the bowel.

This process of selectively focusing on symptoms and misinterpreting normal sensations as signs of illness can occur in us all. The two examples show how common milder health anxieties are. The health fears usually fall away quite quickly over a period of weeks or months. Health fears can occur alongside physical disease or in its absence. The latter situation is called *health anxiety*. You can find out more about health anxiety in Section 4 of the workbook.

You have now completed thinking about how physical ill health is affecting you in four of the five key areas. We have yet to look in detail at the actions through which we try to cope with illness. The next section will help you to consider this final area – how illness has affected your behaviour.

Section 3   Unhelpfully altered behaviour in illness

This section moves on to the fifth and final area of your Five Areas Assessment – altered behaviour. Our actions can both improve or worsen how ill we feel. It does this in three ways – through reduced activity, avoidance, and unhelpful behaviours.

Altered behaviour 1: Reduced activity

When someone feels ill it is normal to find it is difficult doing things. This is because of:
- feeling ill;
- low energy and tiredness (*'I'm too ill/tired'*);
- low mood and little sense of enjoyment or achievement when things are done;
- negative thinking and reduced enthusiasm to do things *('I just can't be bothered')*.

It can sometimes feel as though everything is too much effort. A *vicious circle of reduced activity* can result.

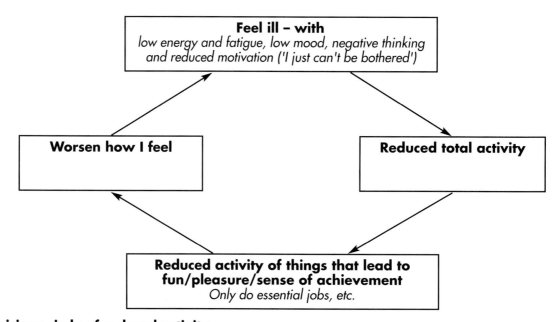

The vicious circle of reduced activity

The result of illness is that we begin to stop doing things. Often the very first things to be stopped are the things that previously we enjoyed, such as meeting friends, socialising, going out, or pursuing hobbies. Instead we may try to focus on keeping up with those things that we see as being more important (things which we *must* do), such as work, or doing things about the house. Unfortunately, the result of this is that we may remove many or all of the things from our lives that would normally have led to feelings of pleasure and a sense of achievement. This reduction in pleasurable activities can end up making us feel even worse. Life can begin to become emptier and emptier. Soon even the everyday core things such as housework, jobs, and looking after ourselves feel like too much to do.

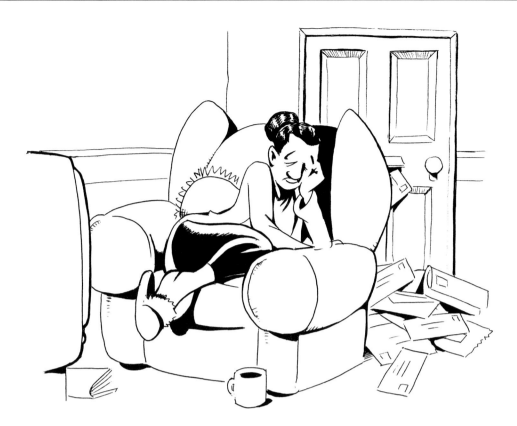

A second aspect of this vicious circle is that it also results in muscle wasting. When we reduce our activity levels, this means that we do not use our muscles and joints as much as normal. Think about the symptoms seen during flu. Here, the person usually recovers after a week or so. As they recover they feel exhausted and weak. Part of this weakness is the result of the viral infection and high temperature. Part of the weakness is also the consequence of being in bed for a week. When we lie in bed, we do not use our muscles as normal. **Muscles that are not used waste and weaken.** This means that when we do use them they will be weak. Also, joints and muscles that haven't been used as much as normal will be painful. Studies show that people lose a significant amount of their muscle bulk after a week in bed. In situations where long-term underactivity has caused wasting, pain and weakness will be greater than this.

The vicious circle of reduced activity therefore can be an important factor keeping you feeling unwell. The good news is that once you have noticed if this is true for you, then you can begin to start working on regaining the pleasurable activities and increasing your activity levels again. The best way to overcome this is to plan to increase your activity levels. This must be done in a planned and paced way. As you do so, you should avoid any temptation to overdo things too quickly. Don't try to rush things. Planning a step-by-step approach is the key to success. As you use your muscles and joints more, they may well hurt. As long as you pace things over a number of days and weeks this does not mean that you are causing any harm – instead it just means you are using the muscles again, often for the first time in months. Take the advice of your doctor as to the right pace for your plan.

Now you can work out whether this problem is affecting you at the moment.

Checklist: Identifying the vicious circle of reduced activity

As a result of how I feel am I:	Tick here if you have noticed this
Going out or socialising less?	
Paying less attention to my self-care or personal hygiene (e.g. washing less, less bothered about my appearance, leaving clothes on for longer, not shaving or combing my hair)?	
Eating poorly (e.g. eating less or tending to eat more 'junk' food, or food that takes little preparation)?	
Stopping or reducing doing hobbies/interests such as reading or other things I previously enjoyed or did to relax?	
Failing to keep up with housework (e.g. am I 'letting things go' around the house)?	
Not always answering the phone or the door when people visit?	
Leaving letters/bills unopened or not replying to them because of a lack of energy or interest in actively dealing with them.	
Less interested in sex (e.g. pushing my partner away physically because of a lack of enjoyment/energy for sex)?	
Staying inactive or lying in bed so that I am far less physically active than before.	

Q. Have I reduced or stopped doing any other things?

Write them in here:

```



```

Summary: Altered behaviour 1: Reduced activity

Having completed these questions, reflect on your answers using the three questions below:

Q. Have I reduced or stopped doing things? Yes ☐ No ☐

Q. Has this reduced my sense of pleasure/achievement in things? Yes ☐ No ☐

Q. Overall, has this worsened how I feel? Yes ☐ No ☐

If you have answered **Yes** to all three questions, you are experiencing the vicious circle of reduced activity. Before moving on, think back on what you have learned and think about how any reduced activity may be affecting your life.

Altered behaviour 2: Avoidance

Anxiety can sometimes be present as part of illness. As discussed in the last section of the workbook, there may be worries or concerns about the illness itself, your ability to cope, the reactions of others, and what will happen in future. Anxiety of any sort tends to cause the person to avoid any situation they see as threatening. This can include any situations that seem to make you either more anxious, and also those that make you feel physically worse. You may therefore find yourself avoiding certain situations, objects, people or places because of how you feel.

Example: Someone with anxious fears about having a heart attack will avoid situations or activities that they think might put them 'at risk'. They may therefore avoid exercise or making love with their partner.

Try to identify ways in which you might be avoiding things. Stop for a minute or so and consider what – if anything – you might be avoiding.

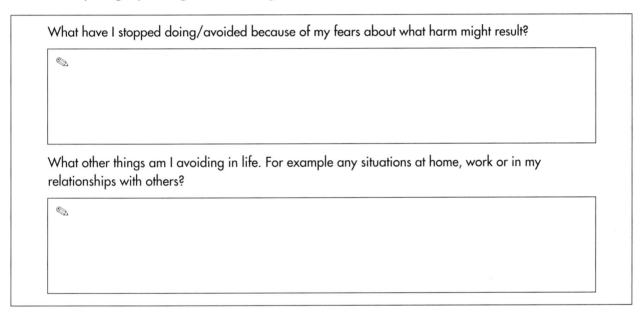

What have I stopped doing/avoided because of my fears about what harm might result?

What other things am I avoiding in life. For example any situations at home, work or in my relationships with others?

The result is often an increasingly restricted lifestyle and additional distress. A *vicious circle of avoidance* may result, and this is summarised below.

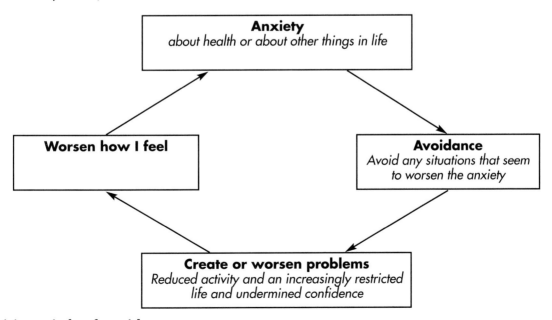

Anxiety
about health or about other things in life

Worsen how I feel

Avoidance
Avoid any situations that seem to worsen the anxiety

Create or worsen problems
Reduced activity and an increasingly restricted life and undermined confidence

The vicious circle of avoidance

To see if this applies to you, ask yourself '*What have I stopped doing because of how I feel*?' You may have had to stop some of these things appropriately as a result of your illness. However, have you **also** stopped some of these things because of anxiety? Remember, sometimes avoidance can be quite subtle. The following checklist will help you consider any areas of avoidance in your life.

Checklist: Identifying the vicious circle of avoidance

As a result of feeling anxious am I:	Tick here if you have noticed this
Avoiding physical activity or exercise as a result of concerns about my physical health?	
Avoiding dealing with important practical problems (both large and small)?	
Not really being honest with others. For example saying Yes when I really mean No?	
Trying hard to avoid situations that bring about upsetting thoughts/memories?	
Brooding over things and therefore no longer living life to the full?	
Avoiding opening or replying to letters or bills?	
Sleeping in to avoid doing things or meeting people?	
Avoiding answering the phone, or the door when people visit?	
Avoiding sex?	
Avoiding talking to others face to face?	
Avoiding being with others in crowded or hot places?	
Avoiding busy or large shops, or finding that I have to think about where and when I go shopping etc.?	
Avoiding going on buses, in cars, taxis etc., or any places where it is difficult to escape?	
Avoiding walking alone far from home?	
Avoiding situations, objects, places or people because of fears about what harm might result?	

Q. Am I avoiding things in other ways?

Write in here how you are doing this if this is applicable to you.

Summary: Altered behaviour 2: Avoidance

Having completed these questions, reflect on your answers using the three questions below:

Q. Am I avoiding doing things as a result of anxiety?　　Yes ☐　　No ☐

Q. Has this reduced my confidence in things and led to an increasingly
restricted life?　　Yes ☐　　No ☐

Q. Overall, has this worsened how I feel?　　Yes ☐　　No ☐

If you have answered **Yes** to all three questions, you are experiencing the vicious circle of avoidance. Take time to think this through and take a break now to do this if you wish to before moving on the third way that altered behaviour can affect how you feel.

Altered behaviour 3: Unhelpful behaviours

When somebody feels ill it is normal to try to do things to feel better. This altered behaviour may be *helpful* or *unhelpful*. The purpose of both types of activity is to improve how you feel – at least in the short term.

Helpful activities may include:
Talking with friends or relatives and receiving helpful support.
- Reading or using self-help materials to find out more about the causes and treatment of the problems.
- Doing activities that provide pleasure or support such as meeting friends, reading or attending religious activities.
- Challenging anxious thoughts by stopping, thinking and reflecting rather than accepting them as true.
- Going to see your doctor or health care practitioner or attending a self-help support group.

Write down any *helpful* things you have done here:

```


```

You should aim to try to maximise the number of helpful activities you do. Sometimes however, we may try to block how we feel with a number of **unhelpful behaviours**. These actions may improve how we feel in the short term, but they can worsen how we feel in the longer term.

Unhelpful behaviours

The following are a list of actions that can be part of the problem rather than part of the solution. These actions tend to make you feel worse and are therefore a key target for change.

Excessive awareness/checking for illness

You have already discovered that becoming overly aware of specific physical symptoms can bring them into the spotlight of the mind. When we notice symptoms we also tend to try to monitor them. This is especially true of symptoms that we are scared of. So, for example, if we find a lump we are likely to keep touching it and checking its size in case it gets larger (as would happen in cancer for example). However, this checking can also *create* symptoms if it is excessive.

Experiment 1: Examine your own forearm and see if you can find a lumpy piece of muscle. Tap this gently with your hand for a minute. This action is trying to reproduce what would happen if you did a 'crash course' in checking behaviour. Now compare that area with the same area on the other arm.

Q. Does the lump feel the same as before? Yes ☐ No ☐

Q. Has it altered in size? Yes ☐ No ☐

Q. Does it feel the same as your other arm? Yes ☐ No ☐

What is the worst-case scenario that could explain a lump that has increased in size/feels hotter/more painful, etc?

Key point: After touching it repeatedly, it is likely that the 'lump' now feels bigger, more tender, and may be more sensitive. The same would occur if you repeatedly checked any lump over a number of days or weeks. Checking can make you more aware of the symptom, and actually worsens it.

Experiment 2: Sometimes people become concerned that they have a problem with their throat. It is quite understandable to therefore check how your throat looks and to be especially aware of any sensations there. You might do this by looking into the mirror and saying 'Aaah'. You may also check your throat by swallowing. Let's try and experiment. What happens if you swallow again and again? Take three large swallows one after another.

Does your swallowing seem easy? Does it become difficult swallowing? Write what you notice here:

What is the worst possible explanation that can explain these symptoms – e.g. that swallowing is becoming difficult?

Of course, sometimes lumps are caused by cancer, and all sorts of throat problems can occur. These experiments, however, make the point that some of the things we do that we think are being useful, can actually become part of the problem.

Key point: Although you need to keep an eye on your body – for example by regular self-examination of your breasts or testicles, it is the extent of this checking that can become inappropriate. Anxious over-examination of your body not only focuses unhelpfully on symptoms, but also the checking itself can begin to create or worsen symptoms. Checking behaviour can include a wide range of things, such as measuring your temperature or blood pressure again and again. The problem isn't doing this just once or twice. It is the excessive focus on the checking that itself becomes part of the problem. It doesn't reassure you, and indeed reinforces any underlying health fears.

Conclusion: sometimes checking behaviour can worsen how you feel.

Q. Write down any excessive checking behaviour here:

Reassurance seeking from others again and again

At one extreme we may choose not to talk at all about how ill we feel. Keeping our problems to ourselves may be because of a belief that '*it is a sign of weakness to be ill or to be seen as not coping*'. At the other extreme, we may recurrently seek support and *excessive reassurance* from those around us. This is again a good example of an action that in moderation can be helpful, but which can become unhelpful when taken to excess. The result is a feeling of dependency on others and a further loss of confidence in yourself. The more reassurance you get the more you seek.

Excessive self-medication

When we are ill, we are often prescribed medication to treat the disorder. It can be tempting sometimes to take an extra dose if you feel worse at a particular time. This raises the possibility of taking too high a dose. The danger is of serious side-effects. For example, some medications prescribed for pain can lead to kidney or liver problems if taken for too long or at too high a dose. Tablets should always therefore be taken as indicated on the prescription and the dose reviewed with your doctor from time to time.

Trying to block how you feel by using drugs/alcohol, etc.

Sometimes people try to block how ill they feel by:

- Misusing alcohol or drugs. This may start out as just having an extra drink to help you cope or to get off to sleep. The danger is of escalating amounts being taken more and more frequently. The risk is alcohol or drug dependency.
- Eating too much (*comfort eating*) – particularly sweet foods/carbohydrates. This may result in weight gain.
- Trying to spend your way out of how you feel by visiting the shops and buying new clothes/goods. The purpose is to cheer you up (so-called *retail therapy*).
- Sleeping with a number of people in an attempt to block how you feel or with the aim of making you feel needed or attractive.

Pushing others away or becoming angry about your illness

Another natural but unhelpful reaction is resolving our feelings by turning against those around us. We may become angry, gossipy, and undermine others by spreading rumours or become bitter and critical. This particularly can occur towards people who are easy targets and less likely to hit back, such as close relatives and friends. Sometimes this behaviour is a form of testing out the love, friendship and support of others. The consequence may be isolation, rejection and loneliness.

Quickly stopping doing activities because of sudden feelings of anxiety

We can feel suddenly physically worse for a number of reasons. Sometimes we may have sudden fears that what we are doing will worsen how we feel physically. In Patrick's case he has sudden rushes of fear that he will have a heart attack. This is where clear medical advice can be really helpful. Anxious fears are often very catastrophic and unrealistic. In Patrick's case, these fears are exactly that. He will not bring on a heart attack by walking with his wife, but whenever he stops what he is doing and sits down to rest this just confirms him in his belief that it is only by stopping all activity that he is avoiding a heart attack.

Over-committing yourself to doing things

Sometimes we unwisely try to fill every part of the day to avoid noticing how ill we feel. This may involve deliberately staying up late watching films, or sleeping in during the day to avoid seeing others. It also could include spending hours on computer games or watching television. Other common activities are listening to music, chatting/surfing on the Internet or texting others all the time. This is not to say that such activities are always unhelpful – but we need to ask why they are done. Doing these things because they can help us to avoid life has a very different motivation from doing them because they are fun.

Posture, aids and mobility

When long-term physical illness occurs, there is a risk of physical disability. This may have a number of causes, including the physical disease process and symptoms themselves (for example, arthritis, or muscular problems after a stroke). Long-term reduced activity also can play a part. This leads to muscle weakness and possibly even contractures of underused muscles and joints. Another important factor is that when we have problems such as pain we alter our posture to attempt to 'protect' painful joints or muscles. There are clear and understandable reasons for this. However, sometimes this attempt to improve things can backfire.

Reflection: Think about your own posture. Are you holding your own muscles in a very tense and 'unnatural' way? If you are, you may be making yourself more prone to muscle strains. This can create or worsen pain symptoms by creating excessive pressures on your back, arms and legs. Similarly, walking with a stick or using a wheelchair can sometimes add to difficulties. If possible, plan to reduce such aids unless advised otherwise by your health care practitioner. Specialist advice is sensible here so that, if you do need such aids, they are the correct ones for you and you know how best to use them.

Key point: Remember that the purpose of the unhelpful behaviours is to make us feel safer/better, at least in the short term. This is a normal reaction in the face of physical illness. What defines them as unhelpful is that although each action causes a short-term relief in symptoms, this doesn't last. They can instead worsen the problems for yourself, your family and your friends.

These actions also teach an unhelpful lesson – *that it is only by checking /avoiding/drinking or leaving the situation etc. that you manage to cope.* In the longer term this behaviour therefore backfires and adds to your problems. This can further worsen how you feel by confirming negative beliefs about yourself, your illness or others. A **vicious circle of unhelpful behaviour** can occur.

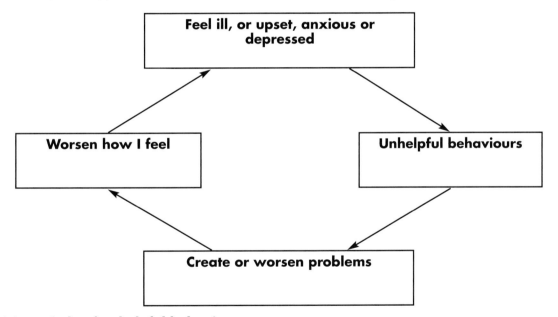

The vicious circle of unhelpful behaviour

A useful question in order to identify unhelpful behaviours is to ask '*What am* I *doing differently to cope with how I feel?*'

The following checklist will help you to identify any unhelpful behaviour in your life. At times these actions can be quite subtle.

Core unhelpful behaviours in physical health problems	**Tick here if you have noticed this**

Being overly aware and excessively checking for symptoms of ill health.

Excessively changing the way I sit or walk to reduce symptoms of physical discomfort. The altered posture then creates or worsens the physical problem.

In addition, a number of other unhelpful behaviours may occur as a means of blocking how you feel.

Checklist: Identifying the vicious circle of unhelpful behaviour

As a result of how I feel, am I:	**Tick here if you have noticed this**

Misusing drink/illegal drugs or prescribed medication to block how I feel in general or improve how I sleep?

Eating too much to block how I feel (*comfort eating*), or over-eating so much that this becomes a binge?

Trying to spend my way out of how I feel by going shopping (*retail therapy*)?

Becoming very demanding or excessively seeking reassurance from others?

Looking to others to make decisions or sort out problems for me?

Throwing myself into doing things so there are no opportunities to stop, think and reflect?

Pushing others away and being verbally or physically threatening/rude to them?

Deliberately harming myself in an attempt to block how I feel?

Taking part in risk-taking actions for example crossing the road without looking, or gambling with money I don't really have?

Compulsively checking, cleaning, or doing things a set number of times or in exactly the 'correct' order so as to make things 'right'?

Carrying out mental rituals such as counting or deliberately thinking 'good' thoughts/saying prayers to make things feel 'right'?

Sleeping with a number of people as a means of blocking how I feel or to feel needed, attractive or relaxed?

Sometimes unhelpful behaviours can lead to quite subtle avoidance. Do you notice any of the following in your own life?

Unhelpful behaviours leading to subtle avoidance of anxiety-provoking situations.

Am I:

Quickly leaving anxiety-provoking situations?

Rushing through a task as quickly as possible? (e.g. walking or talking faster).

Trying very hard not to think about upsetting thoughts/memories? Trying to distract myself to improve how I feel?

Only going out and doing things when others are there to help?

Taking the easiest option (for example joining the shortest queue in the shop as a result of anxiety, or turning down opportunities that seem scary)?

Deliberately looking away during conversations and avoiding eye contact? Bringing conversations to a close quickly because of not knowing what to say?

Q. Am I avoiding things in other subtle ways?

Write in what you are doing here if this applies to you.

Summary: the vicious circle of unhelpful behaviours

Having completed these questions about unhelpful behaviours, reflect on your answers using the three questions below:

Q. Am I doing certain activities or behaviours that are designed to improve how I feel?　　Yes ☐　No ☐

Q. Are some of these activities unhelpful in the short or longer-term either for me or for others?　　Yes ☐　No ☐

Q. Overall has this worsened how I feel?　　Yes ☐　No ☐

If you have answered **Yes** to all three questions, you are experiencing the vicious circle of unhelpful behaviour.

Having completed these questions, think back on what you have learned and then answer the questions below.

The purpose behind the unhelpful behaviours is to help improve how you feel. The following questions will help you see how well it achieves this.

Q. Does carrying out the action(s) make me feel better **in the short term?**   Yes ☐   No ☐

If **Yes,** how long do I feel better for?

Less than 30 mins ☐   30–60 mins ☐   1–3 hours ☐   All day ☐   All week ☐

All month ☐

It lasts forever ☐

Q. Overall, does carrying out the behaviour make me feel better **in**   Yes ☐   No ☐

the long term?

Q. What impact does the behaviour have on my confidence and ability to live my life as I would want?

If you have ticked Yes to Question 1, this could be one thing that is keeping your unhelpful behaviour going. Feeling better (even if for only a short time) can be a powerful reinforcer for what you do. The good news is that you have now identified an important area you can focus on changing.

Key point: Remember that the purpose of the reduced activity, avoidance and unhelpful behaviours is to feel better – at least in the short term. Although they do lead to a short-term relief in symptoms, this doesn't last. **Anxieties or symptoms usually quickly return to the same or an even higher level.**

Summary for Area 5: Altered behaviour (reduced activity, avoidance or unhelpful behaviours)

Having answered the questions in this section:

Q. Overall, do I have any problems in this area?   Yes ☐   No ☐

These difficulties are potential targets for change. You will find out more about what steps to take to tackle these in Section 5 of the workbook.

You have now finished your Five Areas Assessment. Before you move on, please stop for a while and consider what you have learned. How does what you have read help you to make sense of your symptoms?

Q. How well does this assessment summarise how you feel?

Poorly ———————————————————— Very well

0   10

The purpose of the Five Areas Assessment is to help you plan the areas you need to focus on to bring about change. The workbooks in the course can help you begin to tackle each of the five problem areas.

Section 4   Health anxiety – anxiety about physical health

In health anxiety, worrying thoughts are focused upon a fear of physical health problems. The person feels ill, and believes they have a potentially dangerous disease. Because what they think affects how they feel emotionally and physically, they feel anxious and notice a number of the physical symptoms of anxiety. Because what they believe also affects what they do, they understandably go to see the doctor.

These reactions are all very similar to a normal response to illness. The key difference here is that there is either no physical disorder present at all, or the extent of physical disorder cannot explain why they feel so ill. In spite of normal physical investigations and tests, the person is not reassured. Reassurance in fact just makes things worse. They go again and again to the doctor and are often referred on to other health care practitioners for further reassurance. Throughout this they continue to feel ill.

Does this apply to me?

The following checklist will help you identify if you are experiencing any of the main problems seen in health anxiety.

Health anxiety checklist

Q. Do I feel very anxious whenever I think about my physical health?   Yes ☐   No ☐

Q. Am I going to the doctor far more than I used to?   Yes ☐   No ☐

Q. Am I thinking again and again about how ill I feel, yet my doctors' tests seem to show no strong evidence of a physical illness?   Yes ☐   No ☐

Q. Am I finding it difficult accepting that the physical tests and investigations show little or no strong evidence of a physical illness?   Yes ☐   No ☐

Q. Am I constantly examining myself (e.g. taking my pulse or temperature or checking myself for lumps or looking at myself in the mirror)?   Yes ☐   No ☐

Q. Am I constantly aware of how my body feels and paying particular attention to symptoms that especially worry me?   Yes ☐   No ☐

Q. Has my own health care practitioner or someone else that I would usually trust told me that they think I am too worried about my health?   Yes ☐   No ☐

Choice point: If you have answered **Yes** to several of these questions, then you may have problems of health anxiety. Continue to read the rest of this section to find out more.

If you answered **No**, you can skip this section if you wish and move to the start of the final section of the workbook.

What causes health anxiety?

Health anxiety is usually caused by a combination of factors:

- The person is overly aware of normal symptoms in the body. They may also misinterpret symptoms of everyday common diseases such as colds as evidence of severe ill health. For example, if you are concerned about having a brain tumour, you will be particularly aware whenever you have a headache or feel fuzzy-headed. Because these fears cause tension you may also notice tension headaches. These will then reinforce your fears. If you are concerned about bowel disease you will be aware of any gurgle or bowel pain, and know exactly when you last used the toilet/how your motions appeared, etc.
- People with health anxiety are prone to misinterpret information from health care practitioners, magazines and the media. Even slight comments, such as '*you look pale*' are seized upon and worried about.
- Because of their health concerns, the person goes again and again seeking reassurance from their doctor or other health care practitioner. Yet they are not reassured by the normal results of physical tests. You will find out more about this shortly.

> **Practical problem:** If anyone who is completely well goes to the doctor and has 20 blood tests, one of them will come back falsely showing evidence of disease. This is because all medical tests are prone to something called *false positive* results. Even a very good test is only 95 per cent efficient. This means that in 1 in 20 cases a so-called false positive result will occur. The difficulty in health anxiety is that this will lead to more anxiety. A flurry of further tests result. In health anxiety physical treatments are not needed. However, if they are given they may cause various side effects. These can cause even more problems. The person does have problems, and these problems need to be treated. However, the treatment is not a physical one. Instead it should focus on helping the person challenge their health fears and to alter any unhelpful behaviour that is worsening how they feel.

Let's read about Patrick who has problems of health anxiety. He also has a physical health problem, which originally caused him to start worrying.

> **Example:** After a mild heart attack, Patrick becomes convinced that his heart is not working properly. As a result he constantly feels anxious and is preoccupied with his illness. He feels physically tense and cannot sleep. He is overly aware of any sensations of tension in his chest, and of his heart rate. He keeps checking his pulse rate using a stopwatch. Every time he notices his heart speeding up he is even more convinced that he is seriously ill in spite of 'all-clear' investigations by his specialist. He is now repeatedly arranging to see his GP asking for more tests. He has stopped any activities that he fears may bring on a heart attack such as doing exercise, and making love with his wife. This has led to arguments that have further added to his problems.
>
>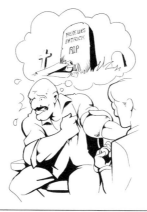

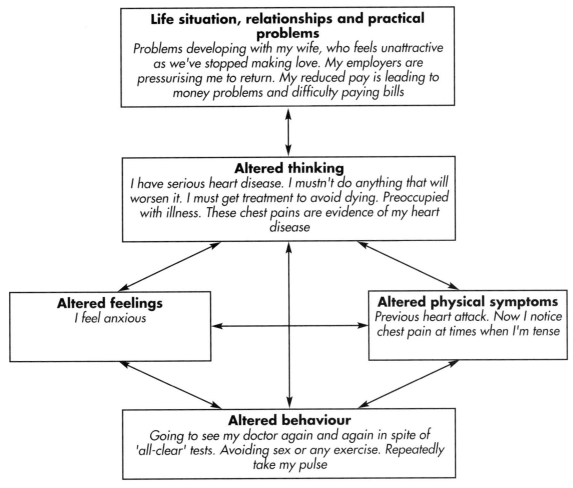

Life situation, relationships and practical problems
Problems developing with my wife, who feels unattractive as we've stopped making love. My employers are pressurising me to return. My reduced pay is leading to money problems and difficulty paying bills

Altered thinking
I have serious heart disease. I mustn't do anything that will worsen it. I must get treatment to avoid dying. Preoccupied with illness. These chest pains are evidence of my heart disease

Altered feelings
I feel anxious

Altered physical symptoms
Previous heart attack. Now I notice chest pain at times when I'm tense

Altered behaviour
Going to see my doctor again and again in spite of 'all-clear' tests. Avoiding sex or any exercise. Repeatedly take my pulse

Patrick's Five Areas Assessment

The Five Areas Assessment shows that what Patrick thinks affects how he feels physically and emotionally, and also alters what he does. The five areas affect each other. Although Patrick has health anxiety, there *has* been a previous heart attack. However, his response to this is excessive and unhelpful. His fears of illness are dominating his life to an unhelpful extent. They are also interfering with his recovery plan after the heart attack.

Think about how well Patrick's reactions in the diagram can be explained using this approach. You may find the diagram difficult to understand at first, or you may not be sure whether it applies to you.

How do Patrick's *thoughts, and physical/emotional reactions* fit together? How do his health fears affect how he feels?

How do Patrick's *thoughts and behaviour* fit together? How do his health fears affect what he does?

What impact do you think Patrick's actions are having on his wife and health care practitioner? How does this fit in with his fears?

How could Patrick alter his health fears and his unhelpful behaviour?

This short description of health anxiety has provided some key information about how the processes described in the workbook can cause someone to feel ill in spite of the absence of disease. **Anxiety about health may occur where there is clear physical disease and where there is none.** It builds upon reactions we are all prone to. If it affects you, then there are some clear things you can do to overcome these problems. The final part of this workbook will help you to identify which additional workbooks you need to read to find out how to plan to move forwards.

Section 5 Choosing your targets for change

The main problem areas seen in physical ill-health are the:

- Current situations, relationship or practical problems
- Altered thinking (with extreme and unhelpful thinking)
- Altered feelings/emotions
- Altered physical symptoms
- Altered behaviour (with reduced activity, avoidance or unhelpful behaviours)

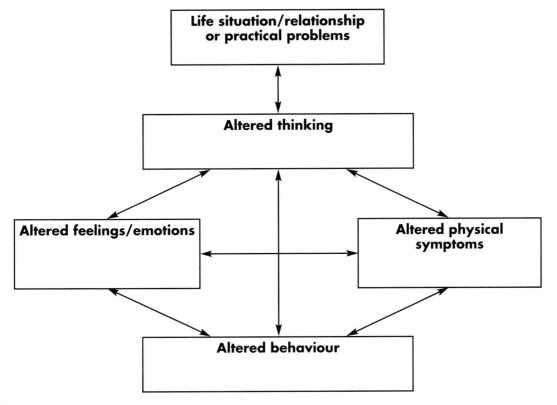

The Five Areas Assessment

You have previously answered questions about each of these five areas. Look again at the answers you gave in your own Five Areas Assessment, in Sections 2 and 3 of the workbook. Your answers summarise the problems you identified in each area. Since there are links between the areas, it is possible by altering any of the areas to bring about changes in others, and help improve how you feel.

> **Key point:** By defining your problems, you have now identified possible target areas to focus on. The key is to make sure that you do things **one step at a time**. Slow steady steps are more likely to result in improvement than very enthusiastically starting and then running out of steam.

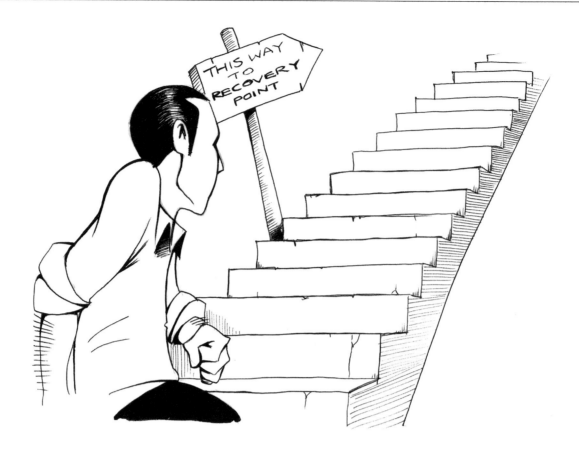

Short-, medium- and longer-term goals

You may have made all sorts of previous attempts to change, but unless you have a clear plan and stick to it, change will be very difficult. Planning and selecting which targets to try and change first is a crucial part of successfully moving forwards. By choosing some specific areas to focus on to start with, this also means that you are actively choosing at first **NOT** to focus on other areas.

Setting yourself targets will help you to focus on how to make the changes needed to get better. To do this you will need to decide:
- Short-term targets: changes you can make today, tomorrow and next week.
- Medium-term targets: changes to be put in place over the next few weeks.
- Long-term targets: where you want to be in six months or a year.

The questions that you have answered in this workbook will have helped you to identify the main problem areas that you currently face. Although this workbook makes up part of The *Overcoming Anxiety* course, it is aimed at people who are facing the challenge of physical health problems even when anxiety is absent. It aims to help you to identify problem areas so that you can make helpful changes in how you feel.

The workbooks can be used either alone or as part of a complete course. The Workbooks 1a to 1e in Part 1 are designed to help you to identify your current problem areas. This will help identify which of the Workbooks 2 to 9 in Part 2 you need to read. Finally, you can summarise what you have learned and plan for the future by completing Workbook 10. This will help you keep putting what you have learned into practice.
- If you have anxieties about your health or concerns about how you are or the future, workbooks 4 and 5, which deal with identifying and changing extreme and unhelpful thinking, may be helpful.
- If you have problems of reduced activity, then workbook 6 in the companion book, *Overcoming Depression*, addresses this area.

- If you have noticed that you experience problems of avoidance as a result of anxiety, read Workbook 6: *Overcoming avoidance*.
- Finally, the Workbook 7: *Overcoming unhelpful behaviours* addresses how to record and then slowly plan how to reduce any unhelpful behaviours in a step-by-step way.

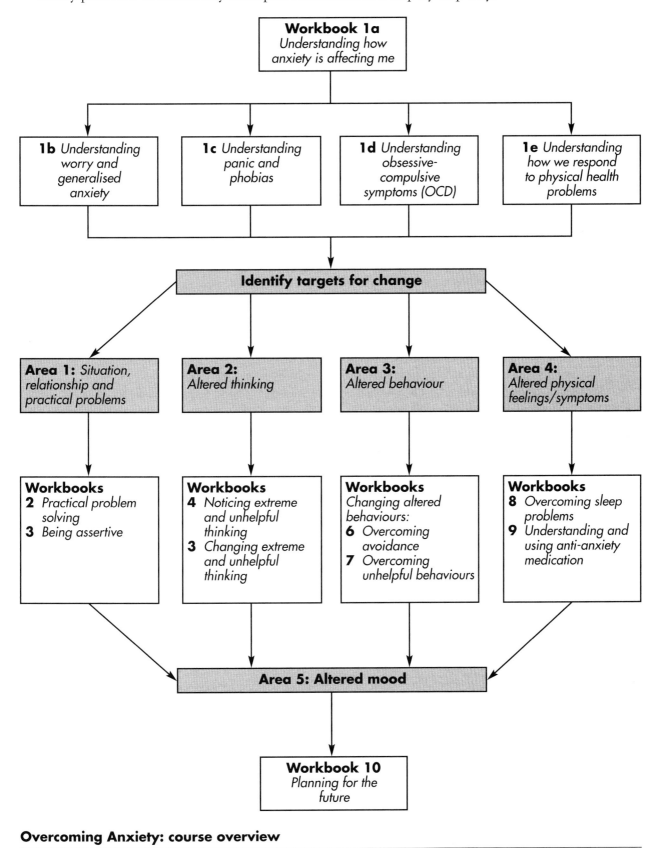

Workbook 1a
Understanding how anxiety is affecting me

1b *Understanding worry and generalised anxiety*

1c *Understanding panic and phobias*

1d *Understanding obsessive-compulsive symptoms (OCD)*

1e *Understanding how we respond to physical health problems*

Identify targets for change

Area 1: *Situation, relationship and practical problems*

Area 2: *Altered thinking*

Area 3: *Altered behaviour*

Area 4: *Altered physical feelings/symptoms*

Workbooks
2 *Practical problem solving*
3 *Being assertive*

Workbooks
4 *Noticing extreme and unhelpful thinking*
3 *Changing extreme and unhelpful thinking*

Workbooks
Changing altered behaviours:
6 *Overcoming avoidance*
7 *Overcoming unhelpful behaviours*

Workbooks
8 *Overcoming sleep problems*
9 *Understanding and using anti-anxiety medication*

Area 5: Altered mood

Workbook 10
Planning for the future

Overcoming Anxiety: course overview

The Overcoming Anxiety course

Understanding anxiety

Workbooks 1a to 1e provide an introduction and overview of anxiety problems. It is recommended that you read these workbooks first to give you an overview of how anxiety can affect you. The five workbooks together cover the common anxiety disorders – worry, panic, phobias, obsessive-compulsive disorder and also how we respond to physical health problems. They will help you identify which of these areas you need to focus on changing and will help you decide which of the remaining workbooks you need to read.

Area 1: Dealing with difficult situations, relationship and practical problems

Workbook 2: *Practical problem solving*

In this workbook you will learn a step-by-step plan that you can use to deal with practical problems. It will provide you with the tools to tackle any practical problems that you face. This will help you to take more control of your life and the decisions that you make. By feeling more in control of your life, you will improve your self-confidence.

Workbook 3: *Being Assertive*

Have you ever thought that no one listens to you, and that other people seem to walk all over you? Have others commented that they think that you always walk over them? You will find out about the difference between passive, aggressive and assertive behaviour and learn how to develop more balanced relationships with others where your opinion is listened to and respected, and you listen to and respect other people.

Area 2: Changing extreme and unhelpful thinking

Workbook 4: *Noticing extreme and unhelpful thinking*

What you think about yourself, others and the situations that occur around you, can alter how you feel and affect what you do. This workbook will help you to learn ways of identifying extreme and unhelpful ways of thinking. You will learn how to notice such thoughts and to understand the impact these have on how you feel and what you do.

Workbook 5: *Changing extreme and unhelpful thinking*

This workbook will teach you the important skill of how to challenge extreme and unhelpful thinking. With practice this will help you change the extreme and unhelpful thinking that is often a major problem in anxiety or depression.

Area 3: Changing altered behaviours

Workbook 6: *Overcoming avoidance*

You will find out more about how avoidance keeps problems going. You will learn ways of changing what you do in order to break the vicious circle of avoidance.

Workbook 7: *Overcoming unhelpful behaviours*

You will learn some effective ways of overcoming unhelpful behaviours such as drinking too much, reassurance seeking and trying to spend your way out of how you feel.

Area 4: Physical symptoms and treatments

Workbook 8: *Overcoming sleep problems*

Often when someone is anxious they not only feel emotionally and mentally low, but they also notice a range of physical changes that are a normal part of anxiety. This workbook will help you find out about these common changes, and in particular will help you to deal with problems of poor sleep.

Workbook 9: *Understanding and using anti-anxiety medication*

When someone is anxious sometimes their doctor suggests they take an anti-anxiety medication. You will find out why doctors suggest this, and also learn about common fears and concerns that people have when first starting to take these tablets so that you can find out for yourself whether this medication may be helpful for you.

Area 5: Altered mood

The fifth and final area, anxious mood, will improve if you work at the other areas where you have problems (the altered thinking, behaviour, physical symptoms and the situations, relationships and practical problems that you face). Once you feel better, the final workbook of the series can be read to help you to summarise what you have learned.

Workbook 10: *Planning for the future*

You will have learned new things about yourself and made changes in how you live your life. This final workbook will help you to identify what you have learned and help you plan for the future. You will devise your own personal plan to cope with future problems in your life so that you can face the future with confidence.

The work you do using the workbooks can supplement the help you receive from your doctor or other health care practitioner or friends. Sometimes more specialist help is needed to help how you feel and your doctor may suggest that you see a trained specialist such as a clinical psychologist, occupational therapist, social worker, psychiatric nurse or a psychiatrist.

Use the following table to help you decide which workbooks are right for you to read now, and over the next few weeks and months. You have already read the current workbook, and it is recommended that you also read Workbook 1a: *Understanding how anxiety is affecting me*. You may find it helpful to discuss this with your health care practitioner or other trusted supporter.

Workbook title	Short-term goals (plan to read in the next week or so)	Medium-term goals (plan to read over the next few weeks)	Long-term goals (plan to read over the next few months)	Tick when completed
Understanding anxiety workbooks				
1a *Understanding how anxiety is affecting me*	✔			
1b *Understanding worry and generalised anxiety*				
1c *Understanding panic and phobias*				
1d *Understanding obsessive-compulsive symptoms (OCD)*				
1e *Understanding how we respond to physical health problems*	✔			
Workbook 2 *Practical problem solving*				
Workbook 3 *Being assertive*				
Workbook 4 *Identifying extreme and unhelpful thinking*				
Workbook 5 *Changing extreme and unhelpful thinking*				
Workbook 6 *Overcoming avoidance*				
Workbook 7 *Overcoming unhelpful behaviours*				
Workbook 8 *Overcoming sleep problems*				
Workbook 9 *Understanding and using anti-anxiety medications*				
Workbook 10 *Staying well*				
Worksheet *Overcoming hyperventilation/over-breathing*				
Worksheet *Understanding depersonalisation*				

In order to help you to review your progress, it can be useful to record how you feel at different times as you work on your problems. Your health care practitioner may work with you to decide what information it might be helpful to record. Don't expect to feel better all at once. Change can take time, however by working at your problems, most people find that improvement is possible.

> **Key point:** In order to change, you will need to choose to try to apply what you will learn regularly **throughout the week**, and not just when you read the workbook or see your health care practitioner. The workbooks will encourage you to do this by sometimes suggesting certain tasks for you to carry out in the days after reading each workbook.
>
> These tasks will:
> - help you to put into practice what you have learned in each workbook;
> - gather information so that you can get the most out of the workbook.
>
> Experience has shown that you are likely to make the most progress if you are able to put into practice what you have learned.

Summary

In this workbook you have learned about:
- how to use this workbook;
- how we respond to physical health problems;
- the key ways that physical health problems can affect your life;
- the Five Areas Assessment: the *situations*, *relationship and practical problems* we face, and the *altered thinking*, *emotional* and *physical feelings* and *behaviour* that make up our response to the challenge of illness;
- how our thoughts and concerns about illness can worsen how we feel;
- the areas you need to tackle in order to overcome your own problems.

Putting into practice what you have learned

- Read through the current workbook again. Think in detail about how illness is affecting your thinking, emotional and physical feelings, and behaviour. Decide which areas you want to change.
- Use the diary sheet at the end of the workbook to record the intensity of your main symptom/problem on the hour throughout the day. Use this to help identify any factors that might helpfully affect your symptoms and put what you learn into practice in your own life. Look back to the example of Patrick doing this on page 1e.14 of the workbook if you feel stuck.
- Choose **two episodes** over the next week when you feel either more physically ill or more anxious. Use the blank Five Areas Assessment that follows this section to record the impact on your thinking, mood, body and behaviour at that time. Try to generate a summary of how you feel in each of the five areas. Use this workbook to identify whether you showed any of the unhelpful thinking styles during these occasions. What impact did your thoughts have on how you felt and what you did during these two episodes? Can you identify any examples of reduced activity, avoidance or unhelpful behaviours? Please photocopy or draw out additional copies of the diagram as you need it and keep the sheet handy.
- Finally, review your list of which workbooks you will choose to use next and move on to work through these in your own time.

If you have difficulties with these tasks, don't worry. Just do what you can. If you have found any aspects of this workbook unhelpful, upsetting or confusing, please can you discuss this with your health care practitioner or someone else whose opinion you trust.

A request for feedback

An important factor in the development of all the Five Areas Assessment workbooks is that the content is updated on a regular basis based upon feedback from users and practitioners. If there are areas which you find hard to understand, or which seem poorly written, please let me know and I will try to improve things in future. I regret that I am unable to provide any specific replies or advice on treatment.

To provide feedback, please contact me via:

Email: Feedback@fiveareas.com

Mail: Dr Chris Williams, Department of Psychological Medicine, Gartnavel Royal Hospital, 1055 Great Western Road, Glasgow, G12 0XH

Acknowledgements

I wish to thank all those who have commented upon this workbook especially Alan Davidson, Anne Joice and Stephen Williams.

The cartoon illustrations in the Workbooks have been produced by Keith Chan (kchan75@hotmail.com) and are copyright of Media Innovations Ltd.

My notes

....

....

....

....

....

....

....

....

....

....

....

....

....

....

Worksheet: A Five Areas Assessment of a specific time when I feel more anxious/worse

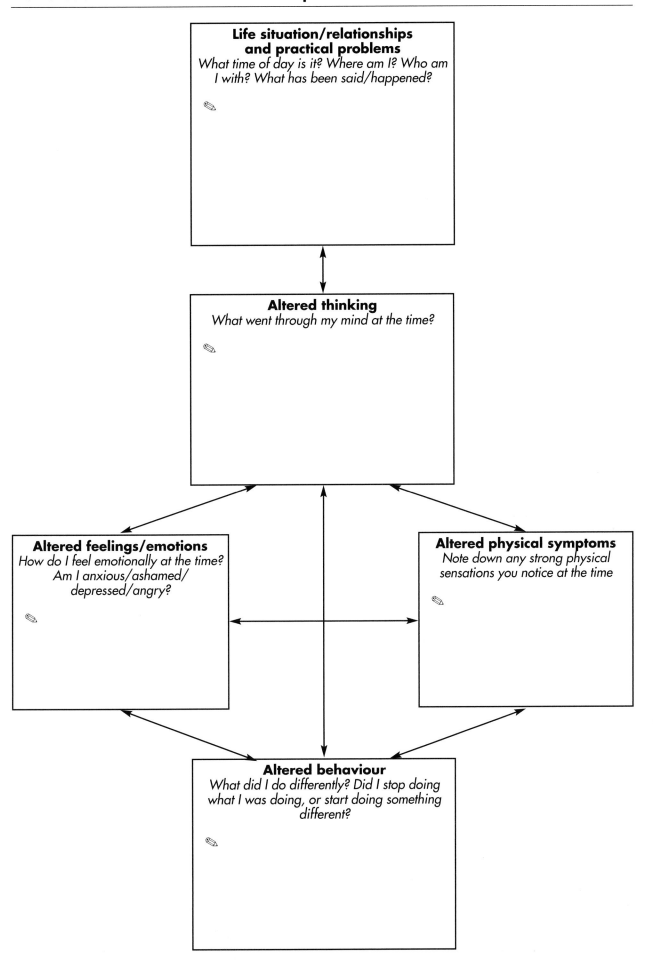

Diary record of the intensity of my main symptom/problem during the day.   Date: . . . .

Time	What am I doing at the moment?	Intensity of the main symptom (0–10)
7 am		
8 am		
9 am		
10 am		
11 am		
12 pm		
1 pm		
2 pm		
3 pm		
4 pm		
5 pm		
6 pm		
7 pm		
8 pm		
9 pm		
10 pm		
11 pm		

Part 2

Overcoming Anxiety self-management workbooks and worksheets

Workbook 2
Practical problem solving

Dr Chris Williams

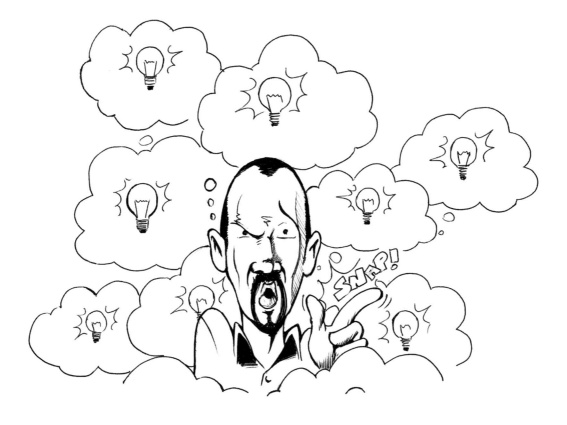

A Five Areas Approach

Introduction

Everyone faces problems from time to time in their lives, and sometimes many problems are faced all at once. Problems are a normal part of daily life. No matter how hopeless you feel right now; in the past you will have faced problems that you have solved.

Task: Make a list of things that you have done well in the past. This will remind you of things you have coped with before and that will help you see your problem in a different perspective.

The reason for not managing to cope with problems is usually because too much has happened at the wrong time. When difficulties occur one at a time, it is usually easier to solve them. But when they happen one after the other, or all at once, it may seem much harder. When someone is finding that everything is 'too much' a common response is to 'do nothing'. In fact, the person never does just nothing. They may not take any practical steps to overcome their problems, but they use plenty of energy worrying about the problem – but in a way that does not help sort it out.

A different approach is to tackle the problem in a planned step-by-step manner. The principles of problem solving include:

- **defining** the problem **clearly**;
- approaching each problem separately **in turn**;
- breaking down each problem into **smaller parts** that are then easier to solve.

The seven steps to problem solving

There are seven steps to problem solving. By working through these you can learn an approach that enables you to overcome your own problems. The first step is to choose the problem you are going to tackle first.

Choosing a clear target

The key is to move from more general problem areas to a clearer target problem. So, for example, if you have a problem area such as '*I don't have enough money*', a clearer target problem could be decided by asking yourself '*In what way does not having enough money cause me problems at the moment?*'. It might cause problems because a credit card payment is due at the end of the month, and you don't have enough money to pay it.

One way of thinking about this process is to think of it as a *funnelling process*. You funnel down from the general problem area to a more specific target that you tackle first.

The funnel process: defining a specific problem

General problem:

'I don't have enough money.'

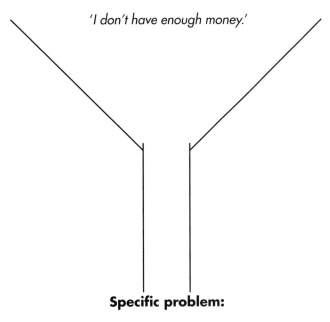

Specific problem:

'I can't pay my electricity bill this month.'

A similar process can be used to help make any problem area clearer. So, for example, if the problem is *'I'm stressed by the behaviour of my neighbours'* you might find it easier to be precise about the problem by asking yourself *'Exactly what is it about my neighbours that is so stressful?'*

Step 1: Identify and clearly define the problem
Use this funnel-type process to start with a general problem area. Work towards getting a clearer target by asking 'Exactly what is it about this problem area that is difficult for me at the moment?'

Task: Try to clearly define your own problem as precisely as possible. Write it down and ask yourself if this is a clear and focused problem.

My problem (*please write in*)

Q. Is this a clear, focused problem?   Yes ☐   No ☐

If you have ticked **No**, re-write it so that it is clear and focused.

Step 2: Think up as many solutions as possible to achieve this initial goal
- The more solutions that are generated, the more likely a good one will emerge.
- Ridiculous ideas should be included as well even if you would never choose them in practice. This can help you adopt a flexible approach to the problem.

Write a list of possible solutions. Useful questions to help you to think these up might include:

- What *ridiculous* solutions can I include as well as more sensible ones?

- What helpful ideas would others (e.g. family, friends or colleagues at work) suggest?

- What approaches have I tried in the past in similar circumstances?

- What advice would I give a friend who was trying to tackle the same problem?

Example: Paul's problem

Paul has a debt problem, and cannot repay his credit card bill at the end of the month. Possible solutions (including ridiculous ideas at first) are:

- Ignore the problem completely – it may go away.

- Mug someone or rob a bank.

- Try to arrange an overdraft from the bank and use this to pay off the bill.

- Pay off a very small part of the money (the minimum asked for).

- Switch credit card payments to another credit card (one with a lower interest rate).

- Speak to a counsellor (e.g. at the Citizen's Advice Bureau) with skills in debt repayments.

- Speak to the credit card company to see if they will agree different repayment terms.

Task: Brainstorming your problem by writing in as many possible solutions as possible. Include ridiculous ideas as well!

Step 3: Look at the advantages and disadvantages of each of the possible solutions

Think about the advantages and disadvantages of each possible solution. This will help you to decide which of the options are likely to be most practical and achievable for you.

Example: Paul's thoughts about how to deal with his debt problems.

Suggested solution	Advantages	Disadvantages
Ignore the problem completely.	*Easier in the short term with no embarrassment.*	*The problem will worsen in the long term. It will have to be tackled sometime.*
Mug someone or rob a bank.	*It would get me some money.*	*It's unethical and wrong. I couldn't do it. I might be arrested. I couldn't harm someone else in this way. That's just ridiculous.*
Arrange a loan or overdraft with my bank.	*It would allow me a better rate of interest than paying off the high rate on my credit card. I could also spread the payments over a longer time.*	*How would I do this? It would be scary seeing the bank manager. They may also say 'no'.*
Pay off the minimum payment possible.	*Good short-term answer. It would prevent me defaulting the payments.*	*The debt wouldn't get any smaller, and the interest rates would make it larger and larger. I would never be able to pay it off.*
Switch to a cheaper credit card.	*This would be a lot cheaper. There are lots of good deals around with cheaper introductory rates.*	*I would need to look at the small print of the different agreements and complete all the paperwork.*
Speak to a debt counsellor.	*I hear they can be very good.*	*I'd feel embarrassed talking to them. How do you contact them?*
Inform the credit card company and ask if they will agree different re-payment terms.	*It would provide the company with clear information. It's in their best interests for me to keep up the payments. They may be flexible and allow a repayment break at lower interest.*	*It seems quite scary to do this.*

Task: Think through the pluses and minuses of all the suggested solutions you came up with in Step 2. Write them below.

Suggested solution	Advantages	Disadvantages

Step 4: Choose one of the solutions

In Paul's example, he decides to try to arrange a loan or overdraft with his bank. This solution should be one that is helpful and achievable. Use your answers from the last step to help decide the solution that seems best for you.

This solution should fulfil the following two criteria:

a) Is it helpful?   Yes ☐   No ☐

b) Is it achievable?   Yes ☐   No ☐

My choice:

Step 5: Plan the steps needed to carry it out and apply the questions for effective change

This stage is a key part in the problem-solving process. The example below shows how Paul plans step 5.

Example: Paul's solution

Paul has decided to arrange a bank loan or overdraft. This seems a reasonable solution. Other suggestions might also have worked, but this one seems to be the most helpful and achievable based on his previous banking record. He now plans the steps needed to carry out his solution.

I could phone my bank. I have the phone number on my bank statement. I'm quite nervous so I'm going to plan out what I am going to say in advance. I will phone up and ask to arrange a time to come in. I will tell them I'm having problems repaying my credit card because I'm off work sick. I'll ask if I can come in to see someone in the afternoon because I feel better then. I think it's best if I also phone them in the afternoon. I'm more likely to get straight through to them then, and also I generally feel more confident after lunch.

Next, Paul applies *the questions for effective change* to his plan to check how practical and achievable it is.

The questions for effective change

Is the planned solution one that:

Q. will be **useful** for understanding or changing how I am?   Yes ☑   No ☐

Q. is a **specific task** so that I will know when I have done it?   Yes ☑   No ☐

Q. is **realistic**: is it practical and achievable?   Yes ☑   No ☐

Q. makes clear **what** I am going to do and **when** I am going to do it?   Yes ☑   No ☐

Q. is an activity that won't be easily blocked or prevented by practical problems? Yes ☑   No ☐

Task: Write down the practical steps needed to carry out your own solution. Be as precise as possible in your plan. Think through **what** you are going to do, and **when** you are going to do it. Try to predict possible problems and work out how to avoid or deal with them.

Task: Apply the questions for effective change to your planned solution to check how practical and achievable it is.

Is my planned solution one that is:

● **useful** for understanding or changing how I am?   Yes ☐   No ☐

● **a specific task** so that I will know when I have done it?   Yes ☐   No ☐

● **realistic**, that is, is it practical and achievable?   Yes ☐   No ☐

● clear about **what** I am going to do and **when** I am going to do it?   Yes ☐   No ☐

● an activity that **won't be easily blocked or prevented** by practical
problems?   Yes ☐   No ☐

If you have replied **No** to any of these questions, revise your plan to try and overcome this. If it is difficult to do, it may be that another solution from Step 2 might be a better choice.

Step 6: Carry out the plan

Task: Write down exactly what happened when you carried out your plan. As part of this summary, record the thoughts and feelings you experienced before, during and after your carried out the plan.

Step 7: Review the outcome

What happened when you carried out the plan?

Task: complete the checklist and answer the questions that follow:

Q. Was the selected approach successful? Yes ☐ No ☐

Q. Did it help deal with the target problem? Yes ☐ No ☐

Q. Were there any disadvantages to using this approach? Yes ☐ No ☐

Q. What have I learned from doing this? Write below any helpful lessons or information you have learned from what happened. If things didn't go quite as you hoped, try to learn from this. How could you make things different during your next attempt to tackle the problem?

Use the questions below to help you review what happened.

● What went well?

● What didn't go so well?

● What have I learned from what happened?

● How can I put what I have learned into practice?

Even if things haven't gone well, you can learn from this and take it into account with your next plan. Also, even if some things haven't turned out right in the approach, much will have gone well.

What happened to Paul?

Paul phones the bank that afternoon as planned. Just before he does this, he feels quite scared. He predicts that the company representative will humiliate him and turn his request down. Paul decides to try to challenge these fears and phones the bank. When he phones the line is engaged. He tries again two minutes later and the phone is answered by an electronic answering service that asks him to make a selection of which service he wants from five options. Paul is surprised by this, becomes flustered and immediately puts the phone down.

His first thought is 'What an idiot – I should be able to do this.' Over the next few minutes, he is able to challenge this thought. He then decides to learn from what happened and try again. He therefore phones the bank again, but plans to have a pen and paper available to write down the different options. He finds that the current option for those with payment difficulties is Option 2. He selects this and arranges an appointment. When he goes to the bank he feels quite scared. He predicts that the manager will humiliate him and turn his request down and that the card company will then demand immediate payment and issue a court summons.

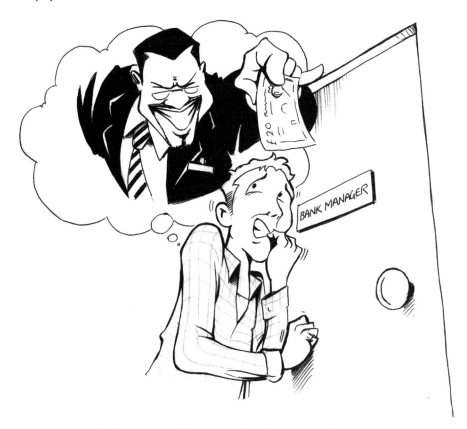

Paul decides to try to challenge these fears and decides to go to the bank anyway.

When he arrives at the bank, Paul is surprised to be met by a friendly bank assistant not the manager. She says that she is his personal account manager. She offers him a cup of tea, and they talk in a separate office so that their discussion is confidential. She tells him that this is a common problem. Because he has banked with them for several years and has a good banking record, she says there will be no problems in offering him a loan at a preferential rate. Paul agrees, and is happy with how things went. His fears were not correct. He was offered a loan, at a rate that he can afford.

Planning the next steps

You have now practised this approach for the first time. The next step is to build slowly on what you have done in a step-by-step way. You have the choice to:

- stop using the approach if you have overcome all your problems;
- work on other aspects of the same problem;
- select a new problem area to tackle.

You must decide for yourself which course is the best for you. Remember, it is not possible to deal with every problem all at once. In fact, if you try to change everything at once you will be potentially setting yourself up to fail. Instead, by focusing on one clear target problem at a time, you can use the 7-step plan to tackle any future problems.

Conclusion

Problem solving is a technique that needs to be practised. You will improve your skills in this approach by using it. Try to learn from anything that goes wrong and keep practising so that using this approach becomes second nature whenever you face a problem.

Putting what you have learned into practice

- Choose one or two problems only and use the seven-step approach to problem solving now and during the next two or three weeks.
- Write down all the steps as you do them, and review for yourself the progress you make. If you have difficulties just do what you can.
- If you have found any aspects of this workbook unhelpful, upsetting or confusing, please discuss this with your health care practitioner or someone else whose opinion you trust.

A request for feedback

An important factor in the development of all the Five Areas Assessment workbooks is that the content is updated on a regular basis based upon feedback from users and practitioners. Please let me know if you have found the content helpful or unhelpful. If there are areas which you find hard to understand, or which seem poorly written, please let me know and I will try to improve things in future. I regret that I am unable to provide any specific replies or advice on treatment.

> **To provide feedback, please contact me via:**
>
> **Email:** Feedback@fiveareas.com
>
> **Mail:** Dr Chris Williams, Department of Psychological Medicine, Gartnavel Royal Hospital, 1055 Great Western Road, Glasgow, G12 0XH

The cartoon illustrations in the workbooks have been produced by Keith Chan (kchan75@hotmail.com) and are copyright of Media Innovations Ltd.

My notes

....

....

....

....

....

....

....

....

....

....

....

....

....

....

....

....

....

....

....

....

....

....

....

....

....

....

....

....

Workbook 3
Being assertive

Dr Chris Williams

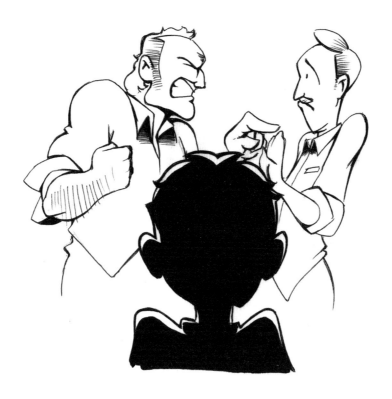

A Five Areas Approach

Introduction

At some time in our lives, however confident we are, we will find it difficult to deal with certain difficult situations. Examples of these could be:

- dealing with unhelpful shop assistants, or with poor service in a restaurant or garage;
- dealing with angry or difficult colleagues at work;
- communicating our feelings to our partner, family or friends.

Sometimes we deal with these situations by losing our temper, by saying nothing or by giving in. This may leave us feeling unhappy, angry, out of control and may not actually solve the problem.

What is assertiveness?

Assertiveness is being able to stand up for yourself, making sure your feelings are considered and not letting other people treat you like a doormat. It is not the same as aggressiveness. You can be assertive without being forceful or rude. It is stating clearly what you expect and insisting that your rights are considered. Assertion is a **skill that can be learnt**. It is a way of communicating and behaving with others that helps us to become more confident and aware of our needs and ourselves.

Where does assertiveness come from?

As we grow up we model ourselves upon those around us, for example parents, teachers and friends, and other influences such as television and the magazines we read. This may teach us to react *passively*, *aggressively* or *assertively*.

What are aggressive, passive and assertive behaviours?

Aggressive behaviour is *expressing your own feelings, needs, rights and opinions in a demanding and angry way*. There is *no respect for other people's* feelings, needs, rights and opinions. Your own needs are seen as being more important than other people's. Their needs are ignored or dismissed. It means focussing on your own rights, but doing so in such a way that you violate the rights of other people. *The aim of aggression is to win*, if necessary at the expense of others.

Task: Try to think of a time when someone else has been aggressive with you and ignored your opinion. How did it make you feel about them and yourself?

✎

In the short term, the aggressive person often feels more powerful. However in the longer term it can cause resentment in others.

Passive behaviour is *not expressing your feelings, needs, rights and opinions*. Instead you see *other person's needs as more important* than your own. You may be frightened to say what you think in case your beliefs are ridiculed. The aim of passive behaviour is to *avoid conflict at all times and to please others*. Everyone else is seen as better or more deserving than you. It involves bottling up your own feelings or expressing them in indirect or unhelpful ways. The effect of passive behaviour is loss of self-esteem, stress, anger and depression. Passive behaviour may cause others to become increasingly irritated at you and to develop a lack of respect for you. This may lead to a pattern where others expect you to give in and do not take your opinion into account.

The good news is that if you have noticed that you tend to respond in aggressive or passive ways, you can learn new ways of communicating. In contrast to aggression and passivity there is a third way to respond – the assertive way.

Assertive behaviour is *expressing your own feelings, needs, rights and opinions with a respect for other people's* feelings, needs, rights and opinions. Assertion is not about winning. It is concerned with being able to walk away feeling that you put across what you wanted to say.

Feelings	When you are being assertive, you are able to express your feelings in a direct and honest way.
Needs	You have needs that have to be met, otherwise you feel undervalued, anxious, angry or sad.
Rights	You have basic human rights and it is possible to stand up for your own rights in such a way that you do not violate another person's rights.
Opinions	You have something to contribute irrespective of other people's views.

Task: Try to think about a time when someone else has been assertive with you and respected your opinion. How did you feel about them and yourself? Write about your feelings.

About me – I felt:

> ✎

About them – I felt:

> ✎

In assertiveness you ask for what you want directly, openly and honestly. You respect your own opinions and rights. You expect others to do the same. You do not:
- violate people's rights;
- expect other people to magically know what you want;
- freeze with anxiety and avoid difficult issues.

The result is improved self-confidence in you and mutual respect from others.

The rules of assertion

I have the right to:

1 **Respect myself** – who I am and what I do.

2 **Recognise my own needs as an individual** – that is separate from what is expected of me in particular roles, such as 'wife', 'husband', 'partner', 'son', 'daughter'.

3 **Make clear 'I' statements** about how I feel and what I think. For example: '*I feel very uncomfortable with your decision.*'

4 **Allow myself to make mistakes**, recognising that it is normal to make mistakes.

5 **Change my mind**, if I choose.

6 **Ask for 'thinking it over time'**. For example, when people ask you to do something, you have the right to say, '*I would like to think it over and I will let you know by the end of the week.*'

7 **Allow myself to enjoy my successes**, by being pleased with what I have done and sharing it with others.

8 **Ask for what I want**, rather than hoping someone will notice what I want.

9 **Recognise that I am not responsible for the behaviour of other adults**.

10 **Respect other people** and their right to be assertive and expect the same in return.

Task: Think about how much you believe each of these rules. How much do you put them into practice in your own life at the moment?

I have the right to:	Do I believe this rule is true?		Have I applied this in the last week?	
1 Respect myself	Yes ☐	No ☐	Yes ☐	No ☐
2 Recognise my own needs as an individual independent of others	Yes ☐	No ☐	Yes ☐	No ☐
3 Make clear 'I' statements about how I feel and what I think	Yes ☐	No ☐	Yes ☐	No ☐
4 Allow myself to make mistakes	Yes ☐	No ☐	Yes ☐	No ☐
5 Change my mind	Yes ☐	No ☐	Yes ☐	No ☐
6 Ask for '*thinking it over time*'	Yes ☐	No ☐	Yes ☐	No ☐
7 Allow myself to enjoy my successes	Yes ☐	No ☐	Yes ☐	No ☐
8 Ask for what I want, rather than hoping someone will notice what I want	Yes ☐	No ☐	Yes ☐	No ☐
9 Recognise that I am not responsible for the behaviour of other adults	Yes ☐	No ☐	Yes ☐	No ☐
10 Respect other people and their right to be assertive and expect the same in return	Yes ☐	No ☐	Yes ☐	No ☐

Assertiveness techniques

It is possible to practise putting these rules into practice by using a number of assertiveness techniques.

1 'Broken Record'

This is a useful technique and can work in virtually any situation, especially when your rights are being ignored. You plan what it is you want to say by repeating over and over again what it is you want or need. During the conversation keep returning to your prepared lines. State clearly and precisely exactly what it is you need or want (e.g. *'I can't lend you any money ... I'm sorry, but I can't lend you any money ...')*. Don't be put off by clever arguments or by what the other person says. Once you have prepared the lines you want to say, you can relax. **There is nothing that can defeat this tactic.**

Example

Anne: *'May I borrow £10 from you?'*

Paul: *'I cannot lend you any money. I've run out.'*

Anne: *'I'll pay you back as soon as I can. I need it desperately. You are my friend aren't you?'*

Paul: *'I cannot lend you any money.'*

Anne: *'I would do the same for you. You won't miss £10.'*

Paul: *'I am your friend but I cannot lend you any money. I'm afraid I've run out.'*

---

2 Saying 'No'

Sometimes 'no' seems to be the hardest word to say. But if we avoid saying this one simple word, we can be drawn into situations that we don't want to be in. The images we recall with saying 'no' sometimes prevent us from using the word when we need it. We may be scared of being seen as mean and selfish, or of being rejected by others.

Q. Do I have problems saying 'no'? Yes ☐ No ☐

If yes, try to practise saying 'no' by using the following principles:
- **Be straightforward but not rude** so that you can make your point effectively.
- **Tell the person if you are finding it difficult.**
- Avoid apologising and giving elaborate reasons for saying 'no'. You are allowed to say no if you don't want to do things.
- **Remember** that it is better in the long run to be truthful than breed resentment and bitterness within you by giving in.

It may be that you have fears of how others may see you if you say no. Use the techniques in Workbooks 4 and 5 (noticing and changing extreme and unhelpful thinking) to challenge thoughts such as these.

3 Scripting

Scripting involves planning out in advance in your mind or on paper exactly what you want to say. A good way to begin to practise scripting is to write down what you want to say before you go into a situation. It uses a four-stage plan that covers the **events, feelings, needs,** and **consequences.**

- **Event:** Say what it is you are talking about. Let the other person know precisely what situation you are referring to.
- **Feelings:** Express how the event mentioned affects your own feelings. Opinions can be argued with, feelings cannot. Expressing your feelings clearly can prevent a lot of confusion.
- **Needs:** People are not mind-readers. It is necessary to tell them what you need. Otherwise people cannot fulfil your needs and this can lead to resentment and misunderstanding.
- **Consequences:** Tell the person that if they fulfil your need, there will be a positive consequence for both of you. Be specific about the consequences.

Example

Anne: *'Hello, how are you?'*

Joan: *'All right, and you?'*

Anne: *'I saw Sandra yesterday. She said she was sorry to hear that I wasn't getting on with my neighbour. I told you about that in confidence. I didn't expect you to go round telling others.'*
[Event]

Joan: *'I thought Sandra was a good friend of yours. I didn't think you would mind. She asked how you were. It seemed natural to tell her – why not?'*

Anne: *'Sandra's okay but she has a tendency to discuss other people's problems with everyone. I feel angry and upset that you have discussed this with her. I feel let down by you as a friend.'*
[Feeling]

Joan: *'I didn't realise. I'm sorry.'*

Anne: *'I value our friendship and the fact that usually I can talk to you about things without you telling everyone else about it.'*

Joan: *'Yes, I feel the same. I don't know what made me say anything to Sandra.'*

Anne: *'I'd like us to remain friends and to be able to share problems but I need to feel I can trust you.'* **[Need]**

Joan: *'I won't make this mistake again. Let's not spoil our friendship over this.'*

Anne: *'We can stay friends but let's agree not to discuss each other's problems with others. Then we can both know a confidence will not be betrayed.'* **[Consequence]**

Task: Identify an area where you could use scripting, then plan out what you want to say:

Event:

Feeling:

Needs:

Consequence:

Conclusion

Assertiveness is an attitude and a way of life. You can slowly learn to be more assertive through practice. **Remember** that although change can seem difficult at first, it is possible.

Putting what you have learned into practice

- Write down and **pin up** the rules for assertion in visible places about the house (e.g. on the fridge door, by your bed).
- Try to put into practice what you have learned. Experiment using the broken record and scripting approaches.
- Begin to say 'No' – politely and assertively. Don't expect to change everything immediately; however, with practice you can gain confidence in your ability to be assertive. If you have difficulties just do what you can.
- If you have found any aspects of this workbook unhelpful, upsetting or confusing, please would you discuss this with your health care practitioner or someone else whose opinion you trust.

A request for feedback

An important factor in the development of all the Five Areas Assessment workbooks is that the content is updated on a regular basis based upon feedback from users and practitioners. Please let me know if you have found the content helpful or unhelpful. If there are areas which you find hard to understand, or which seem poorly written, please let me know and I will try to improve things in future. I regret that I am unable to provide any specific replies or advice on treatment.

To provide feedback, please contact me via:

Email: Feedback@fiveareas.com

Mail: Dr Chris Williams, Department of Psychological Medicine, Gartnavel Royal Hospital, 1055 Great Western Road, Glasgow, G12 0XH

Acknowledgements

I wish to thank all those who have commented upon this workbook, especially Frances Cole.

The cartoon illustrations in the workbooks have been produced by Keith Chan (kchan75@hotmail.com) and are copyright of Media Innovations Ltd.

My notes

....

....

....

....

....

....

....

....

....

....

....

....

....

....

....

....

....

....

....

....

....

....

....

....

My notes

....

Workbook 4
Noticing extreme and unhelpful thinking

Dr Chris Williams

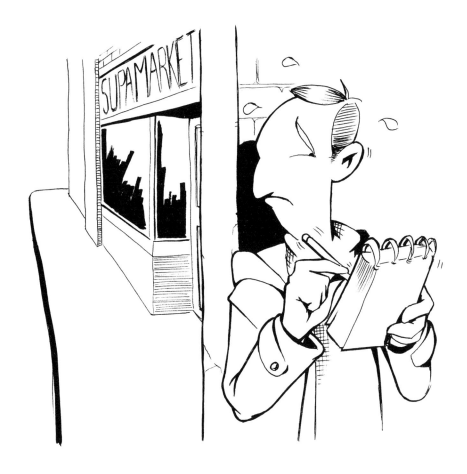

A Five Areas Approach

Introduction

This is the first of two workbooks that will help you find out about and begin to change unhelpfully altered thinking. In this workbook you will learn about:
- identifying unhelpful thinking;
- using a thought investigation worksheet or thought investigation flashcard to carry out an analysis of a time when your mood unhelpfully alters.

Revision

Unhelpful thinking styles

In times of emotional upset such as anxiety and depression, thinking becomes biased and extreme. Low mood leads to unhelpful thinking and, also, unhelpful thinking leads to low mood.

The following unhelpful thinking styles may occur. They can affect how you feel and unhelpfully alter what you do. Do you notice any of these at times when you feel more anxious or depressed?

Unhelpful thinking style	Typical thoughts	Tick here if you have this thinking style
Bias against myself	I overlook my strengths. I focus on my weaknesses. I downplay my achievements. I am my own worst critic.	
Putting a negative slant on things (negative mental filter)	I see things through dark-tinted glasses. I tend to focus on the bad in situations.	
Having a gloomy view of the future (making negative predictions)	I make negative predictions about the future.	
Jumping to the worst conclusion (catastrophic thinking)	Predicting that the very worst will happen.	
Second-guessing that others see me badly without actually checking if this is true (mind-reading)	I mind-read what others think of me. I often think that others don't like me.	
Bearing all responsibility/taking all the blame	I feel responsible for whether everyone else has a good time. I take the blame if things go wrong. I take things personally/to heart. I take unfair responsibility for things that are not my fault.	
Making extreme statements/setting impossible standards	I use the words 'always', 'never' and 'typical' a lot to summarise things. I make 'must', 'should', 'ought' or 'got to' statements to myself.	

Why are extreme thoughts so unhelpful?

Typically, when these sorts of unhelpful thinking styles occur:

1 *Mood changes unhelpfully*: you may become anxious, depressed, upset, ashamed or angry.
2 *Behaviour alters unhelpfully*: by either reducing what you do (avoidance or reduced activity) or causing you to engage in various unhelpful behaviours, such as drinking too much to block how you feel. These changes in behaviour can end up worsening how you feel.

In such ways the unhelpful thinking styles can keep you feeling distressed.

This workbook is designed to help you begin to practise identifying extreme and unhelpful thinking by carrying out a *thought investigation* of the times when your mood alters unhelpfully. This will help you prepare to change these extreme thoughts (Workbook 5).

> **Hint:** In order to identify extreme or unhelpful thinking, try to watch for times when your mood suddenly changes (e.g. you feel sadder, or more anxious, upset or angry). Ask *'what went through my mind then?'*

The questions on the following pages will help you to act like a detective. Piece together bit by bit the factors that led to you feeling worse. First, think yourself back into the situation when your mood unhelpfully altered. Consider the five different areas that might have changed when your mood altered:

1 the situation, relationship or practical problem(s) that occurred;
2 altered thinking (with extreme or unhelpful thinking styles);
3 altered feelings (also called emotions or moods);
4 altered physical sensations;
5 altered behaviour (such as avoidance, reduced activity or unhelpful behaviours).

Take time thinking through what happened by asking yourself detailed questions about the changes that happened in each of the five areas at the time when you felt worst.

Thought investigation: Area 1: The situation/event/practical problem at the time

a) The time

Q. What time of day was it? It was .... o'clock.

b) The place

Q. Where were you at the time? (Please tick)

I was:

● At home	Yes ☐	No ☐
● At work	Yes ☐	No ☐
● At the pub	Yes ☐	No ☐
● At a friend's house	Yes ☐	No ☐
● In a shop	Yes ☐	No ☐
● In town	Yes ☐	No ☐
● On a bus	Yes ☐	No ☐
● Other: I was …		

c) The people

You may have been alone, with only one or two people, or with many people.

Q. Were you alone?	Yes ☐	No ☐

*If **Yes**, skip to d) The current event/situation*

Q. Were you with a relative or relatives?	Yes ☐	No ☐
Q. Were you with a friend or friends?	Yes ☐	No ☐
Q. Were you with anyone else?	Yes ☐	No ☐

If Yes, with whom?

d) The current event/situation

Think about the situation that led to your altered mood. Had anything upsetting or stressful happened? For example, an argument or an upsetting event?

I had been upset by:

● something that was said;	Yes ☐	No ☐
● how someone acted towards me;	Yes ☐	No ☐
● focusing on a practical problem I face;	Yes ☐	No ☐
● a memory of something that had happened;	Yes ☐	No ☐
● worrying about the future.	Yes ☐	No ☐
● Finally, had you had any alcohol to drink or used any illegal drugs?	Yes ☐	No ☐

Other events/situations:

Thought investigation: Area 2: Altered thinking at the time

Q What went through your mind at the time?

At the moment your mood changed, what did you think about:

● Yourself?

● How others see you?

● What might happen in the future?

● Your own situation?

● Your own body, behaviour or performance?

● Were there any painful **memories** from the past?

● Did you notice any **images** or pictures in your mind? Images are an important type of thought and can have a powerful impact on how you feel.

To begin with, sometimes it can be difficult to notice these thoughts. With practice, most people find that a number of negative or extreme thoughts are present at times when their mood unhelpfully alters.

Write any thoughts you noticed here:

Assessing my <u>belief</u> in the most powerful extreme and unhelpful thought.

Choose the thought that seemed to have the greatest emotional impact on you.

Write it here:

Q. Overall, how much did you believe the most powerful thought at that time?

Make a cross on the line below to record how much you believed the thought.

Not at all_____Completely believed
      0%   50%   100%

Q. Were any *unhelpful thinking styles* present when your mood unhelpfully altered?

Am I being my own worst critic? (*bias against yourself*)	Yes ☐	No ☐
Am I focusing on the bad in situations? (*negative mental filter*)	Yes ☐	No ☐
Am I taking a gloomy view of the future? (*making negative predictions*)	Yes ☐	No ☐
Am I jumping to the worst conclusion? (*catastrophising*)	Yes ☐	No ☐
Am I second-guessing that others see me badly without actually checking? (*mind-reading*)	Yes ☐	No ☐
Am I taking unfair responsibility for things that aren't my fault (*taking all the blame?*)	Yes ☐	No ☐
Am I using unhelpful *must/should/ought/got to* statements? (*making extreme statements/setting impossible standards*)?	Yes ☐	No ☐

Thought investigation: Area 3: Altered feelings/emotions at the time

Q. When your mood altered, what emotional changes did you notice?

- I felt low and sad.   Yes ☐   No ☐
- I felt guilty.   Yes ☐   No ☐
- I felt anxious and stressed.   Yes ☐   No ☐
- I felt very panicky.   Yes ☐   No ☐
- I felt angry or irritable about *myself*.   Yes ☐   No ☐
- I felt angry or irritable about *someone or something else*. Yes ☐   No ☐
- I felt ashamed.   Yes ☐   No ☐
- I felt empty with no feelings at all.   Yes ☐   No ☐
- Other: ...

Thought investigation: Area 4: Altered physical sensations at the time

Q. When your mood altered, what physical changes did you notice?

- I felt that I had no energy/sapped of energy.   Yes ☐   No ☐
- I felt a feeling of pressure within me.   Yes ☐   No ☐
- I felt a feeling of heaviness inside.   Yes ☐   No ☐
- I felt tension in my arms or legs.   Yes ☐   No ☐
- I felt tension in my head or neck.   Yes ☐   No ☐
- I felt tension in my chest or stomach.   Yes ☐   No ☐
- I felt restless and wanted to move about.   Yes ☐   No ☐
- I felt slightly dizzy, spaced out or disconnected from things. Yes ☐   No ☐
- I felt sick.   Yes ☐   No ☐
- I felt that I wasn't getting enough air into my lungs.   Yes ☐   No ☐
- I felt that my heart was beating faster.   Yes ☐   No ☐
- Other:

Consider the impact on your behaviour and how this affected you and others.

Thought investigation: Area 5: Altered behaviour at the time

a) My reduced or avoided activity

Q. When your mood altered, what changes occurred in what you said or did at the time?

- I reduced my activity levels when I felt like this. Yes ☐ No ☐

- I avoided doing a planned activity as a result. Yes ☐ No ☐

- I chose to avoid talking to or meeting anyone. Yes ☐ No ☐

- I decided not to go out. Yes ☐ No ☐

- Other:

Q. Were there any unhelpful behaviours leading to subtle avoidance of anxiety-provoking situations?

Examples of subtle avoidance:	**Tick here if you have noticed this**

Quickly leaving anxiety-provoking situations?

Rushing through a task as quickly as possible? (e.g. walking or talking faster).

Trying very hard not to think about upsetting thoughts/memories?

Using distraction techniques to improve how I feel?

Becoming very demanding or excessively seeking reassurance from others?

Only going out and doing things when others are there to help?

Looking to others to make decisions or sort out problems for me?

Taking the easiest option (for example joining the shortest queue in the shop as a result of anxiety)?

Deliberately looking away during conversations and avoiding eye contact? Bringing conversations to a close quickly because of not knowing what to say?

Q. Am I avoiding things in other subtle ways? Write in how you are doing this here if this applies to you:

---

b) My unhelpful behaviours

Q. When your mood altered, did you do anything differently because of what happened?

● I became excessively clingy and dependent.	Yes ☐	No ☐
● I became very suspicious and demanding.	Yes ☐	No ☐
● I did something that set me up to fail.	Yes ☐	No ☐
● I did something that set me up to be let down or rejected.	Yes ☐	No ☐
● I had a drink to block how I felt.	Yes ☐	No ☐
● I overate or binged on food to block how I feel.	Yes ☐	No ☐
● I went and spent some money (retail therapy) to improve how I felt.	Yes ☐	No ☐
● I chose to misuse tablets or used illegal drugs.	Yes ☐	No ☐
● I did something to hurt myself, such as cutting myself.	Yes ☐	No ☐
● I did something risky.	Yes ☐	No ☐

● Other:

Q. Having considered these unhelpful thinking styles in relation to all five areas, what was their impact?

Overall, did the thought(s) have an unhelpful effect on me?   Yes ☐   No ☐

If you find you used one of the unhelpful thinking styles, and it had an unhelpful impact on you, then you have identified an example of an extreme and unhelpful thought. These are the sorts of thoughts that you will learn to challenge in Workbook 5.

Conclusions

Now that you have finished, re-read your answers in your thought investigation. As you do this, try to apply what you know about the Five Areas Assessment model to see how each of these areas might have played a part in how you feel.

Putting what you have learned into practice

- Over the next few days and weeks choose times when you feel worse and carry out a thought investigation. To help you with this, two sheets have been created to summarise this process on one piece of paper that you can carry around with you. One is a **thought investigation prompt card** and the other is a **thought investigation worksheet**. You will find copies of them both at the end of this workbook. Experiment with both and see which you prefer.
- When you feel confident in this task, read Workbook 5: *Changing extreme and unhelpful thinking*. If you have difficulties just do what you can.
- If you have found any aspects of this workbook unhelpful, upsetting or confusing, please can you discuss this with your health care practitioner or someone else whose opinion you trust.

A request for feedback

An important factor in the development of all the Five Areas Assessment workbooks is that the content is updated on a regular basis based upon feedback from users and practitioners. Please let me know if you have found the content helpful or unhelpful. If there are areas which you find hard to understand, or which seem poorly written, please let me know and I will try to improve things in future. I regret that I am unable to provide any specific replies or advice on treatment.

> **To provide feedback, please contact me via:**
>
> **Email:** Feedback@fiveareas.com
>
> **Mail:** Dr Chris Williams, Department of Psychological Medicine, Gartnavel Royal Hospital, 1055 Great Western Road, Glasgow, G12 0XH

Acknowledgements

The cartoon illustrations in the workbooks have been produced by Keith Chan (kchan75@hotmail.com) and are copyright of Media Innovations Ltd.

My notes

....

....

....

....

....

....

....

....

....

....

....

....

....

....

....

....

....

....

....

....

....

....

....

....

....

....

My notes..

....

THOUGHT INVESTIGATION PROMPT CARD

Carry these questions about with you and use them during the day to help you to identify any unhelpful thinking styles.

1 Become aware of your thinking whenever you notice your mood change

At times when you become more anxious, low or sad, guilty, angry or irritable, ashamed, etc. ask yourself **'What is going through my mind right now?'** This might include thoughts about:

- how others see you;
- the events/situations that have just happened;
- what might happen in the future;
- how you see your own body, behaviour or performance.

Remember, thoughts can include memories from the past or mental images.

2 Next, try to work out if you have any extreme and unhelpful thoughts

These thoughts show one of the unhelpful thinking styles.

Useful questions to identify the unhelpful thinking styles:

- Am I being my own worst critic (*bias against yourself*)?
- Am I focusing on the bad in situations (*negative mental filter*)?
- Do I have a gloomy view of the future (*making negative predictions*)?
- Am I jumping to the very worst conclusion (*catastrophic thinking*)?
- Am I second-guessing that others see me badly without actually checking if it's actually true (*mind-reading*)?
- Am I taking unfair responsibility for things that aren't really my fault (*taking all the blame*)?
- Am I using unhelpful *must/should/ought/got to* statements (*making extreme statements/setting impossibly high standards*)?

3 Ask yourself

Q. What is the consequence of believing the thought – does it *worsen how I feel* and *unhelpfully alter what I do*?

If you answer Yes, you have identified an *extreme and unhelpful thought*. This is the sort of thought you can challenge using the *thought challenge prompt card* in Workbook 5.

THOUGHT INVESTIGATION WORKSHEET: Identifying extreme and unhelpful thinking

1 Situation/relationship or practical problem when your mood altered	2 Altered emotional and physical feelings	3 What thoughts are present at the time?	4 What unhelpful thinking style(s) occur?	5 Impact of the immediate thought(s)
Think in detail: Where am I, what am I doing? Consider: ● **The time:** What time of day is it? ● **The place:** Where am I? ● **The people:** Who is present? Who am I with? ● **The events:** What has been said? What events happened?	At that time, am I: ● Low or sad? Guilty? ● Worried, tense, anxious or panicky? ● Angry or irritable? ● Ashamed? **a)** State the feelings clearly. Try to be as precise as possible. If more than one feeling occurs, underline the most powerful feeling. **b)** How powerful is this feeling? (0–100%)? **c)** Note down any strong physical sensations you notice.	What is going through my mind? How do I see: ● Myself? How others see me? ● The current events/situation? ● What might happen in the future? ● My own body, behaviour or performance? ● Any memories or images? **a)** State the thought(s) clearly. Try to be as precise as possible. If more than one thought occurs, underline the most powerful thought. **b)** Rate how strongly you believe the most powerful thought at the time (0–100%).	1 Bias against myself 2 Putting a negative slant on things (*negative mental filter*) 3 Having a gloomy view of the future (*making negative predictions*) 4 Jumping to the worst conclusion (*catastrophic thinking*) 5 Second-guessing that others see me badly without actually checking (*mind-reading*) 6 Bearing all responsibility (*taking all the blame*) 7 Making extreme statements/rules e.g. using *must, should, ought, always, and never* statements. If any of the styles are present, you have identified an **extreme thought**	**a)** What did I do differently? Consider any: ● Reduced activity ● Avoided people, places or situations ● Unhelpful behaviours **b)** What was the impact on: ● Myself? ● My view of others? ● How I felt? ● What I said? ● What I did? ● Others Overall, was the impact helpful or unhelpful? If there is an unhelpful impact, you have identified an **unhelpful thought**
Situation:	**a) My feelings:** **b) Powerfulness:** 0–100%= **c) Physical sensations:**	**My immediate thought(s):** **a)** ✎ State the thought(s) clearly. If you have noticed more than one thought, **underline** the most powerful thought. **b)** Rate your belief in the most powerful thought at the time. 0%　　　　　　　　100% ├─　　　　　　　　　─┤	**Which thinking styles are present?** (please state numbers or types) ✎ No(s):	**a) What did I do differently?** **b)** Overall, is it **helpful** or **unhelpful** for me to believe the thought? Helpful ☐ Unhelpful ☐

Workbook 5
Changing extreme and unhelpful thinking

Dr Chris Williams

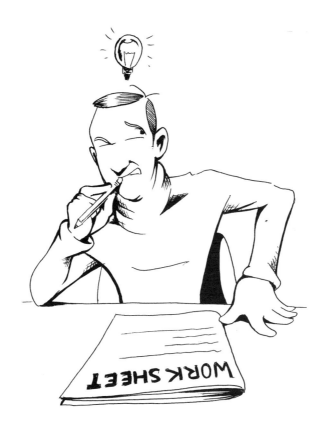

A Five Areas Approach

Introduction

This is the second of two workbooks that looks at the area of altered thinking. In Workbook 4 you discovered that in anxiety and depression, a person is often not completely fair or accurate in the way they judge themself. They often misinterpret what happens to them. You learned to try to notice what is going through your mind at times when you feel more anxious, depressed, upset, ashamed or angry. You also practised using a *thought investigation worksheet* or *prompt card* to identify the thoughts that led up to this mood change.

Examples of extreme and unhelpful thoughts include:

- *'I'm bad.'*
- *'I messed that up.'*
- *'I'll never get better.'*
- *'It's been a terrible week.'*
- *'Just typical – things always go wrong.'*

Such thoughts show one of the unhelpful thinking styles and can worsen how you feel and unhelpfully alter what you do. It is rare for someone who is depressed or anxious to question the *accuracy* of his or her thoughts. But it is important to do so, because many negative thoughts are extreme and inaccurate as well as unhelpful. At the moment it is likely that when you notice thoughts like these you tend to accept that they are true. You may notice that it is easier to believe such thoughts at times of highly negative emotion such as when you feel very low, anxious or upset.

Challenging extreme and unhelpful thinking

One effective way to improve how you feel is to practise skills that allow you to challenge such thoughts. As you become better at this, you will find you are able to challenge the thoughts at more difficult times. The approach uses a 4-step plan to bring about change:

1 **Identify** and rate your belief in the extreme and unhelpful thought(s).
2 **Question** the helpfulness and accuracy of the thought(s).
3 Come to a **balanced conclusion** about the thought(s).
4 **Apply** the balanced conclusion to what you do.

Task 1: Identify an unhelpful thought

a) Identify an extreme and unhelpful thought

It is best at first to choose a thought that is an extreme and unhelpful reaction to something that has happened or that has been said.

- Choose just one thought to question at a time.

- Clearly identify and write down what the thought is.

- For the time being avoid thoughts such as *'I am …'*, *'People are …'*, *'the world is …'* because these sorts of thoughts are often very difficult to challenge at first.

Use your **thought investigation worksheet/prompt card** or recent experiences to identify a thought that is extreme and unhelpful.

Write any extreme and unhelpful immediate thoughts you noticed here:

b) Assess your <u>belief</u> in the most powerful extreme and unhelpful immediate thought

Choose the thought that seemed to have the greatest emotional impact on you.

Write it here:

Rate how much you believed the most powerful thought at that time.

Make a cross on the line below to record how much you believed the thought.

Not at all_____Completely believed

       0%   50%   100%

Task 2: Question unhelpful thoughts: is the thought actually true?

i) Q. What is the evidence a) *for* and b) *against* the extreme and unhelpful thought?

(a) First, ask yourself: **Why** do I believe the thought? Write your reasons here:

Q. Can you show that the thought is correct from what you know to be true?   Yes ☐   No ☐

(b) Now ask: Is there anything to make me think the thought is incorrect?   Yes ☐   No ☐

Write your reasons here:

Q. Are there other ways of explaining the situation that are more accurate?

Other explanations: Yes ☐   No ☐

ii Q. If I wasn't feeling like this, would I believe the thought?   Yes ☐   No ☐

My comments:

> ✎

iii Do I apply one set of standards to myself and another to others?

Q. Are the standards that you set yourself higher than those you expect others to achieve?

Yes ☐   No ☐

My comments:

> ✎

Q. Would you tell a friend who believed the same thought that they were wrong?   Yes ☐   No ☐

My comments:

> ✎

iv Change your perspective: What would other people say?

Q. Have you heard *different opinions* from others about the thought you hold?   Yes ☐   No ☐

My comments:

> ✎

Task 3: Come to a balanced conclusion

Use the answers to the previous questions to come up with a balanced conclusion. A balanced conclusion is based on **all** the information you have available to you at the time.

My balanced conclusion:

Re-rate your belief in the *original extreme thought* and the *balanced conclusion*

My original immediate thought

Write in the thought here:

a My belief in the original thought at the time I had it.
(Make a cross on the line below to record how much you believed the thought)

0%_____**100%**
Not at all   Completely believed

b My belief in the immediate thought now:

0%_____**100%**
Not at all   Completely believed

My balanced conclusion
Write in your balanced conclusion here:

My belief in my new balanced conclusion
Make a cross on the line below to record how much you believe your new balanced conclusion.

0%_____**100%**

Not at all   Completely believed

The series of questions has helped you to **stop, think and reflect** on your thought in a structured way. Look at the rating of the amount you believe the original extreme and unhelpful thought **before and after** this process. If the amount you believe the original extreme thought has dropped, this is a sign that you have been able (at least in part) to challenge the thought. If this proved difficult, don't give up. It takes time to learn skills of effectively questioning extreme and unhelpful thoughts. It may be difficult at first to break the habit of extreme and unhelpful thinking, particularly if you have been depressed or anxious for some time. Keep trying though, and you will find that it becomes easier.

One important way of reducing the strength of your extreme and unhelpful thoughts is to **act against them** and **put your balanced conclusion into practice**.

Putting your balanced conclusion into practice

One helpful approach to find out whether your new balanced conclusion is true and helpful is to **set up a test** to see if it is true in practice. By far the best evidence for or against a thought is found through looking at the consequences of what happens when you choose to act or not act on it. **Reinforce** your balanced conclusions by acting on them. **Undermine** your extreme and unhelpful thoughts by acting against them. Try to create a **plan** to do this. For example, if you are invited to a meal out and have the immediate thought 'I won't enjoy it', you may be tempted not to go. You can undermine this thought and test out whether it is true by going. This will also reinforce any new balanced conclusions that 'Perhaps I'll enjoy the meal a little at least, and it will also get me out meeting others again.'

Please write below your own plan to a) **undermine** the immediate thought and b) to **reinforce** the new balanced conclusion.

Task 4: Create a plan for putting my balanced conclusion into practice

To undermine the immediate extreme and unhelpful thought:

>

To reinforce my new balanced conclusion:

>

Have you created a **plan** to put your balanced conclusion into practice?   Yes ☐   No ☐

If **Yes,** put this into practice and discuss what you learn with your health care practitioner or someone else whose opinion you trust. If you have not been able to think up a plan, discuss this with your health care practitioner. They will help you think how you may be able to reinforce your balanced conclusion and put it into practice.

Conclusion

The questions you have worked through can be applied to any extreme and unhelpful thoughts. By examining, questioning and challenging these thoughts, you will begin to change the way you see yourself, your current situation and the future. Doing this will help you develop more balanced, moderate and helpful thinking.

Putting what you have learned into practice

In order to help you practise the skills of questioning and challenging unhelpful thoughts, two sheets have been created to provide you with a list of prompts for this task. They summarise this process on one piece of paper that you can carry around with you. One is a **thought challenge prompt card** and the other is a **thought challenge worksheet**. Both summarise the key steps of challenging thoughts. You will find copies of them at the end of this worksheet. You can tear them out or photocopy them if you wish. Experiment with both and see which you prefer.

- Carry one of them with you as a resource to help you with this task.
- With practice, you will find that this approach becomes easier to do and you will be able to develop more balanced, moderate and helpful thinking. If you have difficulties just do what you can.
- If you have found any aspects of this workbook unhelpful, upsetting or confusing, please would you discuss this with your health care practitioner or someone else whose opinion you trust.

A request for feedback

An important factor in the development of all the Five Areas Assessment workbooks is that the content is updated on a regular basis based upon feedback from users and practitioners. If there are areas that you find hard to understand, or seemed poorly written, please let me know and I will try to improve things in future. I regret that I am unable to provide any specific replies or advice on treatment.

To provide feedback, please contact me via:

Email: Feedback@fiveareas.com

Mail: Dr Chris Williams, Department of Psychological Medicine, Gartnavel Royal Hospital, 1055 Great Western Road, Glasgow, G12 0XH

Acknowledgement

The cartoon illustrations in the Workbooks have been produced by Keith Chan (kchan75@hotmail.com) and are copyright of Media Innovations Ltd.

My notes

....

....

....

....

....

....

....

....

....

....

....

....

....

....

....

....

....

....

....

....

....

....

....

....

....

....

....

My notes

....

THOUGHT CHALLENGE PROMPT CARD

Useful questions to challenge extreme and unhelpful thoughts.

1 Does the thought show one of the unhelpful thinking styles?
What is the consequence of believing this thought – on how I feel and what I do?

2 What is the evidence *for* and *against* the thought?
a First think about **why** you believe the thought.
b Next identify and write down all the reasons **against** the thought being true. The following questions can help you with this task:

- Is there anything to make me think the thought is incorrect?
- Are there any other ways of explaining the situation that are more accurate?
- If I wasn't feeling like this what would I say?
- Would I tell a friend who believed the same thought that they were wrong? Do I apply one set of standards to myself and another to others?
- What would other people say? Have I heard different opinions from others about the same thought?

3 Create an alternative balanced and helpful thought.
Use your answers to the above questions to try to come up with an alternative thought that is more ***balanced and helpful***. Try to find a conclusion that you can believe.

- Try to **act on** the new balanced thought.
- **Act against** the old extreme and unhelpful thought. This will help undermine it.

By doing this you will build your confidence in using the approach.

THOUGHT CHALLENGE WORKSHEET (Choose one thought to challenge at a time)

Reasons supporting the immediate thought	Evidence against the immediate thought	Come to a balanced conclusion	My plan for putting the balanced conclusion into practice
List all the reasons why I believed the immediate thought at the time.	• Is there anything to make me think the thought is incorrect? • Are there any other ways of explaining the situation that are more accurate? • If I wasn't feeling like this, what would I say? • Would I tell a friend who believed the same thought that they were wrong? • What would other people say? Have I heard *different opinions* from others about the thought?	Use the answers from the first two columns to try to come up with a **balanced** and **helpful** conclusion. Create a balanced conclusion that you can believe. This should be based on **all** the information you have available to you and bear in mind the reasons for and against believing the immediate thought.	• How can I change what I do to **reinforce** my balanced conclusion? • How can I **undermine** my original extreme and unhelpful thought by acting against it? – to overcome reduced anxiety – to overcome avoidance – to reduce unhelpful behaviours
My evidence supporting the immediate thought: ✏	**My evidence against the immediate thought:** ✏	**My balanced conclusion:** ✏ a Rating of my belief in the balanced conclusion 0% ──────── 100% ⊢─────────────⊣ b Re-rating of my belief in the original immediate thought 0% ──────── 100% ⊢─────────────⊣	**My plan** to put the balanced conclusion into practice: ✏ **My plan** to undermine my original extreme and unhelpful thought: ✏

Workbook 6
Overcoming avoidance

Dr Chris Williams

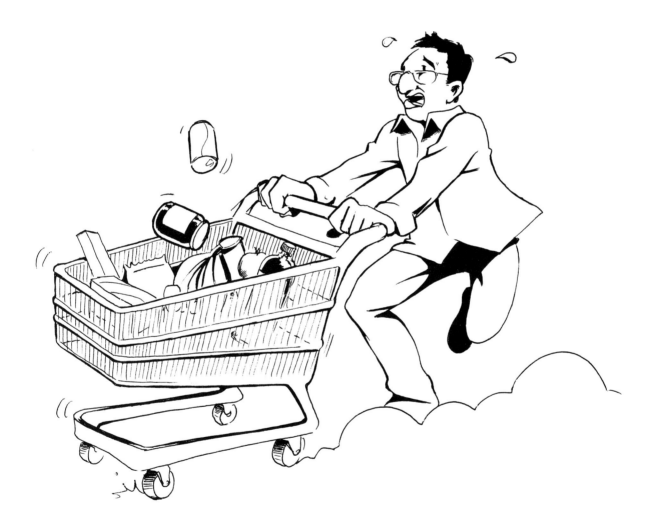

A Five Areas Approach

Introduction

The workbook will cover:
- The vicious circle of avoidance and how to identify your own vicious circle.
- A description of Harvinder who plans a step-by-step approach to overcome his fear of shopping in large shops/supermarkets.
- The chance to practise a seven-step approach to overcome avoidance.
- How to create a further step-by-step approach to overcome your own avoidance.

Don't be concerned if any of these words seem new or difficult to understand. All the terms will be described clearly as you read through the workbook.

Understanding avoidance

Anxiety causes a number of different symptoms and problems. The Five Areas Assessment approach provides a clear summary of the range of difficulties faced by the person in each of the following areas:

1　Life situation, relationships, practical problems
2　Altered thinking (with extreme and unhelpful thinking styles)
3　Altered feelings (also called emotions or moods)
4　Altered physical symptoms/feelings in the body
5　Altered behaviour or activity levels (with avoidance, reduced activity or unhelpful behaviours)

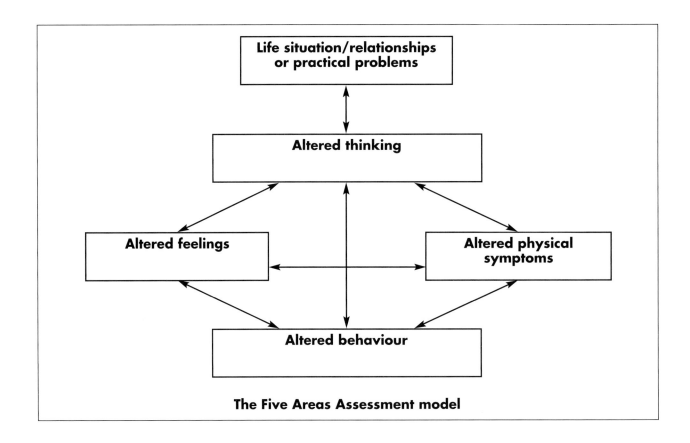

The Five Areas Assessment model

The Five Areas Assessment model indicates that what a person thinks about a situation or problem may affect how they feel emotionally and physically. It also alters what they do. These five areas exert an influence over each other.

Because of the links between each of the areas, the actions that people take when they are anxious can act to worsen or keep their symptoms of anxiety going.

This workbook focuses upon the altered behaviour that occurs in anxiety, and in particular upon avoidance – stopping doing things because of anxious fears.

The vicious circle of avoidance

When somebody becomes anxious, they start to avoid going into places and situations where they predict anxiety will occur. For example, people who have a fear of being in shops will avoid going into larger, busier shops. Similarly, someone who has an intense fear of spiders will try to avoid any situations where spiders may be present. Finally, someone who experiences high levels of anxiety in social settings will try very hard to avoid such situations.

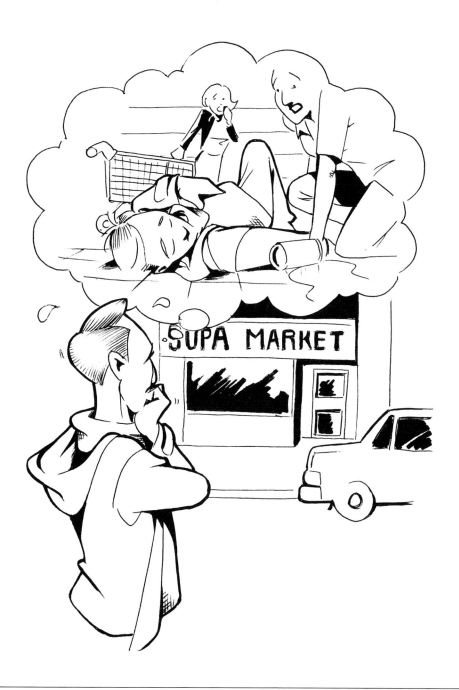

This avoidance adds to the person's problems because although they may feel less anxious in the short term, in the longer term such actions worsen their problem. A **vicious circle of avoidance** may result. The problem with avoidance is that it teaches you the unhelpful rule that the only way of dealing with a difficult situation is through avoiding it. The avoidance also reduces the opportunities to find out that the worst fears do not occur. It therefore worsens anxiety and further undermines your confidence. This process is summarised in the diagram below.

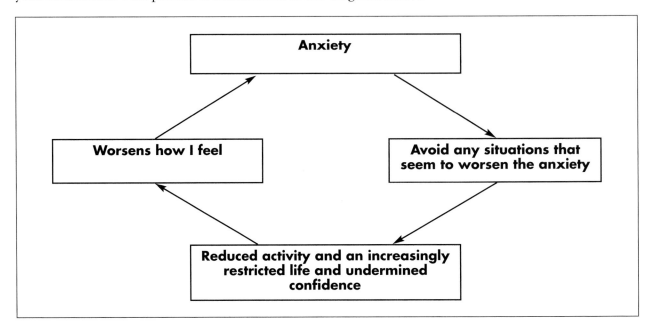

The vicious circle of avoidance

To see if this applies to you, ask yourself '*What have I stopped doing because of my anxiety?*' Remember that at times the avoidance can be quite subtle: for example, choosing to go to the shops at a time you know they are quiet, and then rushing through the shopping as quickly as possible.

Question: what am I avoiding?

The following questions will help you to identify the things you have stopped doing as a result of anxiety.

- Are there situations at work or in my relationships with others that I am avoiding?

- Is there anywhere I can't go or anything I can't do because of anxiety?

- Do I avoid mixing with others because of anxiety?

- Is there anyone I am avoiding? Is this because of anxiety or do I have other issues with them?

- What would I be able to do if I wasn't feeling anxious?

- Am I avoiding things more subtly? For example, choosing a time or place when I think the anxiety-provoking situation will be easier to deal with, or choosing the easiest option when making decisions.

Things I am avoiding:

The checklist below has been designed to help you to think about your avoidance in greater detail. It summarises common areas that are avoided as a result of anxiety. If avoidance is a problem for you, it is likely that you will have noticed changes in at least some of these areas.

Checklist: Identifying your own vicious circle of avoidance

As a result of feeling anxious am I:

Tick here if you have noticed this

Avoiding dealing with important practical problems (both large and small)?

Not really being honest with others. For example saying Yes when I really mean No?

Trying hard to avoid situations that bring about upsetting thoughts/memories?

Brooding over things and therefore not longer living life to the full?

Avoiding opening or replying to letters or bills?

Sleeping in to avoid doing things or meeting people?

Avoiding answering the phone, or the door when people visit?

Avoiding sex?

Avoiding talking to others face to face?

Avoiding being with others in crowded or hot places?

Avoiding busy or large shops, or finding that I have to think about where and when I go shopping etc.?

Avoiding going on buses, in cars, taxis etc., or any places where it is difficult to escape?

Avoiding walking alone far from home?

Avoiding situations, objects, places or people because of fears about what harm might result?

Avoiding physical activity or exercise as a result of concerns about my physical health?

Q. Am I avoiding things in other ways?

Write in here how you are doing this if this is applicable to you.

Sometimes the avoidance can be quite subtle and difficult to recognise. The following checklist gives examples of more subtle avoidance. These actions can undermine attempts to overcome avoidance. Do you do any of these?

Unhelpful behaviours leading to subtle avoidance of anxiety-provoking situations

Am I:

Quickly leaving anxiety-provoking situations?

Rushing though a task as quickly as possible? (e.g. walking or talking faster)

Trying very hard not to think about upsetting thoughts/memories? Trying to distract myself to improve how I feel?

Only going out and doing things when others are there to help?

Misusing drink/illegal drugs or prescribed medication to block how I feel in anxious situations?

Taking the easiest option (for example joining the shortest queue in the shop as a result of anxiety, or turning down opportunities that seem scary)?

Deliberately looking away during conversations and avoiding eye contact? Bringing conversations to a close quickly because of not knowing what to say?

Q. Am I avoiding things in other subtle ways?

Write in what you are doing here if this applies to you:

Summary: the vicious circle of avoidance

Having answered these questions, reflect on your responses using the three questions below:

Q. Am I avoiding things or doing certain actions that are designed to improve how I feel?   Yes ☐   No ☐

Q. Has this reduced my confidence in things and led to an increasingly restricted life?   Yes ☐   No ☐

Q. Overall has this worsened how I feel?   Yes ☐   No ☐

If you have answered **Yes** to all three questions, then avoidance or unhelpful behaviours are a problem for you.

The next section of the workbook will help you to understand how to overcome this avoidance in a planned step-by-step way.

Overcoming an initial area of avoidance using a 7-step plan

During times of anxiety or depression it can seem as if you are standing at the foot of a huge mountain of problems. You may not quite know where to start in order to overcome them. However, even a large mountain can be climbed if you tackle it one step at a time. The best way to overcome avoidance is to do so in a planned step-by-step way. **Pacing is the key.** Do not try to achieve too much too quickly or you may be setting yourself up to fail.

By working through the seven steps outlined below you can learn an approach that will help you to overcome your avoided activity.

The 7-step approach

Step 1: Identify and clearly define the problem as precisely as possible. In this case, this is the precise area of avoidance you wish to tackle. Tackling this will be your goal.
Step 2: Think up as many solutions as possible to achieve this initial goal.
Step 3: Look at the advantages and disadvantages of each of the possible solutions.
Step 4: Choose one of the solutions.
Step 5: Plan the steps needed to carry it out and apply the questions for effective change.
Step 6: Carry out the plan.
Step 7: Review the outcome to see how well you have achieved your goal.

Before you start to look at the plan

You may have made many previous attempts to change. However, unless you have a clear plan and stick to it, change will be difficult. Planning which areas to try and change first is a crucial part of moving forwards. Choose which one problem area to focus on first. This means that you are actively choosing **not** to focus on other areas.

Setting targets will help you to focus on the changes needed to get better. To do this you will need to identify:

● **Short-term targets.** These are the changes you can make today, tomorrow and next week. This will be the first step that you want to achieve in your plan to overcome avoidance.
● **Medium-term targets.** The changes you want to put in place over the next few weeks.
● **Long-term targets.** Where you want to be in six months or a year.

Think about the following questions.

Q. What might be the advantage of planning to change just one problem area at first?

Q. What are the potential dangers of trying to change everything at once?

Important principle: It isn't possible or sensible to try to deal with all your problems at once. You need to prioritise and focus on changing just one area to begin with. The first step is to decide on your eventual target – where you want to get to over a few weeks, and to then think through how best to get there. The very first step in the 7-step plan therefore involves choosing a single clear initial target area for change.

This principle is illustrated by the example of Harvinder. He has several areas of avoided activity. Although this example focuses on Harvinder's fears of shopping in supermarkets, the same principles can be applied to any avoided activities.

Example: Panic attacks when going shopping – agoraphobia

Harvinder has panic attacks whenever he goes to a supermarket. Before making any changes to tackle his avoidance, Harvinder needs to identify the areas of avoidance he wants to tackle first. When he fills in his Avoidance checklist, Harvinder identifies several areas of avoidance:

Identifying Harvinder's avoidance

As a result of feeling anxious am I:	Tick here if you have noticed this
Avoiding dealing with important practical problems (both large and small)?	
Not really being honest with others. For example saying Yes when I really mean No?	
Trying hard to avoid situations that bring about upsetting thoughts/memories?	
Brooding over things and therefore not longer living life to the full?	
Avoiding opening or replying to letters or bills?	
Sleeping in to avoid doing things or meeting people?	
Avoiding answering the phone, or the door when people visit?	
Avoiding sex?	
Avoiding talking to others face to face?	
Avoiding being with others in crowded or hot places?	✓ *My anxiety means I haven't gone to the cinema for ages, I wouldn't want to feel trapped in the middle of a row.*
Avoiding busy or large shops, or finding that I have to think about where and when I go shopping etc.?	✓ *I'm not going to large shops at all now. I definitely couldn't go to a supermarket because I'd get panicky. I'd feel really hot and sweaty and start breathing very fast. I'd be scared I'd collapse.*
Avoiding going on buses, in cars, taxis etc., or any places where it is difficult to escape?	
Avoiding walking alone far from home?	
Avoiding situations, objects, places or people because of fears about what harm might result?	
Am I avoiding things in other ways?	
Write in here how you are doing this if this is applicable to you.	

He also thinks about whether he is avoiding things in more subtle ways.

Unhelpful behaviours leading to subtle avoidance of anxiety-provoking situations.

Am I:

Quickly leaving anxiety-provoking situations?

✓ I have left one shop really quickly. I just left the trolley in the middle of the store and ran.

Rushing through a task as quickly as possible? (e.g. walking or talking faster).

✓ I definitely rush round the shop to get it over with as soon as possible.

Trying very hard not to think about upsetting thoughts/memories? Trying to distract myself to improve how I feel?

Only going out and doing things when others are there to help?

Misusing drink/illegal drugs or prescribed medication to block how I feel in anxious situations?

Taking the easiest option (for example joining the shortest queue in the shop as a result of anxiety, or turning down opportunities that seem scary)?

✓ I go to the small local shops at the quietest possible time. I always choose the shortest queue because of anxiety rather than because it is the obvious choice.

Deliberately looking away during conversations and avoiding eye contact? Bringing conversations to a close quickly because of not knowing what to say?

Q. Am I avoiding things in other subtle ways?
Write in what you are doing here if this applies to you.

✓ I grip hard onto the trolley when I feel anxious.

On answering the following three questions Harvinder determines that he is experiencing a *vicious circle of avoidance*.

	Harvinder's answer	
Q. Am I avoiding doing things as a result of anxiety?	Yes ☑	No ☐
Q. Has this reduced my confidence in things and/or led to an increasingly restricted life?	Yes ☑	No ☐
Q. Overall, has this worsened how I feel?	Yes ☑	No ☐

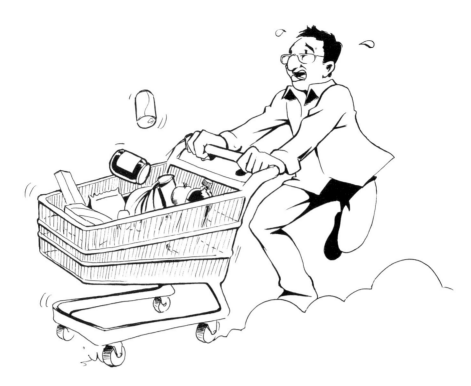

Harvinder has very clear areas of avoidance (going into larger shops/supermarkets and also the cinema). He has also identified some more subtle problems of avoidance that need to be built into his plan.

Harvinder uses the 7-step approach to overcome his avoidance.

Step 1: Identify and clearly define the problem as precisely as possible

The important first step is identifying a **single** initial target area that he wants to focus on. This should be *clearly defined*. This step is particularly important as he has identified two main problems of avoidance (going to large shops/supermarkets and to the cinema). It is not possible to overcome both these areas at once. Instead he needs to decide which **one** area to focus on to begin with. This means putting the other area on one side for the time being.

He should choose a target problem that:

- will be *useful* for changing how he is;
- is a *specific* target problem so that he will know when he has done it;
- is *realistic*, that is, practical and achievable.

Harvinder has decided that the specific area of avoided activity that he is going to focus on to start with is:

> **Harvinder's target area:** *Tackling my avoidance of large and busy shops/supermarkets.*

Step 2: Think up as many solutions as possible to achieve this initial goal

One difficulty that people often face after they have chosen the initial problem area is that it can often seem too large to even start tackling. One way around this is to try to step back from the problem and see what approaches could be used to tackle it. This approach is called *brainstorming*.

In brainstorming:

- The more solutions that are generated, the more likely it is that a good one will emerge.
- Ridiculous ideas should be included as well, even if you would never choose them in practice. This can help you to adopt a flexible approach to the problem.

Useful questions to help you to think up possible solutions might include:

● What *ridiculous* solutions can I include as well as more sensible ones?
● What helpful ideas would others (e.g. family, friends or colleagues at work) suggest?
● What approaches have I tried in the past in similar circumstances?
● What advice would I give a friend who was trying to tackle the same problem?

The purpose of brainstorming is to try come up with as many ideas as possible. Amongst them Harvinder hopes to be able to identity a realistic, practical and achievable first step towards overcoming his problem.

Harvinder sits and thinks about possible ways he could begin to start going into large and busy shops again:

1 Contact the manager of the supermarket and pay them a lot of money to arrange a personal evening opening when I can shop alone.
2 Go into the largest busiest shop I can find and stay there until I feel better.
3 Take part in a sponsored shop for charity.
4 Plan a slow increase in going to shops. Go to a local smaller shop first. Begin to face my fears by slowing down my shopping and not racing round the store.
5 Go to the post office at the busiest time and join the longest queue.

Step 3: Look at the advantages and disadvantages of each of the possible solutions

Harvinder assesses how effective and practical each potential solution is. This involves considering the advantages and disadvantages for each potential solution.

Suggested solution	Advantages	Disadvantages
1 Contact the manager of the supermarket and pay them a lot of money to arrange a personal evening opening when I can shop alone.	I'd be able to go shopping without anyone else there. It would make me feel like a VIP.	That's one of those ridiculous ideas you're supposed to think up in brainstorming. It would cost a fortune. I can't afford that sort of thing. Anyway, I'd feel like a right idiot asking for this. I'm not at all sure the shop would go along with this sort of arrangement.
2 Go into the largest busiest shop I can find and stay there until I feel better.	There don't seem to be many advantages I can think of!	Although I've heard that sort of approach can sometimes work, there is just no way I am going to do this. It is just too scary.
3 Take part in a sponsored shop for charity.	It would raise some money for charity.	I just don't fancy this at all. Everyone would know what I was doing. I'd let people and the charities down if I couldn't do it. That would just make me feel like I'd failed. It's just too scary to do.

Suggested solution	Advantages	Disadvantages
4 Plan a slow increase in going to shops. Go to a local smaller shop first. Begin to face my fears by slowing down my shopping and not racing round the store.	This is something I can do without getting too panicky. It would be a really good first step. I could build up my confidence doing this first and then begin to go to larger busier shops and the supermarket. It would boost my confidence. This could be the first small step in getting back to normal.	The local shop doesn't stock all the food I like. It also costs a lot more than the supermarket. I don't want to have to keep shopping there. I want to be able to go to the supermarket.
5 Go to the post office at the busiest time and join the longest queue.	I want to be able to do that. I post a lot of letters to friends.	It might be a little too scary. I go there anyway, but the idea of going when it is really busy and then joining the longest queue is too much at the moment. It's just too ambitious.

Step 4: Choose one of the solutions

The chosen solution should address his problem. It should be realistic and likely to succeed. Harvinder's decision is based on the answers to Step 3. Harvinder decides on **option 4:** *Plan a slow increase in going to shops. Go to a local smaller shop first. Begin to face my fears by slowing down my shopping and not racing round the store.*

This solution should fulfil the following two criteria:	**Harvinder's answer**	
a) Is it helpful?	Yes ☑	No ☐
b) Is it realistic, practical and achievable?	Yes ☑	No ☐

> **Key point.** The initial target that is chosen should be something that helps Harvinder tackle his avoidance. It needs to seem at least a little scary. He must be realistic in his choice so that the target does not appear impossible for him. You will see later how Harvinder can build upon this initial target for change with subsequent additional targets that will help him to move towards his goal of shopping in large supermarkets.

Step 5: Plan the steps needed to carry it out and apply the questions for effective change

This is a key stage. Harvinder needs to generate a clear plan that will help him to decide exactly *what* he is going to do and *when* he is going to do it. It is useful for Harvinder to *write down* the steps needed to carry out the solution. This will help him to plan what to do and allows him to predict possible blocks and problems that might arise.

The *questions for effective change* can help Harvinder to re-check how practical and achievable his plan really is.

The questions for effective change

Is the plan one that:
- will be *useful* for understanding or changing how I am?
- is a *specific task* so that I will know when I have done it?
- is *realistic*, that is, practical and achievable?
- makes clear *what* I am going to do and *when* I am going to do it?
- is an activity that won't be easily blocked or prevented by practical problems?

Review of plan using the questions for effective change

Will it be useful for understanding or changing how I am?
I can go to small local shops at the moment. I try to go at quieter times like the early afternoon, and then rush round. If I could change that rushing around, that would be an important first step.

Is it a specific task so that I will know when I have done it?
I need to be clear about what I am going to do. I will go shopping as I normally do. Instead of just shooting round the shop and grabbing the things I need, I will try to walk round it at a slower pace. I'll know I've done this if I look at my watch just before I go into the shop, and again just after I leave. I want to stay in there at least 10 minutes to begin with.

Is it realistic: is it practical and achievable?
Is it realistic? Yes, I can do that. It's really only a little bit scary. I'm sure I can do that.

Does it make clear what you are going to do and when you are going to do it?
I have a clear idea of what I need to do. I will spend at least 10 minutes in the shop. I need to think about how I can spend the extra time there. I could look for some other provisions, or read the ingredient labels. Even better, I could stop at the video stand and look at what videos they have in. That's something that could take a few minutes. I need to decide when I am going to do this trip to the shops. I think I should do it on Tuesday at 2pm.

Is it an activity that won't be easily blocked or prevented by practical problems?
Now then, what might block it? If the shop was very busy, I might want to leave more quickly. I could plan to go at a quieter time of day, and even if there are a few people there, I could choose to stay in. The only other thing that I can predict could prevent me doing this is if I lose my nerve and try to start rushing round when I get there. If I have that temptation, I just need to make sure I slow down my breathing, and also my walking. I'll deliberately not leave the shop, and just stay there for a few more minutes before leaving. I know from before that I'm going to notice my usual fear that I will collapse. I need to be aware of that and try to challenge these fears.

Harvinder's goals are *clear, specific and his target is realistic*. He knows *what* he is going to do and *when* he is going to do it. He has predicted potential difficulties that might get in the way. This seems like a well thought through plan.

Step 6: Carry out the plan

Once Harvinder's plan is complete, he should carry it out. He should pay attention to his thoughts about what will happen *before, during* and *after* completing the activity.

Harvinder goes to the shop the next day. Before he enters the shop, he notes his anxious thoughts down on a piece of paper and records how much he believes them. He reminds himself that as he carries out the plan this will help undermine the old fears.

Before he goes into the shop, he notices the fear that '*I will collapse*'. He believes this 30 per cent at the time. He records his anxiety as being about 30 per cent too. He challenges it by reminding himself that he never has collapsed. When he goes into the shop, there are three other people already there. They are an older couple and a school child. His belief that he will collapse shoots up to 80 per cent. He rates himself as 70 per cent anxious. He thinks about leaving and begins to feel hot and sweaty. He notices an increase in both his heart rate and breathing. He begins to walk faster to try to get all his shopping done as quickly as possible. He then remembers that he had decided that if he felt like this he would try to control his breathing and slow down his walking. Harvinder makes a big effort and stops in the aisle by the videos. He picks one up and looks at the description on the back. He does this for a couple of minutes, and begins to feel much better. His anxiety and belief that he will collapse both slowly drop to around 40 per cent. He is able to complete the rest of his shopping at a normal pace. When he leaves the shop, he is surprised to find that he has been in there for almost 15 minutes.

Step 7: Review the outcome

Harvinder should next review what happened when he carried out his plan. Did it go smoothly, or were there any difficulties along the way? What has he learned from carrying out the plan?

Harvinder's review of what happened

Q. Was the selected approach successful? Yes ☑ No ☐

Q. Did it help start to overcome the problems of avoidance during shopping (the target problem)? Yes ☑ No ☐

Q. Were there any disadvantages to using this approach? Yes ☐ No ☑

Q. What have I learned from what happened?

> That went really well. I was almost thrown though when there were three people already in the shop. That hardly ever happens.
> The three things I have learned are:
> 1 Just how useful it is to have predicted what to do if I began to feel worse. When that happened I felt really scared. I remembered that I had planned to slow down my breathing and my walking if that happened. It worked! I felt a lot better – especially after looking at the video.
> 2 All my concerns about collapsing if I stayed in just weren't true. I did feel anxious when I went in – especially when I noticed the others there. However, the anxiety quickly began to fall as time passed. It didn't just keep going up and up like I thought it would.
> 3 Although at the time when I felt most anxious, I believed the fears that 'I'm going to collapse', the fear and physical sensations did not continue rising. I didn't collapse and when I think back – I never have collapsed while shopping.

Q. What does this say about any fears before or during the activity?

> Well, I didn't collapse. The fears just weren't right. I did feel bad at one stage, but I stuck with it and nothing bad happened. Amazing! I certainly believe that I'll collapse far less than before.

Harvinder reviews what happened to his fears and level of anxiety as he went round the shop. He writes down his extreme and unhelpful thoughts and records how much he believed them (from 0: not at all, to 100: believing them fully).

What happened as I carried out my plan

My fearful thought: *I will collapse.*

I believed this: 30%   **before** going into the shop.

80%   **during** the time in the shop when I saw all those people there. It then slowly dropped to 40%.

10%   5 minutes **after** leaving the shop.

My level of anxiety:

30%   **before** going into the shop.

70%   **during** the time in the shop when I saw all those people there. It then slowly dropped to 40%.

15%   5 minutes **after** leaving the shop.

In spite of the high levels of anxiety that arose because of the people present in the shop, Harvinder succeeded in his plan. He also noticed something else that is very important. Even though he felt 70 per cent anxious just after entering the shop, after only a few minutes the level of anxiety quickly began to fall. His fear that he would collapse also dropped to only 40 per cent. By the time he left the shop and reflected on what happened, his belief in the original fearful thought had dropped to only 10 per cent. Facing up to his fearful thoughts was a very good way of testing and challenging them.

Key point: A key part of this approach is being aware of any extreme and unhelpful thinking *before, during* and *after* entering the shop. These thoughts are the cause of the anxiety. The best way to undermine an extreme and unhelpful anxious thought is to act against it. This provides an excellent way of testing out how accurate and helpful the anxious fears are.

By repeating the same activity **again and again** over the next week, Harvinder's fear becomes less and less intense. It also lasts for shorter and shorter lengths of time. By repeatedly facing his fears he is able to challenge his fearful thoughts and reduce his anxiety. You can read more about this in Workbook 4: *Noticing extreme and unhelpful thinking* and Workbook 5: *Changing extreme and unhelpful thinking.*

This same pattern happens no matter what fear is being tackled. Facing up to fear causes it to slowly lose its impact. This is illustrated in the diagram below.

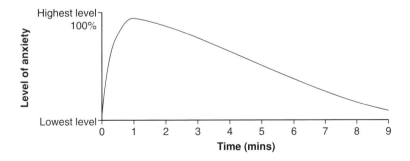

First time Harvinder faces his fears: Tuesday at 2pm

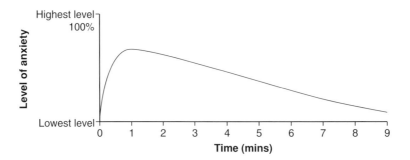

Second time Harvinder faces his fears: Wednesday at 11.30am

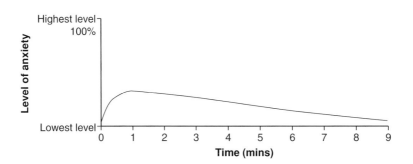

Third time when Harvinder faces his fears: Friday at 3pm

Building on the initial change using a step-by-step approach

The next stage is for Harvinder to build upon this initial success by making a clear plan to move things forward. To do this, he needs to think about his *short-, medium- and longer-term* targets/goals. The key is to go forward step by step, one target at a time, using the 7-step approach at every stage to help plan the next target. Each step/target should move him closer to his eventual goal of going shopping in the supermarket. Without this sort of careful and gradual step-by-step approach he may find that although he makes some attempts to tackle his fears, these are all moving in different directions and he will lose his focus and motivation as a result.

Harvinder makes a step-by-step plan of targets/steps he needs to complete over the next few weeks. His plan includes reducing and stopping doing any of the more subtle types of avoidance he has noticed. In Harvinder's case this is rushing round the shop and gripping hard onto the trolley.

Harvinder's step-by-step approach: weekly targets

Target/step	Initial fear level (0–100%)	Time scale
1 Going into the local shop for a paper. Walking round slowly, and staying there for at least 10 minutes.	Hardly scary at all – 5–10%	Week 1 and then repeat at least twice that week.
2 Going into the local shop. Deliberately choosing a busier time of day, and again to walk round slowly, staying in the shop for at least 20 minutes each time.	A little scary – 15%	Week 2 and then repeat at least twice that week.
3 Queuing in the Post Office and deliberately choosing the longest queue.	Quite scary – 35%	Week 3 and then repeat at least twice that week.
4 Going into the supermarket foyer area to buy a newspaper and staying there for at least 20 minutes.	Pretty scary – 50%	Weeks 4 and 5 and then repeat at least twice that week.
5 Going into the supermarket at a quieter time and shopping for at least 20 minutes. Relaxing my grip on the trolley.	Moderately scary – 75%	Week 6 and then repeat at least twice that week.
6 Going shopping in the supermarket at a busier time by myself for at least 20 minutes. Having a relaxed grip on the trolley all the time.	Very scary – 85%	Week 7 and then repeat at least twice that week.
7. Eventual goal. Going shopping in the supermarket at a busier time and deliberately choosing the longest checkout queue by myself. Spend at least 20 minutes in the shop.	Very very scary – 100% scary at first	Week 8 and then repeat at least twice that week.

Each new target builds upon the previous one to help Harvinder to move forwards. At each stage he is able to further test out and disprove his original fear that he will collapse. *Each next target on the way can be planned out in detail using the 7-step approach.* Step 5 (see page 6.14) is particularly helpful for planning each new target.

Over a number of weeks following his plan Harvinder will see a very significant total change in what he is able to do. By facing his fears he will find that his anxiety level slowly begins to fall. Each time he repeats the same step his anxiety will be less intense. It will also last for a shorter time than the time before.

You can see that the steps taken are rated in terms of how scary and difficult they seem when he first creates the plan. The plan helps Harvinder to face up to his fear in a planned and paced way. This means that he never feels so anxious that he wants to give up. By repeating each new stage several times each week, Harvinder can build up his confidence before moving on to the next step/target. If he found that a particular stage is too difficult, he could always take a step back, and re-plan the task. Each step should be realistic, practical and achievable. By succeeding in these planned steady steps, real progress can be achieved.

> **Key point.** A key part of this is approach is being aware of any extreme and unhelpful thinking both *before, during* and *after* each step of the plan. Workbooks 4 and 5 will help you to identify and challenge any fears. Remember that the best way to undermine anxious thoughts is to act against them. This provides an excellent way of testing out how accurate and helpful these fears really are.

Harvinder needs to be careful that he doesn't subtly avoid facing up to his fear when he is in the shop. For example, he may be tempted to rush around the shop as quickly as possible, try to distract himself from his fears while in the shop, or only go shopping when accompanied by a friend so that he feels safer. Instead, he should walk round each shop deliberately slowly. He should plan to have some pauses and relax his grip on the trolley.

You will see from the plan below that Harvinder is facing up to his more subtle areas of avoidance. His plan to reduce these subtle ways uses exactly the same principles as his plan to deal with the more obvious ways of avoidance.

'Subtle' avoidance	Plan to tackle this avoidance
Deliberately to go shopping only when the shop is likely to be empty.	Slowly plan to go to the shop at busier times. Eventually to go to busier and larger shops.
Rushing round the shop as quickly as possible.	Slow down the walking round the shop. Plan to deliberately stand and look at some of the goods. At a later stage deliberately choose to talk to an employee about a product.
Choosing the smallest queue at the tills. The motivation here is to leave the shop as quickly as possible because of anxiety rather than just to be efficient.	Choose to use longer queues.
Using *distraction techniques* to avoid noticing the anxiety when in the shop. For example by doing mental arithmetic while in the shop, or completing a physical activity (such as clenching his fists tightly).	Choose to stop doing the distraction technique and pay attention to the task he is doing.
Seeking reassurance and support from others when out shopping.	Create a reassurance-free zone by beginning to do things with less and less reassurance from others.

You will have a chance to practise this same 7-step plan yourself after you have looked at how the same approach can be used to overcome other common areas of avoidance.

Overcoming other common areas of avoidance

You have now seen an example of how Harvinder has begun to tackle his own avoidance of shopping in larger shops/supermarkets. The example illustrates the key elements of overcoming avoidance.

The key elements of overcoming avoidance

- Break the problem down into smaller parts and clearly identify your first target/step to change.
- Use the 7-step approach to plan this first step towards your eventual goal.

- Use the *questions for effective change* to help plan what you will do. Make sure the plan is practical and achievable.
- Build upon this by identifying short-, medium- and longer-term goals. Use the 7-step plan to plan each target/step along the way.
- There can be as **many** or as **few** steps as you want in your plan.
- Set yourself practical, realistic and achievable goals. Do not try to move too quickly from one step to the next.
- Repeat each step several times before moving on.
- Pacing is the key. If you find any step is too difficult, *go back a stage and regain your confidence.* Then, decide on a different next step that is not quite so difficult. Plan this new step using the questions for effective change.
- Make sure your plan includes ways of reducing any subtle forms of avoidance.
- Each step of the plan allows the opportunity to challenge your belief in any worrying or fearful thoughts before, during and after the activity.
- The main reason why a plan might be ineffective is if you are too ambitious or allow yourself to believe that change is impossible.
- Any avoided activity can be overcome using this planned approach.
- **Review** what happens at every step. Use everything (good and bad) as an opportunity to learn.

The next few pages give some other examples of how this same approach can be applied to some other examples of avoidance. Please skip those examples that are not of interest to you.

Social anxiety/social phobia: anxiety when talking to people or going into social situations

Severe anxiety in social situations occurs when the person is fearful that others think badly of them. This is described as social phobia.

> **Choice point:** If this is a problem for you, please read this section.
> If not, move on to page 6.24.

Example: Dawn has problems of intense anxiety in social situations. This has worsened since adolescence when she had bad acne. Even though the acne has now cleared, her anxiety in social situations has got worse and worse. When she talks to others she notices strong physical symptoms of anxiety. She feels hot and flushed, sweaty and slightly shaky. She becomes very aware of her dry mouth and notices a frog in her throat. She is very sensitive of these physical symptoms and constantly predicts that the person she is speaking to will be aware of her discomfort. She believes they will judge her even more negatively as a result. In the past she has found it difficult meeting people of the opposite sex, and has increasingly withdrawn from going out socially.

Dawn's first step
- **Eventual goal to be achieved.** I want to have some friends round for a meal.
- **Main fear to be challenged.** They will think I'm boring and see how bad at conversation I am.
- **Subtle avoidance to take into account in the plan.** Avoiding eye contact while I talk. Cutting conversations short.

Dawn's step-by-step approach: weekly targets to overcome fear of social situations

Target/step	Time scale
1 Phone my friend Sarah and speak by phone to catch up. Ask her at least one question about how she is and let her talk.	Week 1 and repeat later in the week.
2 Contact two other friends by phone and speak for a longer time.	Week 2
3 Arrange to meet Sarah at my flat for coffee. Make sure I allow her to talk by asking her at least two questions about her week.	Week 3
4 Go for a walk with Sarah and her children. Make eye contact with her at least twice as we talk.	Weeks 4 and 5 and repeat once with another friend.
5 Arrange to meet Sarah by herself for a meal. Ask her at least four questions and make eye contact at least five times.	Week 6
6 Meet Sarah and two other friends at the park and have a chat while the children play.	Weeks 7 and 8
7 Eventual goal Be able to have three friends round to my flat for a meal.	End of Week 8

Additional useful things to consider

The following are some tasks that can be useful when planning to overcome problems of social phobia.

- **Learn useful techniques for small talk.** Several techniques can be used to keep the other person talking. Have planned a series of questions you can ask when the conversation seems to flag. These can include questions starting *Why, What, Where, When, How*. For example, *How* was your holiday? *Why* did you choose to go to Turkey? *Where* did you stay? *What* was the beach like? etc. This approach can help you to small talk your way around any topic. Remember to allow the person to answer. Don't interrupt them or cut them off. Also listen to what they say. Don't spend so much time rehearsing your next question that you overlook that they have already answered it!
- **Learn how to look just past people.** If you find that making eye contact with people is difficult, then practise looking into the middle distance just past their heads. For example, look at a picture on a wall just behind the person, but so that it appears that you are looking at them. Practise making brief eye contact and gradually increase the amount and length of this.
- **Role-play.** A good way of reducing anxiety in social situations is to practise small talk with someone you trust. For example, ask a friend to help you to practise conversations. A number of self-help groups offer regular drop-in groups or specific groups for people with social phobia. Consider attending an anxiety management group. Everyone else there will also have problems with anxiety, and this could be built in as part of your own plan of self-treatment.
- **Video yourself talking to others.** This will provide you with powerful feedback and allow you to test out fears that you are dripping with sweat, shaking like a leaf, or look in some way 'odd'. It will also help you to check out how others react to you. You could do this yourself with a friend if you have access to a video. Health care practitioners sometimes offer this approach if you jointly agree that it will be helpful.

Be sure to try to **reduce or act against subtle avoidance** as part of your plan. For example:

● Relax your posture and allow yourself to move/walk more freely.
● Relax your hands rather than gripping them tightly.

Finally, **watch your alcohol intake.** Make sure you don't use alcohol as a means of building false confidence with other people. This will just add to your problems.

The following are two experiments to try to work out how helpful or unhelpful such behaviours are.

Experiment 1: Discovering the impact of trying to control trembling shaking hands[1]

Background. If a person has a fear that others may see trembling hands, they may try to control this by gripping their hands very tightly. They may make a fist or place their hands deep into their pockets. Sometimes they may try very hard to stand straight and stiff.

Task. Place your hands by your sides. Spread your fingers and now try as hard as you can to prevent your fingers from trembling. Use all the muscles of your hands and arms to keep each hand/finger as still as possible. Then try this again, this time putting you hand into a tight fist. Repeat both actions this time looking at the impact on your overall posture. Does your posture look normal or hunched/strained?

Review. Sometimes trying hard not to shake actually worsens the shakiness. Trying hard not to let symptoms of tension be seen by rigidly controlling your posture can end up with you looking exactly that – tense and rigid. If this applies to you, try to reverse this by relaxing your hands and posture as you talk to people. Moving around slightly or adopting a relaxed posture can be helpful.

Experiment 2: The impact of swallowing/clearing your throat to excess[2]

Background. A common experience in social phobia is to notice a dry throat/frog in your throat and to be concerned about how your voice sounds. In response to these fears the person may swallow or clear their throat repeatedly to try to overcome this. Let's do an experiment to try to find out about the impact of these actions.

Task. Swallow four times in a row one after another. Notice what happens.

Review. What did you notice? Often what is noticed is that a) it becomes increasingly difficult to swallow, and b) doing this moves your mental focus onto swallowing for a short time. There is an important lesson here – that paying especial attention to our bodies can make something that is usually done without problem begin to seem a little 'odd/strange'.

Think about your own reactions to these experiments and what you found. Reflect on whether you have discovered anything that might be relevent to your own problems of social phobia. Part of the answer to overcoming social phobia is to try to identify, reduce and then stop doing any unhelpful behaviour. This is important because such actions add to your problem by reinforcing underlying fears. Use Workbook 4: *Noticing extreme and unhelpful thinking* and Workbook 5: *Changing extreme and unhelpful thinking* to help challenge such fears.

---

1 Do not do this experiment if you have a bone, muscle or nerve problem such as arthritis in your hands or arms. If in doubt, please discuss this with your doctor.
2 Do not do this if you have a throat or oesophageal/swallowing problem. If in doubt, discuss this with your doctor.

A specific phobia of heights

Some people have a specific fear of heights or of falling and avoid any situations with drops such as escalators, or walking near edges as a result.

> **Choice point:** If this is a problem for you, please read this section. If not, move on to page 6.25.

Example: John has a lifelong fear of heights. He has never experienced a fall, however he remembers that his mother was always very wary of going near drops. His fear of heights is in fact a fear of falling. As a child and teenager he could face heights to some extent, but always tried to avoid such situations if possible. He now walks a long way to avoid walkways, or staircases with open railings. He also avoids using lifts with glass walls and always keeps as far away from drops as possible. He walks faster than usual to leave such situations and often tenses his muscles in order to steady himself. This may actually backfire by making him feel even unsteadier on his feet. When anxious he tends to overbreathe and this adds to his feelings of dizziness. It also makes him feel disconnected from things. Together these sensations reinforce his fear of falling.

John's first step
- **Eventual goal to be achieved.** I want to be able to go round the city museum walls with my daughter.
- **Main fear to be challenged.** I'll fall and die.
- **Subtle avoidance to take into account in the plan.** I stay as far away as possible from any drop. I also grip onto handrails very tightly and hold myself in a very tense posture to make sure I don't fall.

John's step-by-step approach: weekly targets to overcome fear of heights

Target/step	Time scale
1 To walk up some stairs with a solid edge to it which can be looked over. To deliberately walk and look over the drop for at least 10 seconds. To increase this time through repeated practice. By the end of this practice, to relax my posture and not hold on to anything while looking safely over the edge.[3]	Week 1 (start of week)
2 To identify some stairs with metal rails where you can see through to the floors below. To repeat the same actions as at the start of the week.	Week 1 (end of week)
3 To travel in a see-through glass lift. To go up and down initially one floor at a time and then build this up to four floors in the local shopping centre. To make sure that I look out of the lift and look down for increasing times. By the end of this step to be able to do this for at least 10 minutes non-stop. Let's wear that lift out!	Week 2 (start of week)
4 Eventual goal To go to the local museum and walk round the open walls outside which only have low metal railings. To stop and look over the edge. Not to grab on to anything. To relax my posture. To keep doing this until the anxiety subsides. To then return and do the trip with my daughter.	Week 2 (end of week)

3 A balance needs to be achieved where fears are faced up to, but at the same time no actual danger occurs. This principle applies to all such plans to overcome avoidance.

Anxiety about physical health problems

> **Choice point:** If this is a problem for you, please read this section.
> If not, move on to page 6.27.

Example. After a mild heart attack, Patrick becomes convinced that his heart is not working properly. As a result he constantly feels anxious and is preoccupied with his illness. He feels physically tense and cannot sleep. He has stopped any activities that he fears may bring on a heart attack such as doing exercise, and making love with his wife. This has led to arguments that have further added to his problems. His doctor has advised him that he needs to do some exercise in order to stay fit.

Patrick's first step
- **Eventual target to be achieved.** I want to be able to jog to the park.
- **Main fear to be challenged.** I will bring on a heart attack if I overdo things.
- **Subtle avoidance to take into account in the plan.** I look in the mirror to see if I look pale. I only go places when someone else is around.

Patrick's step-by-step approach: weekly targets to increase the level of physical exercise

Target/step	Time scale
1 Go for a walk with my partner at a leisurely pace down the road for 200 yards. Over the week repeat twice, increasing the distance slightly. Continue to walk at this slow pace. By the end of the week aim to be able to walk to the park. To start reducing looking at myself in the mirror so I do this no more than five times a day.	Week 1 and repeat the walk on two more occasions this week.
2 Go at a brisker pace for the first five minutes of the walk to the park with my partner. Then have a more leisurely walk home. Reduce looking in the mirror to four times a day.	Week 2
3 Walk to the park by myself, briskly for the first 10 minutes. At home use the exercise bike or climb up and down stairs for two minutes.	Week 3
4 Use the bike for 10 minutes each day and by week 5 increase to using this twice a day. Stop using the mirror apart from to comb my hair, once or twice a day.	Weeks 4 and 5
6 Eventual goal Jog to the park with my partner, then by myself.	Week 6

Additional useful things to consider
First, go to see your doctor and ask for specific guidance as to how fast to pace this plan. You need to also confirm what target you should realistically be aiming for. Build their advice into this plan.

Identify and challenge health fears
Use the principles in Workbooks 4 and 5 (on identifying and then changing extreme and unhelpful thinking) to help challenge any extreme and unhelpful health fears.

Identify unhelpful behaviours that you can then slowly reduce

- Scanning your body for any signs of illness can continue to reinforce fears about ill health.
- Sometimes walking in a way designed to protect against pain and stiffness actually worsens this by creating additional stresses on your body. Holding your muscles stiffly can lead to pulled muscles or cramps.
- Only going out with someone else 'just in case' you become ill. This teaches you the unhelpful rule that you can only cope if you have this support.

Be aware of a range of similar actions – each prompted by anxious fears

- Taking a mobile phone because of anxious fears that you may need to call for help if you become ill.
- Misusing inhalers or tablets such as an anti-angina tablet or painkillers. For example, taking them before exercise even though this was not why they were prescribed.
- Walking more slowly or exercising less than usual as a result of health fears.
- Feeling your pulse to check it is strong and regular. Other ways of checking how you are can include looking in the mirror, feeling for lumps etc.
- Doing daily health checks, for example of blood pressure, temperature and pulse rate.
- Going to the doctor over aches or pains that have been investigated fully before.
- Asking for reassurance from others about how you look.
- Spending time either paying especial attention to news items or information about health, or trying to avoid it altogether. Your aim should be a healthy balance here.
- Selectively listening to what other people say and picking out any small thing that might just relate to your health.
- Expecting others to do things for you that you are capable of doing yourself.
- Walking with a stick or using a wheelchair can sometimes add to difficulties. If possible, plan to reduce such aids unless advised otherwise by your health care practitioner. Specialist advice is sensible here.

If any of the above activities or actions is present, they need to be slowly reduced. Don't try to change everything at once. Learn from Harvinder's approach of having short, medium and longer-term goals, and try to do this in a paced way.

Overcome unnecessary inaction

Muscles that are underused for a time become weak (for example by staying in bed, or seated in one place all day). This means that when they are used they will feel sore and painful. There may also be stiffness and feelings of weakness. Pace your activity to overcome this. This will build up your muscles and prevent you from 'seizing up'. It will also reduce the dangers of deep vein thrombosis – DVT. This can occur when blood clots form in your legs or pelvis after prolonged inactivity. You may have heard press reports with suggestions of possible links to so-called 'economy class syndrome' on long-haul flights. Staying in bed or in the same position all day fails to keep your blood circulating, as it would do if you were more active. You can overcome this by gradual, planned increases in activity, remembering that although this may hurt at first it will not do any harm. Again, specialist advice is sensible here from your healthcare practitioner.

Obsessive-compulsive disorder

> **Choice point:** If this is a problem for you, please read this section.
> If not, move on to page 6.34.

General principles for a self-treatment plan

Remember, in Workbook 1d: *Understanding obsessive-compulsive disorder (OCD)* you discovered that the problem with OCD is not the actual thoughts themselves, but instead it is how the person interprets them. Because the thoughts are distressing they cause the person firstly to try not to think them and, secondly, to try to prevent or reverse harm by carrying out compulsive actions or other unhelpful behaviours.

The targets of treatment are to help the person not to feel distressed about the obsessional thoughts, and also to plan to reduce any compulsive actions that are acting to keep the fears going.

Overcoming obsessional thoughts

Many people with obsessive-compulsive disorder try to challenge their thoughts or try to think them through to some sort of conclusion. However they find this isn't very effective. Obsessional fears always focus on a topic that is very distressing to the person (their 'Achilles heel'). The key problem is that the person becomes frightened by their thoughts and will do anything to avoid them. The result is a situation where the person develops a phobia of their obsessional fears. In the same way as overcoming a phobia by facing up to fears bit by bit, it is far more effective to just **let the thoughts be** rather than trying hard not to think them.

A key target is therefore for you to aim to **get used** to the thoughts and **become less anxious** about them. To illustrate this, imagine if a large bluebottle was in the same room as you. If you ran around trying unsuccessfully to catch it, this will only make it more excited so that it buzzes around even more noisily than before. Sometimes the best approach is just to ignore it and let it be. Although this does not remove the bluebottle from the room, it causes a lot fewer problems. Together with reducing compulsive actions, this is the approach that is most successful in treating Obsessive Compulsive Disorder.

To help you allow the thought to 'just be', try to think it more than usual. Instead of trying hard not to think it, do the reverse. Deliberately bring on the thought again and again. To help you do this, try the following:

- Write it down in detail again and again, thinking about it as you do so.
- Speak out the thought in great detail describing what would occur if the worst were to happen. Consider recording this with a tape recorder. Play back your tape again and again. Pay attention to what you think and feel. Don't avoid anything in your description no matter how scary, obscene or nasty the obsessional fear is. Saying the thought or fear will not cause it to occur.
- If the fear is very high to begin with, you may need to choose to pace how much is written down/said to begin with. Choose a small part of the fear (e.g. someone might be ill) and think this again and again, slowly adding in the areas that seem too frightening to begin with (e.g. that you or a loved one will become ill and die).
- As you do so, be aware of any attempts to neutralise or 'make good' the thought such as saying prayers to yourself or carrying out any compulsive actions. Try to increase this for increasing lengths of time.
- The purpose of doing this is to realise that having the thought does not cause the feared event(s) to occur.

Eventually by doing this you will find that the thought makes you feel less and less anxious, and that this anxiety lasts for shorter and shorter periods of time. **Try to aim to spend so much time with the thought that you become bored by it.** The aim is to be able to say to yourself '*It's just that silly little thought again*'. Notice it as if from a distance and then carry on with life.

Overcoming compulsive actions

Acting on an obsessional fear reinforces it. It is therefore very important to identify and plan to reduce any unhelpful compulsive actions. At the same time, slowly reduce and stop any examples of subtle avoidance that may be present (for example drinking too much to block how you feel, using mental rituals or other so-called 'distraction' techniques.).

Example. Sarah finds that she cannot leave the house without being troubled by obsessional fears that it will be burgled. She tries hard not to think these thoughts, but this just seems to make the fears worse. She notices tension headaches and eventually goes back to check the door. The result is that over months she has found it almost impossible to get out shopping. She is now asking friends to do her shopping for her. Recently, she has begun to sleep downstairs so that she can actually see the door. She has not been able to go into the back garden for long without checking the door, and as a result the garden is getting overgrown.

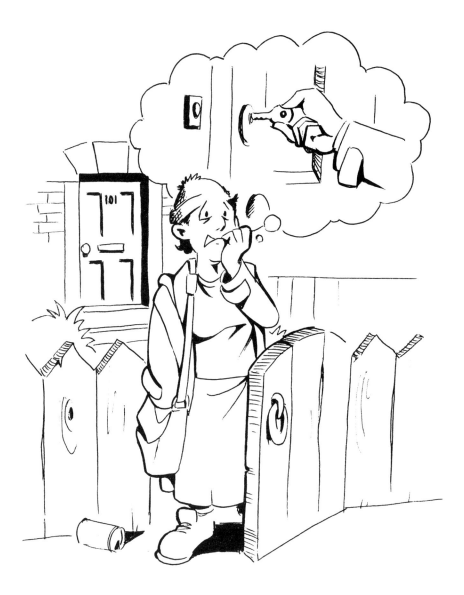

Sarah's first step

- **Eventual target to be achieved.** I want to be able to just lock the door and go shopping without stopping to check the door.
- **Main fear to be challenged.** Burglars will get into the house and take everything. It will be all my fault.
- **Subtle avoidance to take into account in the plan.** Asking others to do the shopping.

Sarah's step-by-step approach: weekly targets to overcome her obsessional fear

Target/step	Time scale
1 To lock the door and go upstairs without checking it. To allow the thoughts that I'll be burgled to *'just be'*. To choose not to go down and check the door for at least 10 minutes to begin with.	Week 1
Over the week to repeat this again and again increasing the time each time by 5 minutes. By the end of the week aim to be able to stay upstairs without checking for one hour.	
In the evenings to spend increasing amounts of time bringing on the thoughts by writing them down and speaking them out loud and observing them in detail.	
2 To lock the door and go to the back of the house to do my gardening. To allow the thoughts to *'just be'*. Over the week to build up the amount of time in the garden without checking to at least one hour at a time.	Week 2
3 To lock the door and go shopping for at least 30 minutes without going back to check the door. Do my own shopping this week for the first time in ages. To allow the thoughts to *'just be'* when out of the house. By choosing not to act on the obsessional thoughts this will undermine them.	Week 3
Over the week to build up the amount of time out of the house and away from home to at least one hour.	
4 Eventual goal Be able to go shopping for two hours without going back home once.	Weeks 4 and 5

This same technique can be used to overcome any obsessional thoughts and compulsive actions.

> **Key point.** In avoidance the key areas that need to be faced are:
>
> - Allowing the obsessional thoughts to *'just be'*. Not to go over them again and again trying to convince yourself that there is no problem. Once you have done this once that is enough.
>
> - Slowly reducing the compulsive actions (such as checking, cleaning etc.). This will also test out and undermine your obsessional fears.

Creating your own plan to overcome avoidance

In order to create a clear plan of how to slowly overcome your own avoided activities, the key is to apply the principles you learned by looking at Harvinder's plan earlier.

First, complete again the avoidance checklist that has been designed to help you to identify any activities that you are avoiding as a result of anxiety.

Checklist: Identifying your own vicious circle of avoidance

As a result of feeling anxious am I:	**Tick here if you have noticed this**

Avoiding dealing with important practical problems (both large and small)?

Not really being honest with others. For example saying Yes when I really mean No?

Trying hard to avoid situations that bring about upsetting thoughts/memories?

Brooding over things and therefore no longer living life to the full?

Avoiding opening or replying to letters or bills?

Sleeping in to avoid doing things or meeting people?

Avoiding answering the phone, or the door when people visit?

Avoiding sex?

Avoiding talking to others face to face?

Avoiding being with others in crowded or hot places?

Avoiding busy or large shops, or finding that I have to think about where and when I go shopping etc.?

Avoiding going on buses, in cars, taxis etc., or any places where it is difficult to escape?

Avoiding walking alone far from home?

Avoiding situations, objects, places or people because of fears about what harm might result?

Avoiding physical activity or exercise as a result of concerns about my physical health?

Q. Am I avoiding things in other ways?

Write in here how you are doing this if this is applicable to you.

Step 1: Identify and clearly define the problem as precisely as possible

The important first step is to make sure that you have identified a **single focused target** that is **clearly defined**. In doing this, it is important that you choose a target problem that:

- will be *useful* for changing how you are;
- is a *specific* target problem so that you will know when you have done it;
- is *realistic*, that is, practical and achievable.

Please select only **one** problem of avoided activity that you wish to work towards changing at the present time. This means putting the other areas on one side for the time being. Remember in Harvinder's case this was the problem of going into larger, busier shops/supermarkets. Once you have chosen one target activity, write below.

> **My target area is:** ....

Step 2: Think up as many solutions as possible to achieve this initial goal

Try to brainstorm as many possible solutions to overcoming this area of avoided activity as possible. This can help you to adopt a flexible approach to the problem. In brainstorming, the more solutions that are generated, the more likely it is that a good one will emerge. Ridiculous ideas should be included as well as more sensible ones even if you would never choose them in practice.

Useful questions to help you brainstorm include:

- What *ridiculous* solutions can I include as well as more sensible ones?
- What helpful ideas would others (e.g. family, friends or colleagues at work) suggest?
- What approaches have I tried in the past in similar circumstances?
- What advice would I give a friend who was trying to tackle the same problem?

Remember, the purpose of brainstorming is to try come up with as many ideas as possible. Amongst them you hope to be able to identity a realistic, practical and achievable first step towards overcoming the problem.

Write your ideas in the box below.

Step 3: Look at the advantages and disadvantages of each of the possible solutions

Assess how effective and practical each potential solution is. This involves considering the advantages and disadvantages for each of your potential solutions. Add additional boxes if you need them.

Suggested solution	Advantages	Disadvantages

Step 4: Choose one of the solutions

The chosen solution should be an option that will address the problem, and also is realistic and likely to succeed. This decision will be based on your responses in Step 3.

This solution should fulfil the following two criteria.	**My answer**	
a) Is it helpful?	Yes ☐	No ☐
b) Is it realistic, practical and achievable?	Yes ☐	No ☐

Step 5: Plan the steps needed to carry it out and apply the questions for effective change

Write down the steps that you will need to take to complete your plan. Make sure the plan is clear, and tells you *what you need to do* and *when* you are going to do it.

My plan

Try to write down **exactly** what you will do and plan to put it into practice this week. Check your plan against each of the questions for effective change.

Checking my plan with the questions for effective change

Is the planned activity one that:

- will be **useful** for understanding or changing how I am?   Yes ☐   No ☐

- is a **specific task** so that I will know when I have done it?   Yes ☐   No ☐

- is **realistic**, that is, practical and achievable?   Yes ☐   No ☐

- makes clear **what** I am going to do and **when** I am going to do it?   Yes ☐   No ☐

- is an activity that won't be easily blocked or prevented by practical problems?   Yes ☐   No ☐

You should be able to answer Yes to each of the questions. If you have noticed that your current plan has failed on one of the questions, try to think why this is. What changes can you make to alter or improve it? Try to change or alter the plan so that any poorly planned aspects are improved.

It may be tempting to be too ambitious to begin with. Before moving on, ask yourself again whether this is a target activity that you can **really** cope with at present. If not, change it for a more realistic target. **Remember**, large changes can be achieved by taking many little steps. There is an old Chinese proverb, 'A journey of a thousand miles begins with the first step.' Do not push yourself too hard by being overly ambitious, as this will risk setting yourself up to fail.

If you can answer **Yes** to each of the five questions, it means that your activity is well planned.

Step 6: Carry out the plan

Carry out your plan, and pay attention to your thoughts about what will happen before, during and after you have completed the activity.

Task: Record any extreme and unhelpful thoughts and their impact
(0 – do not believe at all; 100 – believe fully)

My fearful thought(s): Write in here:

_____

I believe this: _____%   **before** the task

        _____%   **during** the task

        _____%   **after** the task

Task: Recording levels of anxiety
(0 – no anxiety at all, 100 the maximum anxiety possible)

My level of anxiety:

        _____%   **before** the task

        _____%   **during** the task

        _____%   **after** the task

Remember that as you carry out the plan you are undermining your old fears by acting against them.

Step 7: Review the outcome

Review of the plan in operation

Write what happened here:

> ✎

Q. Was the selected approach successful?   Yes ☐   No ☐

Q. Did it help me to tackle the target problem?   Yes ☐   No ☐

Q. Were there any disadvantages to using this approach?   Yes ☐   No ☐

Q. What have I learned from what happened? Write what you learned here:

> ✎

Q. What does this say about any fears I had before or during the activity?

> ✎

Key point: no matter what happens – whether your plan is effective or seems to have failed badly – you can learn from it. Plan to take what you have learned into account in your next attempt.

Having planned and practised making this first change, the next key stage is for you to build upon this initial step so that you have a clear plan to move things forward still further. This is covered in the next section of the workbook.

Planning the next steps

To build upon this initial step you need to think again about your short-, medium- and longer-term targets. The key is to build one step/target upon another, applying the 7-step approach at each stage to help you consider your next step forward. Steps should always be realistic, practical and achievable. Without this sort of step-by-step approach you may find that although you make attempts to overcome your anxiety, these are all moving in different directions and you will lose your focus and motivation as a result.

Remember to build into your plan a reduction in any **subtle avoidance** you have been taking. Plan to reduce this slowly. Review any subtle avoidance using the checklist below:

Checklist: Unhelpful behaviours leading to subtle avoidance of anxiety-provoking situations

Am I:

Quickly leaving anxiety-provoking situations?

Rushing through a task as quickly as possible? (e.g. walking or talking faster)

Trying very hard not to think about upsetting thoughts/memories? Trying to distract myself to improve how I feel?

Only going out and doing things when others are there to help?

Misusing drink/illegal drugs or prescribed medication to block how I feel in anxious situations?

Taking the easiest option (for example joining the shortest queue in the shop as a result of anxiety, or turning down opportunities that seem scary)?

Deliberately looking away during conversations and avoiding eye contact? Bringing conversations to a close quickly because of not knowing what to say?

Q. Am I avoiding things in other subtle ways?

Write in what you are doing here if this applies to you.

After reviewing this, write out the next steps of your step-by-step approach.

My step-by-step targets	Initial fear level (0–100%)	Time scale (weeks)

The key is to do everything at the right pace, so that change happens. It should not be so quickly that it seems too difficult to achieve. Slow sure steps forward are the best way to make progress.

> **Key point: Repeat each step several times** before moving on to the next step. The more times you can practise the better. Doing this will boost your confidence in your ability to change. If you have any problems use the *questions for effective change* to plan the step again, or set a more realistic target.

Do:

- Plan to alter **only one** area of avoidance over the next week.

- Break the problem down into smaller parts that each builds towards your eventual goal.

- Produce a plan to slowly alter what you do in an effective way. Be realistic in your goals.

- Use the *questions for effective change* to help plan each step.

- There can be as many or as few steps as you want in your plan.

- Write down your plan in detail so that you will be able to put it into practice this week.

- If you find any step too difficult, *go back a stage and regain your confidence*. Then, decide on a different next step that is not quite so difficult. Repeat this step successfully several times before trying again with the step you found too difficult.

Don't:

- Choose something that is too ambitious a target to start with.

- Try to start to alter too many areas of avoidance all at once.

- Be very negative and think, *'nothing can be done'*. Try to experiment to find out if this negative thinking is true or helpful.

- Do not try to move too quickly from one step to the next. Make sure you repeatedly succeed at each step first.

Any avoided activity can be overcome using this approach. Remember, the main reason why a plan might be ineffective is if you are too ambitious or allow yourself to believe that change is impossible.

Summary

In this workbook you have covered:
- The vicious circle of avoidance and how to identify your own vicious circle.
- A description of Harvinder who plans a step-by-step approach to overcome his fear of shopping in large shops/supermarkets.
- The chance to practise a 7-step approach to overcome avoidance.
- How to create a further step-by-step approach to overcome your own avoidance.

Putting what you have learned into practice

Please carry out your step-by-step approach over the next few weeks in order to overcome your own problems of avoidance. Do not try to do everything all at once, but plan out what to do at a pace that is right for you. Whether the problem is avoidance of a situation, people or places, try to overcome it using a **step-by-step plan** similar to the one Harvinder created. If you have difficulties just do what you can.

If you have found any aspects of this workbook unhelpful, upsetting or confusing, please can you discuss this with your health care practitioner or someone else whose opinion you trust.

A request for feedback

An important factor in the development of all the Five Areas Assessment workbooks is that the content is updated on a regular basis based upon feedback from users and practitioners. If there are areas which you find hard to understand, or which seem poorly written, please let me know and I will try to improve things in future. I regret that I am unable to provide any specific replies or advice on treatment.

To provide feedback, please contact me via:

Email: Feedback@fiveareas.com

Mail: Dr Chris Williams, Department of Psychological Medicine, Gartnavel Royal Hospital, 1055 Great Western Road, Glasgow, G12 0XH

Acknowledgements

I wish to thank all those who have commented upon this workbook especially Joan Bond, Anne Joice, Susan Shaw, Graeme Whitfield and Stephen Williams.

The cartoon illustrations in the workbooks have been produced by Keith Chan (kchan75@hotmail.com) and are copyright of Media Innovations Ltd.

My notes

....

....

....

....

....

....

....

....

....

....

....

....

....

....

....

....

....

....

....

....

....

....

....

....

....

....

....

....

My notes

....

Workbook 7
Overcoming unhelpful behaviours

Dr Chris Williams

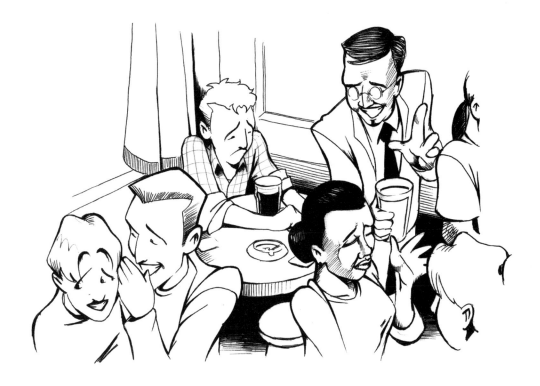

A Five Areas Approach

Introduction

In this workbook you will:
- Revise the vicious circle of unhelpful behaviours.
- Learn a 7-step plan to overcome unhelpful behaviours.
- Practise using the approach to plan a reduction in a single unhelpful behaviour.
- Learn some brief hints and tips of ways to reduce other unhelpful behaviours.

Revision

When somebody is anxious or depressed, it is normal to try to do things to feel better. This altered behaviour may be *helpful* or *unhelpful*. The purpose is to help the person feel safer/better – at least in the short-term.

Helpful activities may include:
- Talking with friends or relatives and receiving helpful support.
- Reading or using self-help materials to find out more about the causes and treatment of the problems.
- Maintaining activities that provide pleasure or support such meeting friends, playing sport, and attending religious activities.
- Challenging anxious worrying thoughts by stopping, thinking and reflecting rather than accepting them as true.
- Going to see your doctor or health care practitioner, or attending a self-help support group.

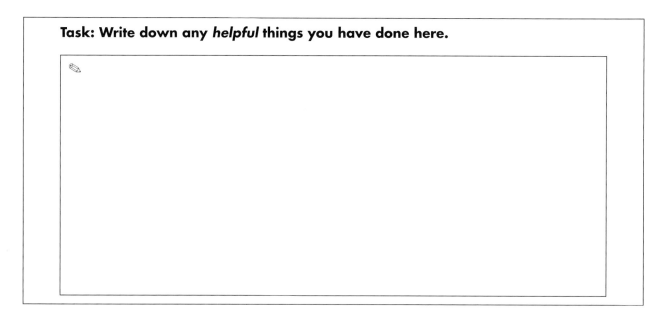

Task: Write down any *helpful* things you have done here.

You should aim to try to maximise the number of helpful activities you do as part of your recovery plan. Sometimes however, we try to block how we feel with a number of *unhelpful behaviours*, such as drinking too much, becoming very dependent on others or pushing people away. These actions can often make you feel better in the short term. However, they can also backfire by creating further problems. This can include immediate or longer-term damage to physical or mental health, or damage to social relationships. These actions therefore act to keep the anxiety and depression going and become part of the problem. A *vicious circle of unhelpful behaviour* may result.

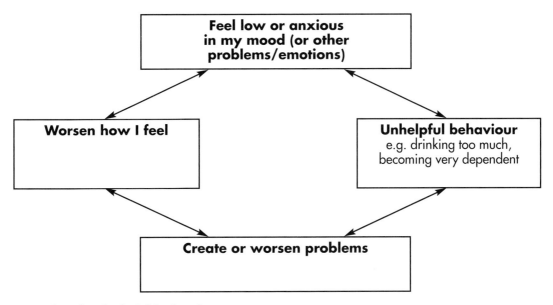

The vicious circle of unhelpful behaviour

Overcoming unhelpful behaviours

Please look at the following list and tick any activity you have found yourself doing in the last week. A wide range of different unhelpful behaviours have been summarised here to help you to think about the changes that are happening in your own life.

Checklist: Identifying the vicious circle of unhelpful behaviour

As a result of how I feel, am I:	Tick here if you have noticed this
Misusing drink/illegal drugs or prescribed medication to block how I feel in general or improve how I sleep etc.?	
Eating too much to block how I feel (*comfort eating*), or over-eating so much that this becomes a 'binge'?	
Trying to spend my way out of how I feel by going shopping (*retail therapy*)?	
Becoming very demanding or excessively seeking reassurance from others?	
Looking to others to make decisions or sort out problems for me?	
Throwing myself into doing things so there are no opportunities to stop, think and reflect?	
Pushing others away and being verbally or physically threatening/rude to them?	
Deliberately harming myself in an attempt to block how I feel?	
Taking part in risk-taking actions for example crossing the road without looking, or gambling using money I don't really have?	

Checklist: Identifying the vicious circle of unhelpful behaviour

As a result of how I feel, am I:	Tick here if you have noticed this
Compulsively checking, cleaning, or doing things a set number of times or in exactly the 'correct' order so as to make things 'right'?	
Compulsively carrying out mental rituals such as counting or deliberately thinking 'good' thoughts/saying prayers to make things feel 'right'?	
Being overly aware and excessively checking for symptoms of ill health?	
Excessively changing the way I sit or walk to reduce symptoms of physical discomfort? The altered posture then creates or worsens the physical problem.	
Sleeping with a number of people as a means of blocking how I feel?	

A range of subtle unhelpful behaviours is also often carried out during times of high anxiety. These are a form of avoidance. If you notice any of the behaviours in the checklist below, it is best to read Workbook 6: *Overcoming avoidance*.

Unhelpful behaviours leading to subtle avoidance of anxiety-provoking situations

Am I:

Quickly leaving anxiety-provoking situations?

Rushing through a task as quickly as possible? (e.g. walking or talking faster)

Trying very hard not to think about upsetting thoughts/memories? Trying to distract myself to improve how I feel?

Only going out and doing things when others are there to help?

Taking the easiest option (for example joining the shortest queue in the shop as a result of anxiety, or turning down opportunities that seem scary)?

Deliberately looking away during conversations and avoiding eye contact? Bringing conversations to a close quickly because of not knowing what to say?

Q. Am I avoiding things in other subtle ways?

Write in what you are doing here if this applies to you.

Overcoming problems of unhelpful behaviour

By working through the seven steps outlined below you can learn an approach that will help you to plan clear ways of overcoming any unhelpful behaviours. The first key step is to choose the problem you are going to tackle first.

Choosing a clear goal

The key is to move from more general problem areas to a clear target problem that you can then work on. So for example if you have a problem area such as '*I am becoming too clingy and dependent on others*' a clearer target problem could be decided by asking yourself '*In what way am I too clingy?*'. In this case a clear target might be to reduce the number of times you phone your friends up for reassurance.

One way of thinking about this process of clearly defining the target problem is to think of it as a *funnelling process*. You funnel down from a general problem area to a clearer target that you then choose to tackle.

The funnel process: defining a specific problem

General problem:

'I drink too much alcohol.'

Specific problem:

'I want to cut down my drinking as I am drinking too much every day.'

A similar process can be used to help make any problem area clearer. So, for example, if the problem is '*I have problems with obsessive-compulsive disorder*', you can be more precise about the problem by asking: '*Exactly what checking/cleaning etc. am I doing?*'

To begin with, **record** the unhelpful behaviour over several days. Make a written note of:
- When the behaviour/activity occurs.
- How often and how much you carry out the behaviour/activity. For example, record how many units of alcohol you drink, how many times you sought reassurance, etc.
- How long it lasts.

Because there are so many possible unhelpful behaviours, you need to use a clear plan to move forwards. The same structured 7-step plan can be used to overcome any unhelpful behaviour. The following example looks at ways of decreasing excessive drinking. Read through this example, and then consider how this approach could be used to tackle your own unhelpful behaviour(s). A short summary providing useful hints and tips for overcoming various different unhelpful behaviours follows after the next example.

Step 1: Identify and clearly define the problem as precisely as possible

The first step of the 7-step plan is to be clear about what area you want to work on, and decide on a clear eventual target.

Example: Paul is drinking too much and has been counting how much he drinks. Currently he drinks 50 pints a week. He decides the eventual goal he wants to aim for is to reduce his drinking to five pints on Fridays and Saturday and nothing over the rest of the week.

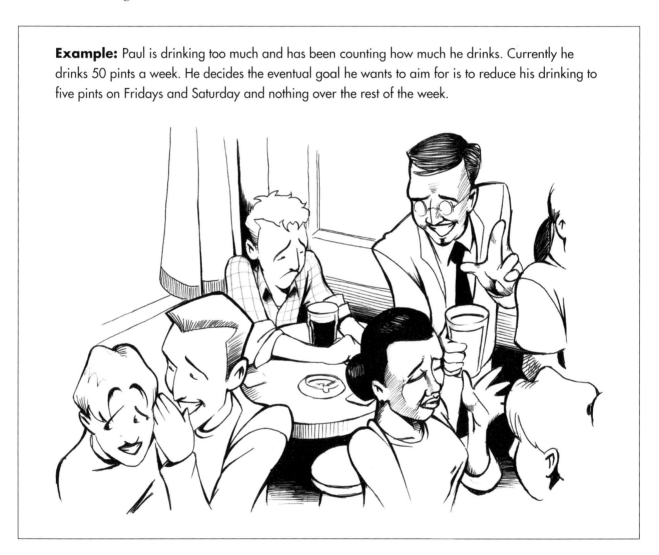

Think about your own problem behaviour and identify a target to aim for. Remember, if you try to change everything at once you will set yourself up to fail.

Once you have chosen one target problem area, write it in the box below.

My initial target is: ....

Q. Is this a clear, focused target for change?   Yes ☐   No ☐

Use this information to help you to clearly define the unhelpful behaviour. This will help you to begin to think about what might be realistic targets for change.

Step 2: Think up as many solutions as possible to achieve this initial goal

Think about things you can do to overcome your chosen unhelpful activity. Useful questions to help you to think up possible solutions might include:

- What *ridiculous* solutions can I include as well as more sensible ones?
- What helpful ideas would others (e.g. family, friends or colleagues at work) suggest?
- What approaches have I tried in the past in similar circumstances?
- What advice would I give a friend who was trying to tackle the same problem?

Example: Paul thinks up as many solutions as possible including some ridiculous ones.

1　I could go away on holiday somewhere where I can't buy drink.
2　I could plan to slowly reduce what I drink in a step-by-step way until I drink 5 pints on Friday and Saturday. My first step will be to cut down to 35 pints a week.
3　I could cut my drinking immediately to 10 pints at the weekend.
4　I could join Alcoholics Anonymous.

Task: Write your own answers in the box below.

Step 3: Look at the advantages and disadvantages of each of the possible solutions

The next step is to think about the pros and cons of each possible option.

Example: Paul's list includes:

Suggested solution	Advantages	Disadvantages
1 I could go away on holiday somewhere where I can't buy drink.	It would be nice to get away from it all.	I can't afford to go away. I bet I'd drink just as much there anyway. It would have to be a desert island – I'd find somewhere to get some beer otherwise!
2 I could plan to slowly reduce what I drink in a step-by-step way. My first step will be to cut down to 35 pints a week.	It would mean that I could plan a slower reduction in what I drink. This might work a lot better. I could cut down to 35 pints.	I'd need to have a good plan that I know I can keep to. It sounds like I could do this. I've tried before and quickly given up when I've set myself unrealistic goals.

Suggested solution	Advantages	Disadvantages
3 I could cut my drinking immediately to 10 pints at the weekend	I would get down to 10 pints a week, as I wanted. I'd save some money and it would be quick.	It just doesn't seem realistic. It would be just too hard to cut down this much all at once. Also, my doctor says I might have problems with withdrawal if I cut down that quickly.
4 I could join Alcoholics Anonymous	Others might encourage me to give up. It would be good to know I'm not on my own.	I want to try on my own at the moment. I don't think my problems are that severe. I don't want to stop drinking completely.

Task: Write your own answers here. Add extra boxes if you need to.

Suggested solution	Advantages	Disadvantages

Step 4: Choose one of the solutions

Decide on an option based upon what you have found out in Step 3. This plan should be an option that is most likely to be helpful and achievable. In many cases this will be to plan to slowly reduce the unhelpful behaviour and to choose a realistic first step as a target.

Example: Paul decides to plan a slow reduction in what he drinks – option 2.

Task: Write your own choice here:

Step 5: Plan the steps needed to carry it out

This is a key part of the plan. Think through in detail what you will do.

> **Example:** *Paul thinks about how his plan could be made up of a number of steps. The very first step needs to be realistic, but also help him reduce what he drinks. He is currently drinking 50 pints a week. He therefore decides that in his plan he will aim to drink 35 pints next week, and slowly reduce his drinking one step at a time from there. Achieving his first step is therefore his goal. He therefore decides to cut his drinking to five pints a night to start with – giving him a total each week of 35 pints.*

Task: Write your own plan here. Try to anticipate any problems/blocks that may interfere or prevent your plan. Your task is to carry this out during the next week. This first step towards your eventual target should be realistic, practical and achievable.

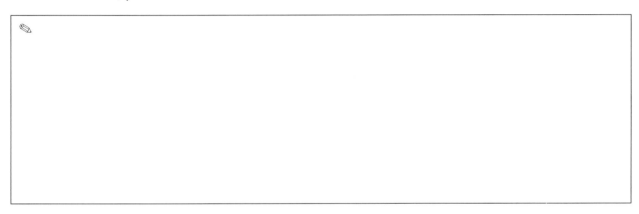

The next thing to do is to check how well thought through your plan is. Do this by applying the questions for effective change.

> **Example:** Paul thinks about how he can apply the **questions for effective change** to review his own plan.
>
> **1 Will it be useful for understanding or changing how I am?**
> *Yes, if I use the right plan. It will get me down to 35 pints this week. That's the first step towards my goal of only drinking 5 pints on Friday and Saturday.*
>
> **2 Is it a specific task so that I will know when I have done it?**
> *I'm clear what I am going to do. I'll have five pints every night instead of the usual seven. That will be my target and I'll spread the reduction over the week.*
>
> **3 Is it realistic; that is, practical and achievable?**
> *Yes, I could do this. I don't want to stop completely, but that seems realistic. It will also prevent the withdrawal problems that my doctor mentioned.*
>
> **4 Does it make clear <u>what</u> you are going to do and <u>when</u> you are going to do it?**
> *Yes, I know what I will do.*
>
> **5 Is it an activity that won't be easily blocked or prevented by practical problems?**
> *What could prevent this? I'm due to go to Bob's party next Saturday so I need to watch what I drink there.*

Task: Check your own plan against the questions for effective change. Is your own planned activity one that:

- will be **useful** for understanding or changing how I am?   Yes ☐   No ☐
- is a **specific task** so that I will know when I have done it?   Yes ☐   No ☐
- is **realistic**, that is, practical and achievable?   Yes ☐   No ☐
- makes clear **what** I am going to do and **when** I am going to do it?   Yes ☐   No ☐
- is an activity that won't be easily blocked or prevented by practical problems?   Yes ☐   No ☐

If you can answer **Yes** to each of these five questions, it means that things are well planned. If your plan has failed on one of the questions, try to think why this is. Change the activity so that any poorly planned aspects are improved. Write down **exactly** what you will do. Plan to put it into practice this week. **Remember**, large changes can be achieved by moving forwards one step at a time. Planning this first step will help you move towards your eventual goal. Do not push yourself too hard by being overly ambitious.

Step 6: Carry out the plan

Carry out your plan. Pay attention to your thoughts about what will happen *before*, *during* and *after* you put the change into practice. Use Workbooks 4 and 5 to help identify and then challenge any extreme and unhelpful thinking. Remember, acting against such thoughts is one of the most effective ways of testing them out and challenging them.

Step 7: Review the outcome

> **Example:** *Paul manages to put his plan into action for the first few days. He feels quite good about how things are going. However, things don't go according to plan. When he goes to Bob's party he has two cans to drink, and then thinks 'What the heck, let your hair down.' He ends up drinking fifteen pints of beer in a binge and has to take a taxi home. The next day he wakes up feeling worse and thinks about giving up the planned reduction in drinking completely. After a few hours, he begins to think about what he has learned about needing a clear plan if he is going to succeed. He also remembers his friend telling him that it is likely there will be occasional hiccups, but that things can still work out. He can learn from what happens and avoid making the same mistake again. Just because a setback occurs doesn't mean that everything is over. Paul therefore re-starts his plan. He is able to succeed in reducing his drinking and achieves the first step of his plan.*

Task: Write what happened to you here.

     © Dr C. J. Williams (text/diagrams) and Media Innovations Ltd (cartoons) (2003)

Q. Was the selected approach successful?   Yes ☐   No ☐

Q. Did it help me to tackle the target problem?   Yes ☐   No ☐

Q. Were there any disadvantages to using this approach? Yes ☐   No ☐

Q. What have I learned from doing this?

```
✎



```

Remember that even if there are problems with your plan, you can learn from what happened.

Planning the next steps

You will need to slowly build on what you have done in a step-by-step way. You can:

- Stop after doing this first step.
- Focus on the same unhelpful behaviour and plan the next step towards your eventual target.
- Or select a new unhelpful behaviour to reduce.

You must decide for yourself which decision is the best for you. It is not possible to deal with every unhelpful behaviour at once. In fact, if you try to change everything at once you will be potentially setting yourself up to fail.

> **Example:** *In Paul's plan, he decides to press on to the second step of his plan. This is to reduce what he drinks from 5 pints a night to 3 pints a night apart from Fridays and Saturdays. This will keep him moving forward towards his eventual target of drinking only 10 pints a week. He plans a number of small steps that he is to achieve over the next three to four weeks. Each week he aims to move one step closer to the target. Eventually he succeeds.*

Task: Once you have chosen one target area as your next step, write it here.

> **My next target is:** ....

Create your own clear action plan for your next step using the 7-step approach. Use a separate piece of paper to write down your plan. Use the questions for effective change to plan clearly **what** you will do and **when** you will do it. Learn from what happens and put this into practice.

Hints and tips on how to apply the 7-step approach to other common unhelpful behaviours

The following table provides some short comments to bear in mind when trying to reduce other unhelpful behaviours. Pick out and read about any unhelpful behaviour that applies to you. If the unhelpful behaviour is one of those that is causing subtle avoidance then you should use Workbook 6: *Overcoming Avoidance* to tackle this. You identified any examples of subtle avoidance in the table on page 7.4.

Unhelpful behaviour	Key hints and tips
Misusing drink/illegal drugs or prescribed medication to block how you feel.	Misusing prescribed medication can be dangerous and may prevent the tablets working properly. Always take medications as prescribed. If you have been over-using medications at a higher than recommended dose for a number of weeks, tell your doctor. He or she will be able to advise you how to safely reduce the dose to the recommended level. Drinking to excess or using illegal drugs can also damage your health. Again, you are best advised to take specialist advise from your health care practitioner as to how to best reduce a very high intake of alcohol, or regular use of illegal drugs.
Eating too much to block how you feel (*comfort eating*), or over-eating so much that this becomes a 'binge'.	Record what you eat, and when. Pay attention to what situations (including thoughts and emotions) are present at times of craving or over-eating. You can help reduce craving for food by eating three regular normal-sized meals a day. If you find you binge on food, you should try to gradually reduce and stop any dieting, self-induced vomiting, missing of meals or misuse of laxatives. If you find that boredom is playing a part, then plan ways of keeping yourself busy at times when you are tempted to overeat. Watch for any extreme and unhelpful thoughts about your shape and weight. Identify and challenge these using Workbooks 4 and 5.
Sleeping with a number of people as a means of blocking how you feel.	What do you want out of a relationship? Answering this question can help you decide what your goal is. For example, if your target is to have a longer-term emotionally fulfilling relationship, then you need to plan ways of achieving this. If you do continue to sleep with a number of people, make sure you have safe sex and use a condom.
Trying to spend your way out of depression by going shopping (*retail therapy*).	In the short term, plan what you spend with a shopping list. Leave credit cards and cheque books at home when you go shopping. Instead only take the money you will need for what you plan to buy. Be aware of times of temptation (e.g. when upset and times when you are in the queue near the till). In the longer term, you need to slowly plan to reduce this behaviour. If you find that you spend a lot of your time 'window' shopping you need to also think about the balance of activities in your life. Plan to increase other activities that previously gave you a sense of pleasure or achievement. If you find that you shop to reduce upset, consider using the workbooks on problem solving (Workbook 2), assertiveness (Workbook 3) and identifying and challenging extreme and unhelpful thoughts (Workbooks 4 and 5).
Deliberately harming yourself in an attempt to block how you feel.	In the short-term try to slowly reduce any self-harming behaviours. If you self-cut try to make the cuts shorter and less deep. Plan to reduce how often and for how long you do this over a number of days or weeks – be realistic in your goal as you plan ways of reducing this. In the meantime, avoid cutting deeply and in areas around tendons, nerves, veins and arteries. Ask your doctor for advice about this if you are not sure. Avoid infection by using antiseptics and dressings.

Unhelpful behaviour	Key hints and tips
	Your self-treatment plan should include keeping a diary to work out what factors cause you to cut. Record the situation, thoughts and emotions that lead to these actions. Use Workbooks 4 and 5 to identify and challenge any extreme and unhelpful thoughts. Use Workbook 2 to consider how to overcome any practical problems – so that you begin to feel less overwhelmed by things. Workbook 3 can help you to be more assertive and help you to act in ways to build your self-confidence.
Throwing yourself into doing things all the time so there are no opportunities to stop, think and reflect.	Plan a slow reduction in this overactivity. Doing this may leave you a chance to stop, think and reflect about upsets and difficulties. This offers an opportunity to use Workbooks 4 and 5 to identify and challenge extreme and unhelpful thoughts. The problem solving approach described in Workbook 2 can help you tackle the problems you face in a slower step-by-step way.
Pushing others away and being verbally or physically threatening/rude.	Play *thought detective* to identify any thoughts, feelings and behaviours that link to these actions. What situations or people bring this on? Are you testing out their friendship or love for you? At the same time as reducing this behaviour, you need to develop more assertive responses to others. Use Workbook 3 to do this.
Taking part in risk-taking actions for example crossing the road without looking, or gambling using money you don't really have.	Risk-taking can be exciting at the time and sometimes can become almost like an addiction. The problem is that these actions can be dangerous for you or for others. As you plan to reduce these actions, you may wish to plan in an increase in other activities that are safer and give you a sense of pleasure or achievement. If you find that you enjoy risk, consider other safer ways of exploring this (for example, cross-country cycling, bungee jumping or outdoor contact sports, etc.).
Being overly aware and excessively checking for symptoms of ill-health.	If you find that you are constantly checking your body for symptoms, or are recording things like your pulse rate, blood pressure, blood sugar or temperature to an excessive degree, plan to reduce these to a 'reasonable' level. Use the step-by-step approach to plan this out at a pace that you can achieve. By acting against this temptation to check you will be undermining any anxious health fears.
Excessively changing the way you sit or walk to reduce symptoms of physical discomfort. The altered posture then creates or worsens the physical problem.	It is natural to try to alter your posture to reduce or prevent symptoms of pain and be more comfortable. Try to identify if you are holding yourself very stiffly or in an unnatural way. Walking with your joints held stiff can worsen symptoms of pain, lead to muscle pulls and strains and even create new pains elsewhere in your body. Consider using a video to watch yourself walking and try to identify any unnatural posture that might be worsening how you feel. See a specialist such as a physiotherapist or consider using massage as part of your plan to slowly reduce these changes. Aim for a more natural and relaxed posture.
Compulsively checking, cleaning, or doing in exactly the 'correct' order or carrying out mental rituals so as to make things 'right'.	These actions commonly occur in obsessive-compulsive disorder but can sometimes occur as a distraction technique in other anxiety problems. As you plan to reduce these actions, do this at a pace you can cope with. In obsessive-compulsive disorder, doing this may cause you to notice fears that something bad may occur to you or others. Workbook 6 (*Overcoming avoidance*) will help you to find out more about how to overcome such fears. Use Workbooks 4 and 5 to challenge any extreme and unhelpful thinking about this.

Conclusions

This planned approach will help you bring about slow but steady changes in your life. This will re-build your confidence, and increase your control over any unhelpful behaviour.

Do:
- Plan to alter **only one** key unhelpful behaviour over the next week. Do this one step at a time until you reach your eventual goal.
- Produce a plan to slowly alter what you do in an effective way.
- Ask yourself the *questions for effective change* to check that the change is well planned.
- Write down your plan in detail so that you will be able to put it into practice this week.

Don't:
- Choose something that is too ambitious a target to start with.
- Try to start to alter too many things all at once.
- Be very negative and think, *'Nothing can be done, what's the point, it's a waste of time'*. Try to experiment to find out if this negative thinking is accurate or helpful.

Putting what you have learned into practice

- Please can you carry out the **action plan** that you created earlier. This will help you reduce one unhelpful behaviour over the next week. If you have difficulties just do what you can.
- If you regularly use illegal drugs or drink excessive alcohol, please discuss this with your health care practitioner. If you are doing this on a regular basis, this may act to prevent you getting better.
- If you have found any aspects of this workbook unhelpful, upsetting or confusing, please can you discuss this with your health care practitioner or someone else whose opinion you trust.

A request for feedback

An important factor in the development of all the Five Areas Assessment workbooks is that the content is updated on a regular basis based upon feedback from users and practitioners. If there are areas which you find hard to understand, or which seem poorly written, please let me know and I will try to improve things in future. I regret that I am unable to provide any specific replies or advice on treatment.

To provide feedback, please contact me via:

Email: Feedback@fiveareas.com
Mail: Dr Chris Williams, Department of Psychological Medicine, Gartnavel Royal Hospital, 1055 Great Western Road, Glasgow, G12 0XH

Acknowledgements

The cartoon illustrations in the Workbooks have been produced by Keith Chan (kchan75@hotmail.com) and are copyright of Media Innovations Ltd.

My notes

....

....

....

....

....

....

....

....

....

....

....

....

....

....

....

....

....

....

....

....

....

....

....

....

....

....

....

....

My notes

....

Workbook 8
Overcoming sleep problems

Dr Chris Williams

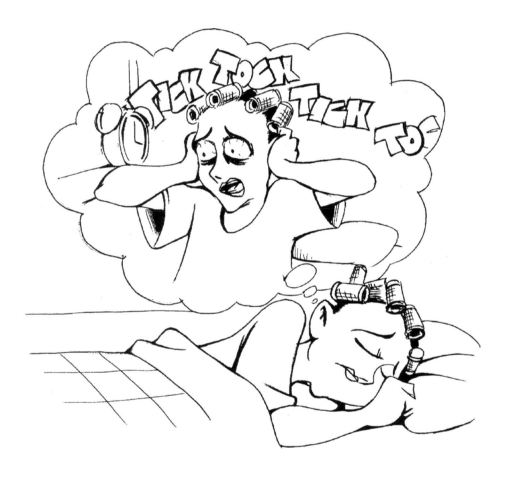

A Five Areas Approach

Introduction: What is sleep?

Sleep problems are common and affect large numbers of people. There is a wide normal healthy sleep range. Some people sleep only 4 to 6 hours a day whereas others can sleep for as many as 10 or 12 hours a day. Both extremes are quite normal. The amount of sleep each individual needs also varies throughout life. Babies and young children need a lot more sleep than older adults. By the time they reach their 60s or 70s, many people find that the amount of sleep they need has dropped by up to several hours a night.

What is insomnia?

Insomnia is an inability to sleep. Many people have problems sleeping from time to time. Insomnia often starts after an upsetting life event or can be caused by a person's lifestyle. A number of different psychological problems can also upset sleep. They include anxiety, depression, and stress at work or in relationships. For example, a person who experiences depression may find that it takes them up to several hours to get off to sleep. They then may wake up several hours earlier than normal feeling unrested or on edge.

A Five Areas Assessment of sleeplessness

The following factors can worsen sleep. Think about whether they affect your own life.

Area 1: Situation, relationship and practical problems

Physical environment. Is your bed comfortable? What about the temperature of the room where you sleep? If the room is either very cold or very hot this might make sleeping difficult. Is the room very noisy? Is there too much light to sleep? If bright lights such as streetlights come through your curtains, this can also prevent sleep.

Q. Do I try to sleep in a poor sleep environment?　　　　　Yes ☐　　No ☐

If Yes: The following are specific things that you can do.

Poor mattress. If your mattress is old, try turning it over, rotate it or change it. Try adding extra support such as a board or old door underneath.

Too hot/cold. If it is too hot open a window or use a fan. If it is too cold, think about insulation, secondary or double-glazing etc., or add an extra blanket or duvet.

Problems with noise. Reduce noise if you can. Speak to noisy neighbours to ask them to turn down their television or music. Have you thought about fitting double-glazing or internal plastic sheeting over windows to reduce noise?

Problems with excessive light. Consider changing your curtains. Add a thicker lining or blackout lining. If cost is a problem, a black plastic bin bag can be an effective blackout blind. Staple or stick it to the curtain rail.

Area 2: Altered thinking

Anxious thoughts are a common cause of sleeplessness. Anxious thoughts may be about worries in general. They can also sometimes focus on worry about not sleeping. You may worry that it will not be possible to sleep at all, or that sleeplessness will reduce your ability to be effective at work. These unrealistic fears prevent you getting off to sleep. Other common fears include worries that your brain or body will be harmed by lack of sleep. In sleep, there is a reduction in tension levels leading your body and brain to begin to relax and drop off to sleep. In contrast, in anxiety the brain becomes overly alert. You end up mulling things over again and again. This is the exact opposite of what is needed to get off to sleep. Worrying thoughts are therefore both a cause and effect of poor sleep.

Q. Do I worry about things in general?

If Yes: Read Workbook 1b: *Understanding worry and generalised anxiety.*

Q. Do I worry about not sleeping?

If Yes: Jot down notes of your worries on a notepad. You will need to challenge any catastrophic fears about the consequences of not sleeping. Studies show that most people do not need very much sleep at all to be physically and mentally healthy. In sleep research laboratories, it has been found that many people who experience insomnia actually sleep far more than they think. Sometimes people who are in a light level of sleep **dream that they are awake**. You therefore may be sleeping more than you think. You also need to know that sleep deprivation does **not** have a catastrophic impact on your brain or body. It is possible to function effectively with very little sleep each night.

Task: If worrying thoughts are problems for you, read Workbook 4: *Noticing extreme and unhelpful thinking* and Workbook 5: *Changing extreme and unhelpful thinking.*

Area 3: Altered physical problems

Symptoms such as pain, itching or other physical symptoms can cause sleeplessness. Tackling these physical symptoms will help sleep problems.

Q. Are physical symptoms keeping me awake?   Yes ☐   No ☐

If Yes: If physical symptoms are keeping you awake, please discuss this with your health care practitioner. Sometimes symptoms of depression or anxiety can worsen symptoms such as pain, in which case treating the low or anxious mood will help reduce the pain.

Area 4: Altered emotions/feelings

A range of different emotions can be linked to sleeplessness.

Q. Do I feel anxious when I try to sleep? Yes ☐ No ☐

If Yes: Anxiety is a common cause of sleeplessness. It is often associated with a triggering of the body's *fight or flight adrenaline response*. This can cause the person to feel fidgety or restless. You may notice physical symptoms such as an increased heart rate, breathing rate, a churning stomach or tension throughout the body. The anxiety therefore acts to keep you alert. This is the opposite of what you want when you are trying to fall off to sleep.

Q. Am I feeling depressed, upset or low in mood and no longer enjoy things as before?

If Yes: Depression is a common cause of sleeplessness. For example, a person who is feeling depressed may find that it takes them up to several hours to get off to sleep. They may wake up several hours earlier than normal feeling unrested or on edge. Treatment of depression can often be helpful in improving sleep.

Other emotions such as shame and anger can also be linked in with sleeplessness.

Area 5: Altered behaviour: Unhelpful behaviours

- **Preparing for sleep.** The time leading up to sleep is very important. Build in a '**wind-down' time** in the evening when you are less active. Physical over-activity such as exercising, or eating too much just before bed can keep you awake. Sometimes people read or watch television while lying in bed. This may help them wind down, but for many people it can make them become more alert and add to sleep problems.

Q. Am I engaging in activities which wake me up when I should be
winding down? Yes ☐ No ☐

If Yes: Keep your bed as a place for sleep or sex. Don't lie on your bed reading, watching TV, working or worrying. This will only wake you up and prevent you sleeping. You need to decide whether listening to a radio or music helps you sleep or not. Don't exercise in the half-hour before going to sleep as it may wake you up.

- **What about caffeine?** Caffeine is a chemical found in coffee, tea, cola drinks, hot chocolate and some herbal drinks. It causes increased alertness. If taken at high levels for several weeks it can cause physical and psychological addiction. Drinking as few as five strong cups of coffee a day on a regular basis is physically addictive. It also reduces sleep quality. There is a real risk that a vicious circle can occur. Tiredness causes the person to drink more coffee to keep alert. Then the coffee itself affects the person's sleep and worsens the original tiredness.

Q. Am I taking in too much caffeine? Yes ☐ No ☐

If Yes: Caffeine-containing drinks should be reduced if you are drinking them to excess. If you regularly drink more than five cups of strong coffee a day, try to reduce your total caffeine intake. Do this in a step-by-step way, or switch slowly to decaffeinated coffees, cola or teas. Definitely avoid having a cup of coffee or a last cigarette before sleep. Both caffeine and nicotine will keep you awake. Some people find that a warm milky drink can help them get off to sleep.

- **What about alcohol?** Sometimes people drink alcohol to reduce feelings of tension and help get off to sleep. One unit of alcohol is about half a pint of beer, one short, or one glass of wine. If you drink more than the recommended levels of alcohol (22 units a week for women and 28 units for men), this can cause problems such as anxiety, depression and sleeplessness. Finally, drinking too much will cause you to go to the toilet more than usual at night. This will keep you awake.

> **Q.** Am I drinking too much alcohol? Yes ☐ No ☐
>
> **If Yes:** Getting up in the night to use the toilet can be avoided by reducing the amount you drink before going to bed. If you take a diuretic (a water tablet), you should aim to take it earlier in the day. Discuss this with your doctor. If you drink above the **healthy drink range**, try to cut down the amount in a slow step-by-step manner. Discuss how best to do this with your health care practitioner.

- **What about your sleep pattern?** If you are not sleeping well it can be tempting to go to bed either **very much earlier** or **very much later** than normal. **Napping** is another habit that can end up backfiring by upsetting the natural sleep–wake cycle.

> **Q.** Do I have a disrupted sleep pattern (time to bed/getting up)? Yes ☐ No ☐
>
> **If Yes:** Set yourself regular sleep times. Get up at a set time even if you have slept poorly. Try to teach your body what time to fall asleep and what time to get up. Go to sleep some time between 10pm and midnight. Try to get up at a **sensible** time between 7am and 9am. Adjust these times to fit your own circumstances. When you cannot get off to sleep, do an activity until you feel 'sleepy tired', and then return to bed.

- **Tossing and turning in bed and clock watching**

> **Q.** Do you find yourself lying awake in bed tossing and turning, waking your partner up to talk ('*Are you awake?*'), or just watching the clock?
>
> **If Yes:** Get up out of bed if you are not sleeping after 30 minutes. Go downstairs and do something else until you are 'sleepy tired' again. Then return to bed.

Task: Look at the Five Areas Assessment diagram. Write in all the factors you have identified that affect you. These are possible targets for change.

My Five Areas Assessment of insomnia

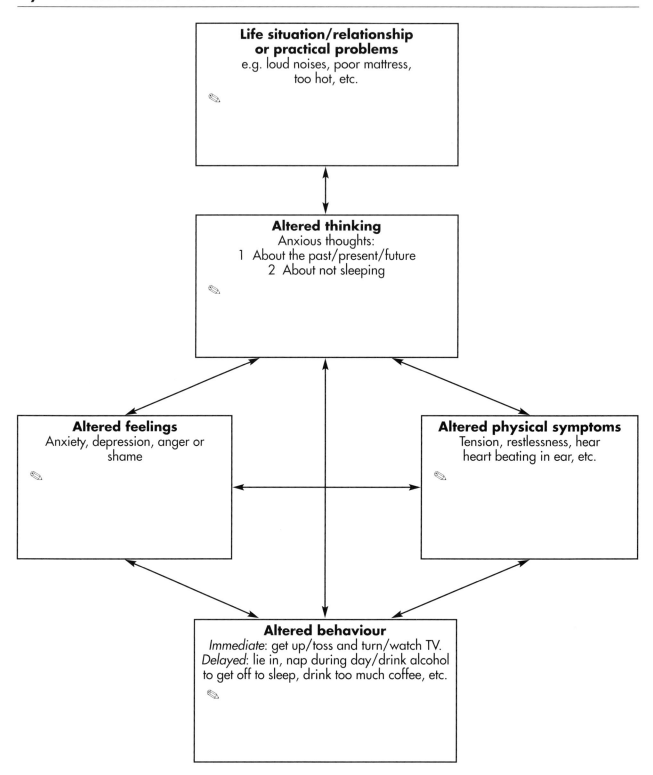

Overcoming sleeplessness

The treatment of insomnia involves two main steps:
1 Identify and challenge any anxious worrying.
2 Identify and reduce any unhelpful behaviours that are worsening your sleeplessness.

Your Five Areas Assessment will have helped you identify the problems you currently face and provided you with hints and tips in each of the main problem areas.

Conclusions

Sleep problems are common. Treatment involves setting up helpful sleep patterns and challenging any anxious thoughts that act to worsen the problem.

Putting what you have learned into practice

1 Try to get into a **routine**. Go to bed and get up at a regular time. Don't drink too much coffee, tea, hot chocolate and cola drinks which contain caffeine. Around five cups or glasses a day of caffeine-containing drinks should be the maximum. Switch to decaffeinated drinks or water for drinks beyond this.

2 **Nicotine** in cigarettes causes sleeplessness. Don't smoke just before bed.

3 **Don't nap** during the day. It upsets your body clock.

4 Watch your **alcohol** intake. Alcohol causes sleep to be shallow and unrefreshing. It also can make you wake up more to use the toilet.

5 Consider the **surroundings** (noise, light levels, temperature, and also the comfort of your bed).

6 If you don't get off to sleep, **get up and leave your bedroom** until you feel 'sleepy tired'. Then return to bed.

● Don't expect to change everything immediately. However with practice you can make helpful changes to your sleep pattern. If you have difficulties just do what you can.

● If you have found any aspects of this workbook unhelpful, upsetting or confusing, please can you discuss this with your health care practitioner or someone else whose opinion you trust.

A request for feedback

An important factor in the development of all the Five Areas Assessment workbooks is that the content is updated on a regular basis based upon feedback from users and practitioners. If there are areas which you find hard to understand, or seem poorly written, please let me know and I will try to improve things in future. I regret that I am unable to provide any specific replies or advice on treatment.

> ## To provide feedback, please contact me via:
>
> **Email:** Feedback@fiveareas.com
> **Mail:** Dr Chris Williams, Department of Psychological Medicine, Gartnavel Royal Hospital, 1055 Great Western Road, Glasgow, G12 0XH

Acknowledgements

I wish to thank all those who have commented upon this workbook, especially Frances Cole. The cartoon illustrations in the Workbooks have been produced by Keith Chan (kchan75@hotmail.com) and are copyright of Media Innovations Ltd.

My notes

....

....

....

....

....

....

....

....

....

....

....

....

....

....

....

....

....

....

....

....

....

....

....

....

....

....

....

My notes

....

Workbook 9

Understanding and using anti-anxiety medication

Dr Chris Williams

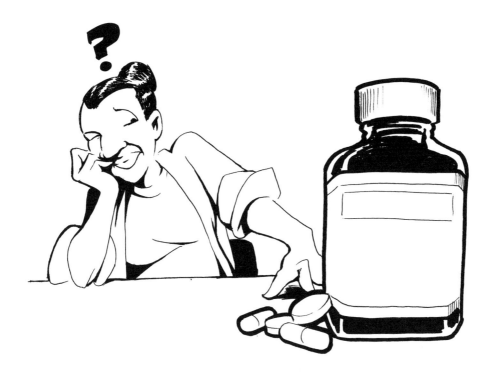

A Five Areas Approach

Introduction

This workbook is written for anyone who is taking one of the different anti-anxiety medications. It will also be of use if you want to find out more about the appropriate use of this treatment approach.

In this workbook you will learn:

- Why anti-anxiety medication can be used as a treatment for anxiety.
- About the advantages and disadvantages of using anti-anxiety medication.
- About your own attitudes towards the use of anti-anxiety medications.
- Ways of using medication more effectively (if you are taking any tablets).

Introductory information

A number of anti-anxiety medications have licences for the treatment of anxiety. They are used for a range of different anxiety problems, such as:

- **Generalised anxiety** where there is anxious worrying about lots of different things. It may even include worry about being worried. The worry causes physical symptoms of anxiety. It also has an impact on the person's behaviour or activity.
- **Panic attacks/disorder** where levels of anxiety reach such a high peak that the person fears something terrible will occur. This causes the person to stop what they are doing and hurry away.
- **Phobic disorders**. Medication is available to help treat *social phobia*. This describes a situation where there is very severe and excessive shyness. Medication can also be used to help treat *agoraphobia*. This describes a situation where there is a fear of being trapped, especially in crowded places such as large shops or buses.
- **Obsessive-compulsive disorder (OCD)**. Here the person is plagued by recurrent intrusive thoughts, impulses or images. They find these distressing and try hard to avoid thinking like this. Obsessive-compulsive disorder often leads to various actions designed to prevent harm occurring. This includes checking or cleaning things again and again, or doing things in a very ritualised way.

Medication should usually only be considered where anxiety is severe or prolonged. There are currently a number of different groups of medications that are used in the treatment of anxiety. No names of any specific medications are mentioned in the workbook. Instead the aim is to inform you about the general principles of using these medications. You can obtain details of the different anti-anxiety medications from your own doctor.

Key information

Why use anti-anxiety medications for the treatment of anxiety?

Links exist between the altered thinking, feelings, behaviour and physical aspects of anxiety. Look at the arrows in the diagram. Each of these five areas affects the others and offers possible areas of change to reduce anxiety.

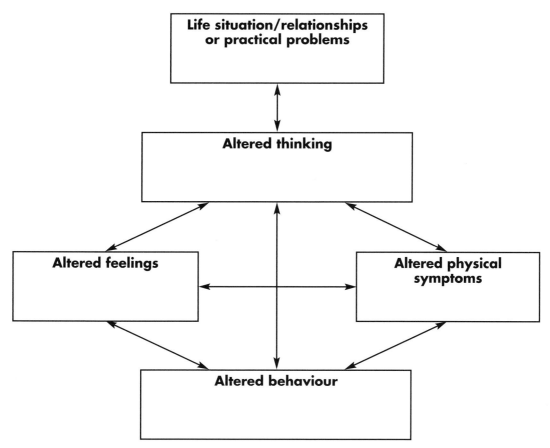

The Five Areas Assessment

Because of the links between each of the areas, the physical treatment offered by medication can lead to positive improvements in each of the other areas as well. Medication aims to relieve the physical symptoms of anxiety. In turn this may make the person feel better, think more positively, and change any unhelpful behaviour.

Where anxiety problems are severe, disabling or prolonged a combined approach of medication and psychological treatment can help you move to a position where you are more able to make changes in other areas of your life.

How long do they take to work?

Most anti-anxiety medications are started at lower doses and slowly increased in dose over a number of weeks. The maximum benefits may therefore take some weeks or months to occur. This is especially true where the anti-anxiety medication is prescribed to treat panic disorder, social phobia and obsessive-compulsive disorder. For example, it can take up to six weeks for the tablets to begin to show any clear benefit in the treatment of panic. It can then take up to twelve weeks to reach full effect. The full dosage is usually then continued for at least another three to six months at this higher dose. It is important therefore to take the tablets regularly and for long enough if they are prescribed. If there is little or no improvement, an increase in dose, change of medication and fresh look at other problems may be needed. Overall, taking anti-anxiety medications helps around half to two-thirds of people.

What happens after the medication is stopped?

A common problem is that the anxiety levels worsen again when the medication is stopped. **Medication is therefore best seen as only part of an overall package of care.** The package should also include learning new ways of tackling anxiety. Overall, treatment with cognitive behaviour therapy and some other psychological treatments seem to be as good as treatment with anti-anxiety medication. There are benefits of using both approaches together. Medication may be helpful when high anxiety makes it difficult for you to achieve change using the psychological approach alone.

Important note about benzodiazepines (minor tranquillisers)

Benzodiazepines have been widely used for the treatment of anxiety. They are commonly called tranquillisers and are also used as sleeping tablets. However, over time, higher and higher doses are often required to have the same effect. Because of this need to take more tablets and the occurrence of problems with withdrawal, they may become addictive. They commonly cause side-effects of tiredness and problems with concentration. When benzodiazepines are taken on a regular basis, about one in three people experience problems of addiction. The risk of addiction is higher if you have had problems of addiction with illegal drugs, other medications or alcohol. If you become addicted to benzodiazepines, suddenly stopping the tablets leads to problems of worsening anxiety. There may also be physical symptoms such as feeling sweaty and shaky with a rapid heart and sleeplessness. This can occur up to three weeks or more after stopping the medication. Due to this problem of addiction, doctors prescribe these medicines much less commonly now. Therefore, the dose should be limited to the lowest possible dose for the shortest possible time. They are short-term medications and not usually for long-term use.

If you have taken benzodiazepines for a long time it is important that any change of medication is done at the right pace and with the agreement of your doctor. **Please do not suddenly stop any regular medication without a discussion with them.** There are some very effective treatment programmes that can help you reduce and stop long-term benzodiazepines use. These treatments usually combine medication and psychological treatments. If you find yourself in this situation, discuss it with your doctor.

Do anti-anxiety medications have side-effects?

All tablets have side-effects. Modern anti-anxiety medications often don't have very severe side effects. Many side-effects disappear within a few days of starting the tablets as you get used to them. Sometimes anxiety can actually worsen when an anti-anxiety medication is prescribed. This especially occurs in the treatment of panic.

If you notice side-effects, your doctor can reduce the dose, or change the tablet to another one. Please discuss this with them.

Can I drive or use machinery if I take tablets?

Many anti-anxiety medications can affect your ability to drive and operate machinery. They can also exaggerate the effects of alcohol. Read the medication advice leaflet that accompanies your prescription to see if this applies to you.

My attitudes towards medication

Anti-anxiety medications are sometimes viewed with suspicion. Think about whether any of the following apply to you.

Do I worry that they are addictive?   Yes ☐   No ☐

Useful information: Benzodiazepines can be addictive. The dose should be kept to as low a dose as possible, and the tablets stopped as soon as possible.

It is **not** possible to become addicted to modern anti-anxiety tablets such as Selective Serotonin Reuptake Inhibitors (SSRIs). These medications do not cause addiction. However, they can lead to a short-term reaction with anxiety and physical symptoms if they are stopped too quickly. To prevent this, the dose of tablets is often reduced slowly over several days or weeks.

Do I think I should get better on my own without taking tablets?   Yes ☐   No ☐

Anti-anxiety medications are one of a number of ways of getting better. They alter some of the physical symptoms that occur in anxiety. They do not replace the need for you to work at changing other aspects of your life. They can be a useful additional way of improving how you feel if your anxiety is at a high level, or other approaches are not helping. If your doctor is recommending anti-anxiety medications, talk to him or her and discuss how they fit in to the overall treatment package.

Do I ever try to cope without my tablets?[1]   Yes ☐   No ☐

When tablets are prescribed to be taken every day it is important to do this, or it may prevent them from being effective. Many people miss their tablets on occasion (or more often) for a variety of reasons. If you decide that the tablets are not for you, it is best to discuss this with your doctor. Then you can jointly agree on how best to work on your problems.

Practical problems taking medication

Remembering to take the tablets

For almost any medication, it may be difficult to remember to take them on a regular basis.

Q. Do you sometimes forget to take your medication?   Yes ☐   No ☐

Helpful hints

The following may help you to remember to take your tablets.

1　Get into a **routine**. Take the tablets at a set time each day.
2　**Place the tablets somewhere where you will see them** when you get up or go to bed. For example, place them by your toothbrush. Make sure children can't take them by mistake.
3　Write **little notes** to yourself saying *Medication*. Use coloured pieces of paper to help remind you if you don't want others to read your notes. Stick them on the fridge, oven and back door so that you are reminded throughout the day.

1　Thank you to Dr David Thomas for teaching me this helpful question.

Getting into a routine to avoid confusion

Q. Do you ever get confused as to whether you have taken the medication? Yes ☐ No ☐

Helpful hints

Anti-anxiety medication generally needs to be taken regularly to be effective. The following can help you be clear when you have taken your medication.

1 Tick off the doses you have taken in a **diary** or calendar.
2 A **dosette box** can help if you are taking lots of tablets at different times each day. These have different compartments for each time of day. You can fill the box up in advance for the whole week. If this is difficult ask a friend, neighbour or health care practitioner. Ask your pharmacist how to get one.

Medication and avoidance – misusing tablets

Q. Do you ever take a higher dose than is prescribed? Yes ☐ No ☐

Medication can be a useful and helpful addition to treatment when anxiety is severe or prolonged. However, there are several possible pitfalls in starting or stopping such medication. For example, it can be tempting to take extra tablets at times of higher anxiety in order to cope even when they aren't prescribed with this in mind. This forms one of the unhelpful behaviours described in Workbook 7. Misusing tablets in this way can backfire and worsen the situation because it teaches you the unhelpful rule that you are only managing to cope because of using the medication. The danger is that you then come to believe that you need the medication and are scared to live life without tablets.

Key point: It is very important **not** to take a higher dose of tablets than your doctor prescribes. Most anti-anxiety tablets usually work over a number of weeks. Taking more on one particular day will have **little or no** impact on your anxiety. Tablets taken at higher than recommended doses can cause unpleasant side effects, or **be dangerous**. If you are concerned that your medication is not working please discuss this with your doctor.

Conclusions

When deciding whether to start or continue anti-anxiety medications, the key questions are whether taking the tablets will help you improve how you feel. Whether you take medications or not, psychological treatments such as the cognitive behaviour therapy approach used in the *Overcoming Anxiety* course are a central part of treatment. Medication should be reserved for when you feel stuck, or when the anxiety is at a distressing level for a prolonged time. Remember if you are taking medication, the best way to move forwards is to also use a cognitive behaviour therapy approach alongside or instead of the tablets.

Summary

In this workbook you have learned about:
- why anti-anxiety medication can be used as a treatment for anxiety;
- the advantages and disadvantages of using anti-anxiety medication;

- your own attitudes towards the use of anti-anxiety medications;
- ways of using medication more effectively (if you are taking any tablets).

Putting into practice what you have learned

If you want to find out more about the use of anti-anxiety medications please discuss this with your doctor or pharmacist. They will be able to suggest other sources of information about the treatments that are available. If you have found any aspects of this workbook unhelpful, upsetting or confusing, please also discuss this with your health care practitioner or someone else whose opinion you trust.

A request for feedback

An important factor in the development of all the Five Areas Assessment workbooks is that the content is updated on a regular basis based upon feedback from users and practitioners. If there are areas which you find hard to understand, or which seem poorly written, please let me know and I will try to improve things in future. I regret that I am unable to provide any specific replies or advice on treatment.

To provide feedback, please contact me via:

Email: Feedback@fiveareas.com
Mail: Dr Chris Williams, Department of Psychological Medicine, Gartnavel Royal Hospital, 1055 Great Western Road, Glasgow, G12 0XH

Acknowledgements

I wish to thank all those who have commented upon this workbook especially Joe Bouch, Celia Scott-Warren and Stephen Williams.

The cartoon illustrations in the Workbooks have been produced by Keith Chan (kchan75@hotmail.com) and are copyright of Media Innovations Ltd.

My notes

....

....

....

....

....

....

....

....

....

....

....

....

....

....

....

....

....

....

....

....

....

....

....

....

....

....

My notes

....

Workbook 10
Planning for the future

Dr Chris Williams

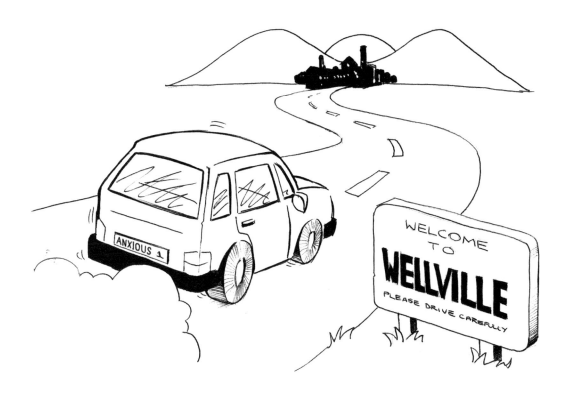

A Five Areas Approach

Introduction

This workbook will help you plan how to face the future. Think of yourself as being on a journey of recovery. Hopefully things have improved in at least some areas since you began your journey down this path.

> **Task:** The following are some questions to help you identify what has been helpful for you and what things have helped you move on.
>
> **Q.** What is different now from before? What gains have I made? How have I improved in each of the five areas (*situation, relationship and practical* problems, *thinking, emotional and physical feelings* and in my *behaviour*)?
>
> [ ]
>
> **Q.** What have I done to make this happen? How can I apply these changes to future problems?
>
> [ ]
>
> **Q.** What things might get in the way of me doing this? How can I deal with these obstacles? What practical steps can I take to overcome them?
>
> [ ]

My rules for life

Try to summarise what helpful things you have learned about recovering from anxiety and depression. Try to write these down as general rules that you can apply in life. You can write as many or as few rules as you want.

Example: Paul's rules for life

1 When I begin to feel anxious and depressed, I need to do something about it before it worsens.

2 I can control my negative thoughts by using the thought worksheets.

3 Don't withdraw from others when I feel down. Other people can really help me pick up.

4 Avoid drinking too much – it only makes things worse.

5 When I feel overwhelmed by problems – just tackle them one at a time.

Task: My rules for life. What have I learned about getting and staying better?

Write your own rules here:

1

2

3

4

5

Watch for early warning signs

One helpful approach is to try to watch out for early signs that problems such as anxiety or depression are returning. This may include changes like:

- *Situation, relationship and practical problems.* Problems begin to build up that seem overwhelming.
- *Altered thinking.* Noticing increased extreme or unhelpful thoughts and no longer challenging thoughts like these.
- *Altered feelings.* Such as beginning to feel anxious, or feeling down and low.
- *Altered physical symptoms.* For example feeling tense, restless or noticing a disturbed appetite.
- *Altered behaviour.* Beginning to withdraw from others or activities (*reduced activity*) or increasingly avoiding things because of anxiety.
- *Altered behaviour – unhelpful activities.* For example, drinking more alcohol to block how you feel.

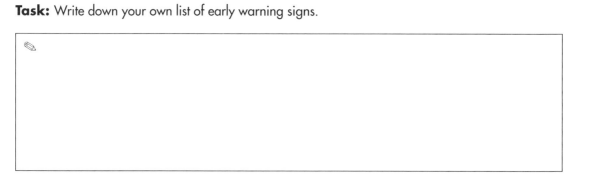

Task: Write down your own list of early warning signs.

Try to identify **one key early warning sign**. If you notice this key early warning sign, this means do something **now** about how you feel.

Sometimes it can help to also talk to others who you know and trust. Ask them if they have noticed that you have any other early warning signs. If they notice any, you could watch for these yourself. You can also ask them to tell you if they notice these returning.

Producing an emergency plan

The purpose of creating this early warning list is to allow you to respond quickly to any future setbacks. Imagine you live in a house that has a smoke detector. One day you hear it beeping. What do you do? Do you ignore it or do you get up, find out if there is a problem and try to deal with it? In the same way, if you notice any of your *early warning signs*, you need to have planned out how you will react.

The following example shows how Harvinder decides to react to his early warning signs.

Early warning sign	Emergency plan
Altered thinking. Negative predictions and catastrophic thinking.	To identify and challenge this unhelpful thinking.
Altered physical symptoms. Feeling physically tense and breathing faster than normal when in shops.	I'll slow down my breathing and take normal-sized breaths. I also need to make sure I don't start walking in a tense way.
Altered behaviour. Avoiding going into larger shops.	Plan to keep going to shops and make sure I don't start going to smaller shops as an easier option.
Altered behaviour. Rushing through the shop as fast as I can.	To slow down my walking and make sure I don't avoid things in other ways like gripping the trolley handle hard to distract myself.
Altered feelings. Feeling anxious about going to the shops.	Do all the above things, and also go back to the support group and discuss how I feel with my friends. Facing up to my fears is the best way to overcome them. If things get worse, I can also arrange to see my doctor.

My emergency plan
What is your emergency plan in the event of a setback? Try to be very clear about the things you will do, and the people you will contact for help.

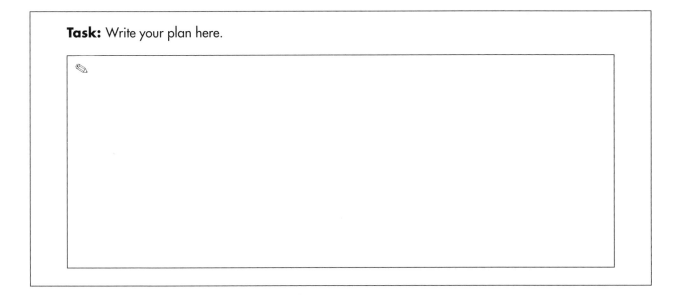

Task: Write your plan here.

Planning a regular self-review session

A regular self-review session during the next few months will help you continue to use the information and skills that you have learned. It will help you to set clear goals, and review how things have gone. Get a pen and mark the last day of each month as a '*review session*' on your calendar or in your diary. During the review session spend 30 minutes thinking back over the previous month.

As you do this, think about things that have gone well and allow yourself to experience pleasure and a sense of achievement as you remind yourself of this. If some areas haven't gone as well, try to work out what it was about the difficult situation(s) that caused this. Was there anything you could have done differently? How could you deal with it differently in future?

From these questions, write an **action plan** for the following month. Try to set clear goals and targets. Plan in some activities that will lead you to have a sense of achievement or pleasure. Plan to tackle problems such as avoidance or any unhelpful activities one step at a time. Remember, you are more likely to succeed if you aim to reach one target to begin with. Plan to move forwards one step at a time.

Be very specific about *what* you are going to do and *when* you will do it. Be realistic in what it is possible to achieve.
- How will you try to make sure that you carry out your plan?
- What can prevent this happening? What might sabotage your plan?
- How can you overcome any problems?

You can complete your review session more often (e.g. every two weeks) if you find this helpful. The purpose is to spend a little time to *stop, think and reflect*, and plan how to move forwards. Finally, remember that you are not alone. Your health care practitioner and others you trust are there as a resource to work with you and help you move forwards.

Putting what you have learned into practice

Read through this workbook again. Summarise your **Rules for life** and put them somewhere you will see them on a regular basis. Remember to keep working actively on continuing to move forwards. Use your review day to watch for early warning signs of slipping back. If you have difficulties just do what you can.

If you have found any aspects of this workbook unhelpful, upsetting or confusing, please can you discuss this with your health care practitioner or someone else whose opinion you trust.

A request for feedback

An important factor in the development of all the Five Areas Assessment workbooks is that the content is updated on a regular basis based upon feedback from users and practitioners. If there are areas which you find hard to understand, or seem poorly written, please let me know and I will try to improve things in future. I regret that I am unable to provide any specific replies or advice on treatment.

To provide feedback, please contact me via:

Email: Feedback@fiveareas.com
Mail: Dr Chris Williams, Department of Psychological Medicine, Gartnavel Royal Hospital, 1055 Great Western Road, Glasgow, G12 0XH

The cartoon illustrations in the Workbooks have been produced by Keith Chan (kchan75@hotmail.com) and are copyright of Media Innovations Ltd.

My notes

....
....
....
....
....
....
....
....
....
....
....
....
....
....
....
....

Worksheet

Overcoming hyperventilation/ over-breathing

Dr Chris Williams

A Five Areas Approach

What is hyperventilation?

Usually, when a person becomes fearful, their body reacts by increasing the heart rate and the speed of breathing. This allows more blood and oxygen to get to the muscles. The purpose is to prepare for either defending yourself or to run away. Sometimes rapid breathing continues long enough to cause a state of *hyperventilation*. This is also known as over-breathing.

It is important to distinguish between *sudden-onset (acute) hyperventilation* – as occurs during panic, and the problem of *longer-term (chronic) hyperventilation* which reflects 'bad habits' of breathing.

In **acute hyperventilation,** fast breathing with the upper part of the chest occurs. *Rapid short breaths* are taken through the mouth. Even though you are getting more than enough oxygen into your body, you may begin to notice a range of unpleasant but harmless physical symptoms. You may feel breathless and dizzy with blurred vision and a dry mouth. This can lead to a tight feeling in the chest. There may be tingling in the tips of your nose, feet, fingers or hands. Over-breathing can occasionally lead to muscle spasms in the hands or face. Finally, it can make you feel dizzy or fuzzy-headed. You may feel 'spaced out', distanced, or strangely disconnected from things.

When somebody develops **chronic hyperventilation** it can cause similar **but milder** symptoms. For example, there can again be feelings of slight dizziness, occasionally blurred vision, a dry mouth, and also sensations of tension or tightness in the chest. Again, it can make you feel dizzy or fuzzy-headed so that you feel 'spaced out' and disconnected from things. You may feel short of breath on occasion when anxious, even if you are not exercising. Finally, it can add to problems with sleep and contribute to longer-term feelings of tiredness. It is important to recognise that although these sensations are unpleasant, **they are not harmful.**

If you over-breathe, which symptoms do you notice?

A sensation of not getting enough air into my body?	Yes ☐	No ☐
A dry mouth?	Yes ☐	No ☐
Blurred vision?	Yes ☐	No ☐
Sensations of increased chest tension or shortness of breath?	Yes ☐	No ☐
Tingling in the nose, mouth, fingers or hands?	Yes ☐	No ☐
Feeling jelly-legged or faint/dizzy?	Yes ☐	No ☐
A strange fuzzy-headed/disconnected feeling where everything seems to go quite distant?	Yes ☐	No ☐

What causes the symptoms of hyperventilation?

The physical symptoms are caused by changes in *carbon dioxide* levels in the bloodstream. When rapid breathing occurs a gas called carbon dioxide is breathed out of your body more than usual. It is the reduced levels of carbon dioxide that causes the bodily symptoms seen in hyperventilation. You may have heard that some people who hyperventilate are given paper bags to place over their mouths for a few minutes while they over-breathe.[1] This helps them to slow their breathing and recapture some of the carbon dioxide so that they quickly begin to feel better again.

1 The use of a paper bag is not suggested in the Overcoming Anxiety course.

Overcoming acute (sudden-onset) hyperventilation

1 **Close your mouth.** It is not possible to hyperventilate for long through your nose. (If you have a cold this can get quite messy!)
2 **Slow down your breathing rate.** Take slow, normal-sized breaths. This is the reverse of the shallow, rapid breaths that are part of the problem in hyperventilation.

Two handy hints:
1 *Count as you breathe*. Count slowly 1, 2, and 3 as you breathe in. Take about a second apart for each number. Then breathe out again counting 1, 2, and 3. This will help you to slow your breathing down to about 7 or 8 breaths a minute. Remember to take normal-sized breaths. If this is difficult at first, start with deeper breaths and then reduce the size of the air intake to normal over a few minutes by using the counting technique.
2 *Visualise a peaceful calm scene*. Perhaps a mental image of the sea lapping on the shore. Choose somewhere you would like to visit or a place where you have happy memories of past holidays. Try to link your breathing to the relaxed movement of the waves. Again aim to slow your breathing to about 7–8 breaths per minute.

These two techniques will help you to stop acute over-breathing. You should follow this up with longer-term practice of the exercises described later to re-establish a healthy breathing pattern.

Overcoming chronic (longer-term) hyperventilation

The key to overcoming problems of longer-term hyperventilation is to develop more relaxed breathing habits. Relaxed healthy breathing uses a muscle called the *diaphragm*. Using the diaphragm creates relaxed, slow, deep breathing. In hyperventilation the normal slower deep-breathing pattern has been lost as a result of anxiety. The result is the shallow, tense upper-chest breathing seen in anxious hyperventilation.

> **Experiment:** When you notice over-breathing you can feel the tension in the chest muscles by pushing on the muscles between the ribs of the upper chest as you breathe in. The muscles will feel tense and tight. Pressing them is painful as a result.

The good news is that it is possible to re-learn healthy habits of breathing – so called diaphragmatic breathing. The diaphragm is based at the bottom of the chest just above the stomach. To feel where the diaphragm is, try to blow up a balloon, or breathe out against a closed mouth. You will notice tension at the top of the stomach just below the chest. Push gently just below the ribs and you will feel a large muscle. This is your diaphragm.

Re-learning how to breathe in a relaxed way using your diaphragm

A number of effective exercises can help your body get back into the way of breathing using the diaphragm. You are then more likely to breathe like this throughout the rest of the day without even having to think about it. Try to persevere. It will take about a week or more of practice to notice a significant change.

Hints and tips to re-establish a diaphragmatic breathing pattern

The following exercises will help you to establish a relaxed diaphragmatic breathing pattern. If you have chest problems such as emphysema, heart disease or chronic obstructive airways disease, please discuss the exercises with your doctor before practising them.

1 Breathe in through your nose while counting silently to 3. Then:
   a Record the length of time you can breathe out saying:

   > s =============→ (i.e. sssssssssssssssssssss)

   Do this once or twice as a baseline to allow comparison later as you practice other exercises. Concentrate on slowly controlling how you breathe out using your diaphragm. You will feel this muscle working as you breathe out. Aim to slowly increase the time you take as you breathe out. An average would be 12–15 seconds with no discomfort and no excessive tension.
   b Breathe out slowly as a sigh:

   > h ============→

   Again, feel your diaphragm gently tense as you breathe out.
2 Breathe in gently through your nose over a silent, slow count of 3.
   Then pause for a count of 3.
   Finally breathe out slowly through your mouth for a count of 3. Take only one or two deep breaths and then relax. Settle your breathing before trying again to avoid any dizziness.

   As you practise this, gently extend the time spent breathing out to a count of 3, 4 and so on. Try to reach 8 to 10. Try to ensure that this is done in a relaxed way and is not rushed. The aim is to re-establish a relaxed rhythm to your breathing.

Helpful hints

Be aware of any tension or excessive movement of your shoulders. This is a useful marker of the shallow rapid breathing that is a problem in anxiety. As you breathe out, relax your shoulders and be aware of tension in your neck, upper back and shoulders.

Do: watch for visible movement of you diaphragm. Remember, the diaphragm is situated just below your ribs at the top of your stomach.

Don't: move your shoulders. You want to reduce any anxious over-breathing and tension in the upper part of your chest.

---

3 Breathe in gently then breathe out slowly through your mouth. Again, correct any shoulder movement and reduce any anxious over-breathing with the upper part of your chest.
4 Produce the following sounds. By doing so you are controlling the rate of air being breathed out by using the diaphragm. Try each exercise on three occasions, but don't necessarily do all of the exercises at one sitting. These exercises teach you how to create gentle variations in volume controlled by the diaphragm.

   ssssSSSSS

   SSSSSssss

   sssssSSSSSsssss

   sssssSSSSSsssssSSSSSsssss

shshshshsh

shshshshsh

sh------sh------sh

sh------sh------sh------sh------sh------sh------sh

By practising each of the exercises several times a day, you should notice that your breathing develops a more natural and relaxed rhythm over several weeks.

Getting further help

Sometimes referral may be helpful. Discuss this with your health care practitioner if you are interested in learning more about this approach and have tried the techniques above for several weeks.

Finally, singing or playing a wind or brass instrument is a very good way to practise breathing diaphragmatically, while doing something enjoyable. Even those who have never thought of themselves as singers or players might find the idea attractive – so follow it up, and see if there is a choir or group around that you could join, for instruction and fun.

> **Important information:** This worksheet is deliberately focused on some practical things you can do to overcome hyperventilation. It is likely however that any problems of over-breathing are only one of the ways that anxiety is affecting you. Anxiety affects your thinking. It also alters your emotional feelings, causes physical symptoms and alters your behaviour and activity levels. It also can affect how you react to others, and the different situation, places and people that you deal with. You may therefore need to also work on overcoming problems in each of these areas.

Acknowledgements

Thank you to Sandra Kinnear for helpful comments and suggested exercises to promote diaphragmatic breathing.

Worksheet
Understanding depersonalisation

Dr Chris Williams

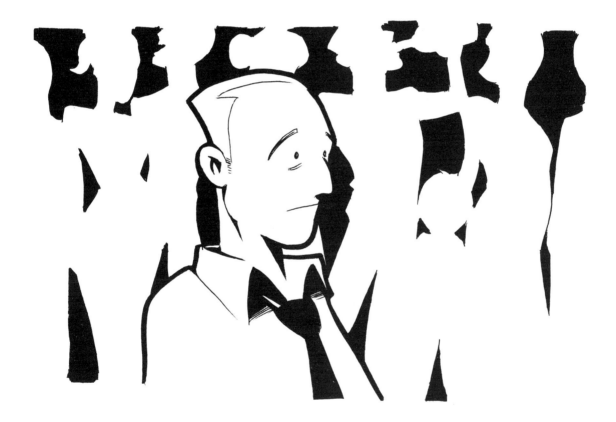

A Five Areas Approach

Depersonalisation: feeling cut-off and disconnected from things

Many people who experience anxiety or depression can feel mentally cut-off from things from time to time. This feeling can last for hours and is called *depersonalisation*. It can be quite difficult to describe what this feels like. You may feel a *fuzzy-headed, spaced-out* sort of sensation. You know that you are fully awake yet you feel distanced from things. You feel like you are a robot acting on automatic. You may seem like being an observer looking at everything from a distance. Also, things around you may not seem completely real – so called *derealisation*. These feelings can be very disturbing. Depersonalisation and derealisation often suddenly start, and just as suddenly stop.

> **Q.** Do you experience this unpleasant 'distancing' from things?   Yes ☐   No ☐

The causes of depersonalisation

A number of different factors can lead to depersonalisation. The following are the most common causes.

High levels of anxiety or panic. High levels of emotion including anxiety or panic can cause depersonalisation. Anxiety may focus upon everyday stresses, or on the experience of depersonalisation itself. For example, common fears during depersonalisation are that we may go mad or lose our mind.

Over-breathing (hyperventilation). Usually, when we become fearful, our body reacts by increasing the heart rate and rate of breathing. In hyperventilation *rapid short breaths* are taken through the mouth. Even though we are getting more than enough oxygen into the blood supply, we begin to notice a range of unpleasant but harmless physical symptoms. This can include depersonalisation as well as other symptoms such as dizziness, blurred vision, a dry mouth, and also sensations of tension or tightness in our chest.

High levels of depression. In depression we feel excessively down and few if any things can cheer us up. Depression is commonly mixed in with feelings of anxiety or panic. A range of physical symptoms of depression such as low energy, reduced appetite and disrupted sleep patterns can occur. Depersonalisation is often experienced during high levels of depression.

Upsetting memories/flashbacks and other upsetting thoughts. Sometimes we may have experienced an upsetting event or trauma in the past. Intrusive recollections of what happened (or what might have happened) can occur. These memories or images cause increased feelings of upset, tension and depersonalisation. Sometimes we are only dimly aware of the thoughts. We are instead more aware of the unpleasant feeling of depersonalisation. The treatment is to try to identify any extreme and unhelpful thoughts or memories, and challenge these. Workbooks 4 and 5 (on noticing and changing extreme and unhelpful thinking) can help you with this.

Physical illnesses and other physical causes can also lead to depersonalisation. These include:
- **Infections** such as colds/flu/viruses and a range of other physical illnesses.
- **Side-effects of medication.** A number of common medications can lead to problems of depersonalisation. These medicines can be prescribed for both mental and physical health problems. They include some antidepressant medications. If you are taking medication ask your doctor if this is a known side-effect.

Are the symptoms a side-effect of medication?

Most medications **do not** cause this problem for most people. If you are experiencing severe depression or anxiety, it is more likely on balance that the cause is the emotional upset. It is therefore important not to stop the medication without an open discussion with your own doctor about this. Useful clues that suggest a possible link are if the depersonalisation *started or worsened* after starting or increasing the particular medication.

If you jointly agree that medication might be a factor in your depersonalisation you can test this out by:

● Changing to another type of medication.
● Reducing the dose of the current medication.
● Having a time off the medication.

These changes can be viewed as an experiment. Record the *severity* and *length of time* you notice the depersonalisation over a week or so **before** and **after** any change in medication. This will help you make a judgement as to whether the medication is affecting your symptoms.

A symptom of epilepsy. A certain type of epilepsy called *temporal lobe epilepsy* can cause symptoms of depersonalisation. Most people think of epileptic fits as causing the person to lose consciousness whilst shaking their limbs. However, some forms of epilepsy can occur while the person is fully awake and otherwise functioning normally. Temporal lobe epilepsy is one of these examples of so-called *partial* epilepsy. The word partial describes the fact that there is a fit, but not so extensive a one as to cause a loss of consciousness.

Are the symptoms caused by epilepsy?

The following questions ask about a number of symptoms that can be present in temporal lobe epilepsy. Please note that a positive response to several of the questions only suggests that temporal lobe epilepsy be *considered*. The questions do not allow a diagnosis of epilepsy to be made. If you have any concerns, please discuss this with your doctor.

Q. Have you ever had a fit or experienced an unexplained loss of consciousness? Yes ☐   No ☐

Q. Do you ever notice strange smells or strange tastes in your mouth that don't seem to have a usual explanation for them? Yes ☐   No ☐

Q. Do you find that sometimes you will visit a place that you know you have gone to before, yet you have no sense of familiarity for it at all? Yes ☐   No ☐

Q. Have you ever experienced the reverse of this – visiting somewhere you know you have never been to, yet the place seems very familiar to you? Yes ☐   No ☐

If you have answered **Yes** to any of these questions, you should discuss this with your doctor. They may suggest further investigations to identify whether temporal lobe epilepsy is present. If epilepsy is present then they may suggest the prescription of anti-epileptic medication. This can be very effective.

Summary

This short worksheet aims to provide you with a brief overview of the main causes of depersonalisation. If you suspect that some of the possible factors that can lead to depersonalisation are present, please discuss this with your health care practitioner so that you can jointly decide how to approach this problem.

Part 3

Using the Five Areas self-help materials: advice for health care practitioners and self-help support groups

Section *1*   Why use self-help approaches?

Cognitive Behaviour Therapy (CBT): an evidence-based form of psychotherapy

Cognitive Behaviour Therapy (CBT) is a short-term, problem-focused psychosocial intervention. A recent report has brought together the evidence base for a range of counselling and psychotherapy treatments (Department of Health, 2001). A number of different psychosocial interventions are identified within this report as being effective. CBT stands out as having the largest evidence base for effectiveness across the widest range of mental health difficulties. It is an effective treatment for depression, panic disorder, generalised anxiety, health anxiety and obsessive-compulsive disorder.

The CBT treatment approach can be used alongside medication. Studies examining depression have tended to confirm that CBT used together with antidepressant medication is more effective than either treatment alone. CBT may have a specific role to play in reducing future relapse.

What makes CBT so effective?

Effective psychosocial interventions share certain characteristics. In summary, they provide:
- a focus on current problems;
- a clear underlying model/structure/plan to the treatment being offered;
- delivery that is built upon an effective relationship with a practitioner.

CBT is founded on these principles, and is essentially a self-help form of psychotherapy. The purpose is for the patient/client to learn new skills of self-management that they will then put into practice in their daily lives. It adopts a collaborative stance that encourages putting into practice what has been learned.

Health care funders and users increasingly request access to effective psychotherapeutic treatments. There are however currently fewer than 900 CBT practitioners accredited by the lead body for CBT in the UK – the British Association for Behavioural and Cognitive Psychotherapies (www.babcp.com). Given the increasing need for treatment, a major challenge is to adapt CBT to make it more widely available. The dilemma is how to offer such treatments effectively within the time, resources and skills available within most clinical settings. One suggested resource is the use of self-help as part of service delivery.

Wider access to CBT treatments

The Department of Health (2001) guidelines review provides a useful synthesis of the current evidence for different psychological therapies. However, what it does not aim to address is how to deliver these psychological services. A key paper concerning effective service delivery models is Multiple Access Points and Levels of Entry (MAPLE). Published in a CBT journal by two respected nurse practitioners and researchers, it asks us to question why we do what we do within mental health services (Lovell and Richards, 2000).

Traditionally most services that deliver CBT do so within secondary or tertiary services that offer specialist CBT to a highly selected number of patients; not many can satisfy the entry criteria to receive this treatment. The result is long waiting lists and limited access to treatment. Thus, these services offer a high-quality and specialist service – but only to a few. There is a huge unmet need and a mismatch of demand and supply. This results in frustrations for patients and their referring practitioners. Lovell and Richards argue that 'services characterised by 9–5 working, hourly appointments and face to face therapy disenfranchise the majority of people who would benefit from CBT'. The evidence base for the effectiveness for CBT is at its strongest in the disorders such as anxiety, panic, phobias, OCD and depression, yet these are disorders which, if present alone, often do not meet the entry criteria needed to access CBT. Instead the services tend to focus only upon the most complex and chronic cases. Not only do such services fail to provide wide access to treatment, they also fail to offer CBT in line with the available evidence. In short, although CBT is an evidence-based form of psychotherapy, we tend to deliver it in services that are themselves not evidence-based.

Providing evidence-based CBT in services

Lovell and Richards argue that the solution required is to routinely deliver services at three broad levels of entry to CBT. These should be flexible and accessible to a far more inclusive range of people than at present, and also address both common and serious mental health problems.

- **Level 1** Less intensive treatments should be the first choice for the majority of patients. Treatments should be routinely initiated by the provision of brief therapies, such as self-help delivered, for example, as structured computer or written self-help materials, or via telephone advice lines. Service-user groups such as Triumph over Phobia (www.triumphoverphobia.com) that base their support through the use of structured CBT self-help materials also deliver this level of input.
- **Level 2** Where the person has more severe or complex problems, or is at risk, more intensive therapist-guided packages of care should be provided. Typically, this would be as focused treatments such as facing up to fears or increasing activity levels in a planned step-by-step way.
- **Level 3** For more complex or treatment resistant, cases, full specialist CBT could be offered by experts. Level 3 input should generally be utilised when there is clear evidence that the person has been unable to benefit from simpler, focused single-strand packages or when such shorter, simpler approaches are inappropriate.

This approach fits with the so-called *stepped care* model. This suggests that patients will respond differently to varying types and intensities of psychosocial interventions. In view of this, it is therefore sensible to provide a range of interventions ranging from self-help to long-term individual treatments (Haaga, 2000).

Why provide self-help treatments within clinical services?

Self-help approaches are popular and used by both users and practitioners. Surveys have shown that between 60 per cent and 90 per cent of practitioners recommend or use self-help materials (Keeley *et al.*, 2002). Self-help approaches are also popular with the general public. Any large bookshop now has a sizeable self-help section addressing a range of mental and physical health issues. Self-help books are frequently amongst the top 100 best-selling books. Large population-based surveys confirm that self-help approaches are rated highly by members of the public. For example, self-help is more positively endorsed than treatment with medication or psychotherapy, or by a health care practitioner (Jorm *et al.*, 1997). Their popularity is seen in the growing number of self-help resources available on the Internet. In November 2002, the 'hits' for self+help+anxiety identified by www.Google.com was 926000. To provide a comparison and to illustrate the rapid rate of growth in the available information, the table below summarises the month-by-month increase in 'hits' for self-help in general.

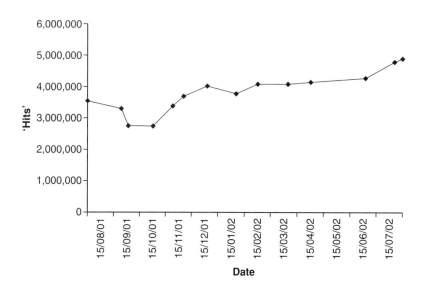

'Hits' identified by the search engine Google.com for 'self-help' from 15 August 2001 to 14 August 2002.

What is self-help?

Clinicians and members of the public use the term self-help in various ways. This includes attending a self-help group. Here, important issues of self-help and support may be offered and received. Another use of the term self-help refers to the use of self-help materials of varying sorts with or without support from a practitioner, friend, relative or support group. One 'research' definition is that in self-help 'the patient receives a standardised treatment method with which he can help himself without major help from the therapist. In (the approach) it is necessary that treatment be described in sufficient detail, so that the patient can work it through independently. Books, in which only information about depression is given to patients and their families cannot be used' (Cuijpers, 1997). This concept of working through materials independently is important because it implies that the structure of the materials provides sufficient clarity to allow this. It also draws attention to a crucial component of self-help – that the person learns how to help him or herself. This is an important distinction from health promotion/education approaches alone. Although the goals of self-help and health promotion/education overlap, there are important differences. A second 'research' definition helps clarify these differences by defining the purpose of self-help as 'gaining understanding or solving problems relevant to a person's developmental or therapeutic needs' (Marrs, 1995).

The term self-help is here used to describe the delivery of materials that employ a media-based format to treatment, such as book, computer or videotape. *However delivered, self-help materials aim to increase the user's **knowledge** about a particular problem, and also to equip them with skills to better **self-assess and manage** their difficulties.* Self-help treatments may be provided independently from (unsupported self-help) or in addition to (supported self-help) sessions with a practitioner or other supporter (Williams, 2001). The purpose of using self-help approaches is to do some (or all) of the work of treatment. The US-term *minimal therapist contact* perhaps best summarises this concept (Gould and Clum, 1993). However, in practice self-help treatments may also be offered flexibly alongside or instead of more conventional face-to-face clinical treatment sessions.

Self-help formats may include written materials (handouts, interactive workbooks and manuals), audio and videotapes, and computer-based materials (CD Rom, hand-held computers, the world wide web, virtual reality applications or interactive voice response – IVR, in which the person phones up a central computer and responds to questions and information verbally or by using a touch-tone phone). In future some self-help services may be available via digital television providers.

The evidence base for self-help

A large number of systematic reviews of the evidence base support the effectiveness of self-help treatments (e.g. Gould and Clum, 1993, Marrs, 1995, Scogin *et al.*, 1990, and Cuijpers, 1997). The consistent findings are that self-help approaches can be effective. Overall, self-help treatments are most effective for skills-based training such as assertiveness, and in the treatment of depression, anxiety and sexual dysfunction. There are, however, significant problems with the quality of some of the studies. There has been an over-emphasis on samples recruited via advertisement coupled with the use of very broad exclusion criteria. There has been a lack of comparison against active treatment groups as most studies to date have used either a waiting list controls or treatment as usual rather than comparison with another active psychotherapy treatment. Also, much of the outcome data has been led by the researchers who have developed the materials themselves. It would be beneficial for additional or collaborative independent evaluation to be completed.

Interestingly, most studies evaluating self-help have used a CBT self-help format. CBT has several advantages as a model for use in self-help treatment. It is a psychoeducational form of psychotherapy, has a clear underlying structure and theoretical model, and focuses on current problems. Finally it encourages the patient to work on changing how they feel by completing various specific tasks. A key component of CBT is to ask a series of effective questions to help the person understand their difficulties differently (so-called Socratic questioning). It also aims to provide the right information at the right time. Of course these questions and this information can be provided within the structure of one-to-one or group treatments, but it can also be written down on paper, or delivered via a video or computer.

The potential advantages of using self-help treatments

Self-help materials provide flexible and ready access to treatment at a time, pace and place the person wishes and with minimum delay. Self-help offers advantages for those who wish to avoid the stigma of formal psychotherapy or psychiatric referral. It also suits those who for reasons of privacy or personal choice prefer to work on their own to deal with their problems. Self-help may enhance the user's sense of control over their illness. There may be added benefits when self-help is offered in addition to individual or group sessions with a practitioner. Here, the self-help materials can build upon what is covered within sessions, reinforcing what has been learned. Finally, the user can return to the material to renew or update their treatment as often as they wish, and at no extra cost.

The potential disadvantages of using self-help treatments

Although self-help treatments can be effective, the choice of self-help materials is rarely based on research evidence. An American survey reviewed which self-help materials were used by clinical psychologists and identified a wide range of materials of which less than 10 per cent had been evaluated in any form of clinical study (Quackenbush, 1991). The finding that some self-help materials are effective does not imply that all self-help materials are effective. It is also clear that although self-help approaches are popular with many people, some prefer more traditional treatment approaches, or prefer not to access such services at all. In the stepped care model one of the main reasons for offering self-help treatments is to increase accessibility. However, this may not always be the case. A certain level of education may be assumed in materials, which often seem to be written by middle-class practitioners for predominantly middle-class audiences. Similarly, relatively few materials are designed to meet the needs of those from ethnic or religious minority groups, for children and adolescents and those with learning disabilities.

An important potential cost of using self-help approaches is the potential for 'side effects' of treatment. Almost all treatments offer disadvantages as well as advantages, yet these are rarely discussed in studies to date, which have tended instead to emphasise effectiveness. There are, however, a number of potential costs. Some people may come with a prior expectation of seeing a practitioner for treatment and can potentially misperceive the offer of self-help as a personal rejection. Users may be misled by the extravagant claims of some commercial packages to provide a definite 'cure'. Users may find the densely packed pages of text found in some self-help books to be overwhelming. The danger is that they might use the self-help approach and then withdraw from treatment as a result, judging themselves as having failed. Drop-out from using the materials may be high – especially when the use of self-help is unsupported by others. This may be from lower estimates of about 7 per cent (Cuijpers, 1997) up to 50 per cent of patients (Glasgow and Rosen, 1978). Drop-out is related to poor motivation and feelings of hopelessness (Whitfield, Williams and Shapiro, 2001). It is not known what impact a partial intervention may have on a person's ability to engage in face-to-face treatment at a later date.

The problem of accessibility to specialist CBT services

The traditional language of CBT is highly technical and often inaccessible. This can also cause problems where concepts such as *negative automatic thoughts, schemata, dysfunctional assumptions, faulty information processing, dichotomous thinking, selective abstraction, magnification, minimisation*, and *arbitrary inference* are used within self-help materials.

The Five Areas *Assessment* model was originally commissioned by Calderdale and Kirklees Health Authority in order to overcome this difficulty. The Authority wanted to develop a more accessible form of CBT for use locally in various training initiatives, and to have this supported by the use of structured self-help materials. The development phase has included extensive piloting of the model and its language in clinical settings to ensure clarity and acceptability of content (Cole, Hardy and Ditchburn 2001). Evaluation and feedback by representatives of these different practitioner groups has led to a continuous process of refinement of the model and its content over the last five years. The model aims to communicate fundamental CBT principles and key clinical interventions in a clear language. It is therefore not a new CBT model, but rather it is a new way of communicating the existing evidence-based CBT approach for use in a non-psychotherapy setting.

Each step of the development of the five areas self-help materials has been linked to the evidence base for CBT. These are summarised in:

1 Williams, C.J. and Garland, A. (2002). A cognitive behavioural therapy assessment model for use in everyday clinical practice. *Advances in Psychiatric Treatment*, 8, 172–9.
2 Wright, B., Williams, C. and Garland, A. (2002). Using the Five Areas cognitive-behavioural therapy model with psychiatric patients. *Advances in Psychiatric Treatment*, 8, 307–15.
3 Williams, C. and Garland, A. (2002). Identifying and challenging unhelpful thinking. *Advances in Psychiatric Treatment*, 8, 377–86.

4 Garland, A., Fox, R. and Williams, C.J. (2002). Overcoming reduced activity and avoidance: a Five Areas approach. *Advances in Psychiatric Treatment*, **8**: 6, 453–62.

Language use and CBT	
Classic 'technical' language: Beck et al. (1979)	**The Five Areas approach 'everyday' language**
Flesch-Kincaid grade 12 (reading age 17)	Flesch-Kincaid grade 7.1 (reading age 12.1)
Thinking errors/faulty information processing	Unhelpful thinking styles
Negative automatic thoughts (NATS)	Extreme and unhelpful thinking
Arbitrary inference	Jumping to conclusions
Selective abstraction	Putting a negative slant on things
Overgeneralisation	Making extreme statements/rules
Magnification and minimisation	Focus on the negative and downplay the positive
Personalisation	Taking things to heart Unfairly bear all responsibility
Absolutistic dichotomous thinking	All or nothing/ black or white thinking

The reading age of the 'classic' CBT language (summarised in the left-hand column of the table) is age 17. In contrast, the reading age of the right-hand column, from the Five Areas Assessment model is age 12.1. However, even if there is a good reading ability, this alone is insufficient to make sense of the classic technical terms. Specialised knowledge is necessary in order to make sense of these concepts.

The reading age required for the *Overcoming Anxiety* course

Two ways in which the complexities of reading materials are communicated are through the concepts of 'readability' and 'reading ages'. Readability refers to all the factors that influence whether someone can read or understand a text. As such, readability includes factors such as the size and the legibility of the print, as well as the motivation of the reader. It is also influenced by the complexity of the words and the sentences relative to the reading abilities of the reader. The reading age is defined as the 'chronological age of a reader who could just understand a text'.

Microsoft Word uses two readability scores, each based on the average number of syllables per word and the number of words per sentence. The Flesch Reading Ease scores rates text on a 100-point scale, the higher the score, the easier it is to understand the document. A score of 60–70 should be aimed for. A second measure is the Flesch-Kincaid Grade Level score rates, based on the US grade school level. In terms of this, an average seventh-grade student could understand a document with a score of 7.0. To transfer this score to a reading age you simply add five (an average seventh-grader would be aged 11–12). It also notes the proportion of sentences that use the passive construction. A sentence such as '*The ball was kicked by John*' would be passive, as compared to '*John kicked the ball*', which is active. Passive sentences are more difficult to understand generally within a text and therefore the aim is to keep their proportion to a minimum.

The easiest way to create readable text is to produce short sentences, in short paragraphs and using short words.

The following table summarises the *Overcoming Anxiety* text as submitted to the publisher.

Readability statistics of the *Overcoming Anxiety* workbooks

Workbook name	Flesch-Kincaid Grade level/ reading age (years)	Sentences/ paragraph and words/ sentence	Flesch reading ease	Passive sentences
Workbook 1a: *Understanding how anxiety is affecting me*	8.0 **13.0**	2.5 14.1	62.2	4 per cent
1b: *Understanding worry and generalised anxiety*	8.0 **13.0**	1.8 12.7	60.0	4 per cent
1c: *Understanding panic and phobias*	7.9 **12.9**	2.0 12.7	60.6	4 per cent
1d: *Understanding obsessive-compulsive symptoms (OCD)*	8.2 **13.2**	2 13.6	59.8	7 per cent
1e: *Understanding how we respond to physical health problems*	7.4 **12.4**	2.2 13.0	64.6	5 per cent
Workbook 2: *Practical problem solving*	5.9 **10.9**	2.1 12.4	74.3	6 per cent
Workbook 3: *Being assertive*	6.4 **11.4**	2.0 11.8	69.7	6 per cent
Workbook 4: *Identifying extreme and unhelpful thinking*	5.9 **10.9**	1.3 7.5	65.5	0 per cent
Workbook 5: *Changing extreme and unhelpful thinking*	5.4 **10.4**	1.1 10.2	74.1	4 per cent
Workbook 6: *Overcoming avoidance*	6.3 **11.3**	2.4 14.6	70.8	5 per cent
Workbook 7: *Overcoming unhelpful behaviours*	7.2 **12.2**	2.0 13.4	67.3	2 per cent
Workbook 8: *Overcoming sleep problems*	7.3 **12.3**	1.5 10.9	61.8	4 per cent
Workbook 9: *Understanding and using anti-anxiety medications*	9.5 **14.5**	2.4 13.2	50.3	18 per cent
Workbook 10: *Staying well*	7.3 **12.3**	2.4 14.6	68.3	5 per cent

All but one of the workbooks have a reading age of 13.2 or below. The only one that is above this is the workbook addressing anti-anxiety medications. The major reason explaining this is the length of the term 'anti-anxiety medications', used repeatedly in Workbook 9.

A useful overview of the issues of readability – and the even more important issue of understandability/usability are summarised by Johnson on the website www.timetabler.com/reading.html.

Individualising the self-help treatment

All sorts of factors affect how individuals respond and make use of any form of psychotherapy – including psychotherapy delivered via self-help materials. Engagement in the use of self-help needs to bear in mind the person's gender, ethnic and religious background, age and other factors unique to them. Effort has been made in the production of the *Overcoming Anxiety* materials to include older and younger case examples, both male and female and representing a variety of ethnic groups. The main way that the materials allow an individualisation of treatments is through the question and answer interactive sections of the self-help resources. This allows the person to summarise how *they* feel, and describe the impact on them.

Section 2 Using self-help approaches in clinical settings

Selecting who will benefit from self-help

Self-help treatments are helpful for some people but not all. Some may be keen to work in this way – others prefer not to. Various factors affect whether the user is able to make effective use of self-help resources. Problems such as poor concentration, low motivation or reduced memory can make the use of self-help materials difficult. Some medications may cause blurring of vision and make it difficult reading small print on a page or computer screen. Attitudes towards the specific self-help delivery format also will affect use. People like to learn in different ways. In the same way that some people like computer games and watching television and others do not, we need to develop a range of ways of offering self-help.

Selection for self-help: the key step

Factors to bear in mind in selection are:
- Preference/motivation to work in this way.
- The practitioners' *enthusiasm* for the approach.
- Client factors: research studies suggest that those people who show high self-belief and think that they can bring about change themselves are most likely to benefit.
- Poor eyesight and an inability to read indicate a need for audio-based materials.
- The severity of distress can rule out self-help approaches at least for a time. For example, severe depression causes poor concentration and reduced memory. High levels of hopelessness predict drop-out from using self-help and the need for supported self-help delivery.

Adequate *preparation* is required. If it is thought that self-help approaches may be beneficial, the role of self-help materials can be discussed a part of the treatment plan and attitudes concerning it evaluated. Useful questions to explore attitudes include:
- *'What is your initial reaction to the idea of using self-help?'*
- *'Have you used any self-help materials before? Were they useful to you?'*
- *'Has anyone else you know used this approach?'*

Doubts and concerns about the use of self-help materials need to be addressed. It is important to emphasise that the use of self-help materials is only one possible component of the whole treatment. Sometimes the person may choose not to take up the offer, or it may be more appropriate to consider their use at a later time.

Engaging people in using self-help

Patients may not know how to get the most out of self-help, so information should be provided to help the person use self-help effectively. Four areas can fruitfully be covered when introducing self-help materials (Richards *et al.*, 2002):

a) The self-help materials used – their purpose, contents and structure: e.g. *'to help you work on your problems'*, *'they will involve answering questions and practical exercises'*.

b) The validity of the programme: why this particular package may help. This covers the formal and informal evidence base for the materials and the legitimacy of those who have written the materials.

c) The overall treatment package/model being offered, including how often and for how long they will be seen in each session.

d) The practitioner's role in the treatment as guide, collaborator and reviewer – checking the person understands what they are doing and reviewing progress.

How often should a progress review occur?

Regular reviews allow materials to be used between sessions and then discussed within a short supportive session. The cycle of using self-help materials at home and then having the opportunity to come back and discuss what aspects were clear/helpful, and which were more difficult/unhelpful provides a structure to the treatment. The session allows a discussion of areas that are going well, identifying areas where there are any problems, and allows the person to obtain the next set of materials to work on at home. This process is summarised in Figure 1.

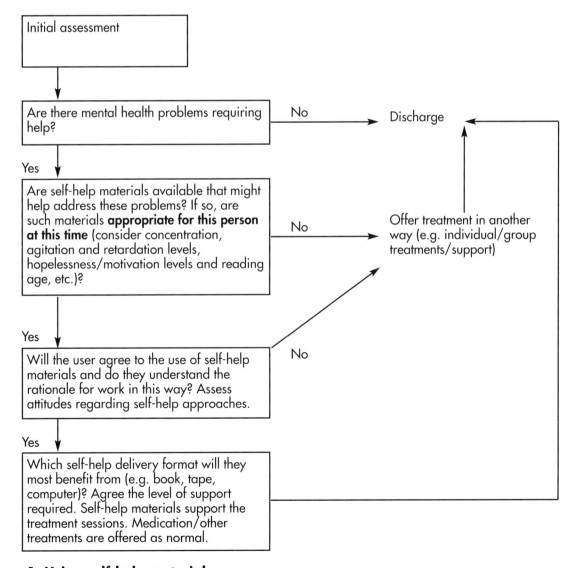

Figure 1 Using self-help materials

Supporting self-help – how long and frequent should sessions be?

When working using self-help the question of how long each session should be and how many sessions should be offered in total can become an issue. There is no right or wrong answer to this and a lot depends on how you see self-help. If self-help is offered with only minimal support from a practitioner (the concept of minimal therapist contact), then few very short sessions would be provided. One recent review of the use of self-help has defined this use of self-help as incorporating 'minimal guidance, defined as one hour or less of professional face-to-face time and up to six, 15 minute telephone calls or independently of professional support'. This approach might be most relevant for shorter and milder difficulties where the person can work through the materials relatively unsupported. Although the *Overcoming Anxiety* materials can be used in this way, they can also be used where the level of support required from the practitioner is higher – for example in more complex or longer-term difficulties, or where the person themselves requires additional support for a range of other reasons.

The use of self-help can most helpfully be considered along a continuum. At one end of the spectrum is 'unsupported' self-help – where the service user uses the materials with no input from a practitioner or other supporter; at the other the 'minimal therapist contact' described above where the self-help materials themselves do the majority of the work of therapy. The amount of support can range from this minimal level to longer lasting and more frequent sessions. At the far extreme you could have CBT offered over 12–16 sessions of one hour with self-help materials acting to help structure 'homework' practice between sessions.

The self-help delivery continuum:

Unsupported   Minimal therapist input   Supported self-help

Time

0 mins   60 mins   Offered as clinically appropriate

To some extent the decisions about how many sessions should be offered and how long they should last for are determined by the practitioner's available time, and the needs of the patient/client.

The 2+1 model

A useful structure to consider using for those with milder to moderate problems is the idea of the '2+1' model of delivering self-help. This model suggests that three sessions are offered in total – two sessions offered a week or so apart and a delayed third final session some 4–6 weeks afterwards. The approach has recently been used in a larger self-help research study (Richards *et al.*, 2003).

The three sessions each lasts a minimum of 20 minutes, but a session of up to 40–50 minutes is preferable.

● **Session 1** This covers a brief assessment of main problem areas, rating of initial symptoms, risk assessment and determination of whether the self-help approach is appropriate for the person and also whether the person wishes to use it. Offer Workbook 1 for them to use between sessions.

This is in the context of providing a brief overview of the materials, model of working, validity of the approach and role of the practitioner in supporting the use of self-help.

- **Session 2** Occurs 1–2 weeks later. The first task is to briefly review Workbook 1 and discuss the Five Areas Assessment. Difficulties in the approach are also discussed and solutions brainstormed. From this, identify which additional workbooks (if any) are jointly agreed as being appropriate. Up to two (on rare occasions three) workbooks are then taken away. The person should attempt to complete each workbook no faster than over a week, again putting into practice the suggested tasks.

- **Session 3** is the final session and is offered after a 4–6 week gap. The purpose of the delayed session is to allow the person time to work on their problems, and also for other factors (time, the impact of any new or altered medication, new supports from elsewhere etc.) to have an impact. This final session provides an opportunity to review what has gone well, not so well, what has been learned and from this plan to put what has been learned into practice. Additional workbooks can be offered at this stage, including the final exit workbook – Workbook 10.

The system can be provided flexibly (for example by adding an additional fourth session if required).

Variants on this approach include having the assessment for self-help completed by a referrer such as a GP. Support may be offered via other routes than directly face-to-face, for example via telephone support. Where resources are limited another option is to offer one rather than three sessions, and the person then works on their own with the materials – perhaps while remaining on a waiting list for treatment. Finally, the 2+1 approach can be offered individually, or within a group treatment setting.

How to get the best out of using self-help approaches

Encouraging the person to stop, think and reflect on the materials as they use them can encourage learning. Evidence suggests that people who interact with the written worksheets and put into practice the tasks suggested do better than those who do not. This is best done by **answering all the questions** that are asked.

The process can be encouraged by asking patients/clients to **write down** notes in the margins or at the back of the materials to help them remember information that has been helpful. They should **review** these notes each week. Once each workbook has been completed, it is best to **put it on one side** and then **re-read it** again a few days later. It may be that different parts of the text become clearer, or seem more relevant on second reading.

Planning self-help treatments into service delivery

Self-help materials can be used in different parts of a clinical service, and are most widely used outside the mental health services completely. For example, self-help is currently offered by:

Self-help groups and organisations
Most self-help groups recommend or make use of extensive self-help materials. The groups themselves also act as an important resource for information, support and advice on a wide range of mental disorders. Some – for example Triumph over Phobia – offer support for the use of self-help materials as their main way of working (www.triumphoverphobia.com).

Other ways that self-help is delivered include:

Direct/open access

- For example, by providing kiosks based in libraries or supermarkets.
- Open access clinics. The first and best known is the Maudsley self-care clinic in London, developed initially by Professor Isaac Marks.

Joint user/service delivery

- Ex-sufferers at East Ardsley in Leeds support a Self-help Resource Room based within secondary care psychiatry.
- A self-help support worker employed in Dumfries is based in both primary care and linked to local voluntary sector groups. She is delivering the *Overcoming Depression* and other self-help materials.
- The START project in Glasgow between Glasgow Institute of Psychosocial Interventions and Depression Alliance Scotland is delivering a large group self-help package using *Overcoming Depression*. This will allow self-referral to an eight session treatment group addressing understanding depression, problem solving and overcoming problems of reduced activity.

Primary care

- A self-help support nurse employed by Glasgow Institute of Psychosocial Interventions delivers the *Overcoming Depression* materials to directly referred General Practice patients. He is based in Drumchapel Resource Centre in Glasgow.

Secondary care

i) Accident and Emergency

- The *Overcoming Depression* self-help materials are offered to people after overdose in Liverpool.

ii) Psychiatry

- Malham House Day Hospital self-help room in Leeds provides access to self-help to patients on the waiting list or seeing members of the secondary care community mental health team (Whitfield, Williams and Shapiro, 2001).
- Ward-based Patient Activity nurses are using the *Overcoming Depression* materials with patients in inpatient settings in some sites in Glasgow.

Such resources can also support individual or group work with a health care practitioner

Developing a self-help room

One way that self-help delivery can be encouraged within a clinical service is to introduce a focus for self-help delivery. One such approach has been developed at Malham House Day Hospital in Leeds. Here, a specific self-help room was set up within an adult acute day hospital setting. This provides a central resource for use by day hospital staff, outpatients (including waiting list patients) and also for patients seen by members of the multidisciplinary sector psychiatric service. This is illustrated in Figure 2. Self-help approaches can be integrated to support other treatments already offered within the different clinical settings (e.g. at a day hospital or resource centre, and within both inpatient and outpatient settings). This has the advantage to the team and the patient of allowing a consistent management plan to be offered across these different settings.

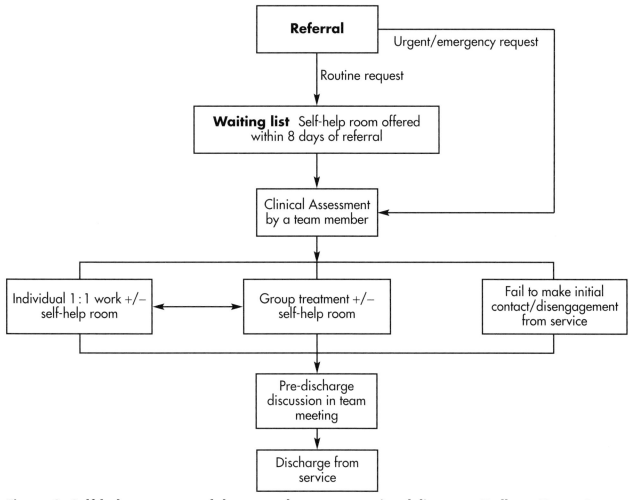

Figure 2 Self-help as a part of the secondary care service delivery at Malham House Day Hospital in Leeds

Setting up a self-help room

The setting up of a self-help room means that decisions need to be made about several issues:
● which materials to offer in the room;
● how to support the room (e.g. consider the cost and practicalities of providing the photocopied worksheets used and/or original copies of the materials);
● how to provide an atmosphere that encourages self-help approaches.

Perhaps the easiest way of delivering self-help is to offer copies of a book or photocopies of materials within the room. Some units ask for a returnable deposit for the chance to borrow books.

Plants, rugs and attractive pictures ensure a relaxing atmosphere. A desk, pens and paper maintain a central focus on the materials. Only one person uses the room at a time to ensure privacy and a booking system allows users to spend sessions of up to one hour. Patients are encouraged to use the room once or twice a week, and to keep all their completed workbooks and worksheets so as to create their own personalised treatment pack. The room is kept neat and tidy, and one of the secretaries has a role in ensuring that pens, paper and photocopied workbooks/worksheets are available at all times that the room is open.

Introducing self-help into a service

When introducing self-help into a clinical service, the following are some issues to bear in mind.

1 **Staff training** Training of staff is required to offer supported self-help. Currently only around one in three (36.2 per cent) of accredited CBT practitioners are trained in the use of self-help. The level of training in the wider workforce is not known (Keeley, Williams and Shapiro, 2002).

2 **Clear models of service delivery** are required, thus providing integrated (or 'stepped') care pathways that build upon existing services.

3 **The level and type of support required by the practitioner needs to be clarified** These might include a psychology assistant, practice nurses (Richards *et al.*, 2002), fellow users/user groups or a generic self-help support worker. How often and for how long this support should be offered is unclear. In many cases only minimal or no support may be needed.

4 **Capacity issues are important** Shared rooms may be disruptive and a room-booking system can be helpful. Rooms also may be offered for use out of normal hours thus allowing easier access to those in employment. This also has staffing implications.

5 **Investigate process issues** Studies to date have examined outcomes in key domains, such as mood and social functioning. There has been no investigation of the sub-components of the packages that may be more or less effective/helpful, or how they are best used. This should be examined within future research and audit.

6 **Changing attitudes** In spite of the promising results of reported studies, mental health staff can sometimes be reluctant to work using self-help. These issues can be partially addressed within staff training, however wider issues concerning the structure of services also need to be considered.

Further details of the issues arising in the setting up and evaluation of a self-help arm to a clinical service are included in Williams and Whitfield (2001), Whitfield and Williams (2003) and Williams (2001).

Training in the use of self-help

The SPIRIT (Structured Psychosocial InteRventions In Teams) course has been designed to address the need to train practitioners to work effectively at service level 1 of CBT delivery. It aims to keep the strengths of the CBT model (its structure, focus on current clinical problems) and to do so in ways that build upon the relationship with the practitioner, and to support this delivery by the use of structured CBT self-help materials *with the support of* the health care practitioner.

Training needs vary, depending on which level of CBT delivery is provided. The SPIRIT course offers jargon-free training in Cognitive Behaviour Treatment to staff working within the health service. The aim of the training is to teach the CBT model in a pragmatic user-friendly style (the Five Areas Assessment model). The course does not aim for staff to become experts in CBT working at levels 2 or 3; instead it offers skills-based training in certain focused areas of CBT (level 1 working) and does this in ways that build upon multidisciplinary and multi-agency team-based working.

The course develops clinical skills for use in busy everyday clinical practice and uses a range of proven educational techniques:

- *Team-based small group training* to encourage attendees to apply what they learn in their own clinical settings.
- *Supervised role-play* to practise clinical skills.
- Each session starts with the *clinical supervision session*, reviewing the use of the approach over the previous week. Each session ends with a '*Putting into practice what you have learned*' component.

- In addition, teams are provided with a *specially commissioned interactive skills-based CD Rom* produced by the University of Leeds Calipso (Computer-Aided Learning in Psychiatry www.calipso.co.uk) unit. This builds upon the training in each session and provides a mixture of text, video and sound clips that help the practitioner practise and assess their learning of the Five Areas Assessment model in clinical practice. In addition, self-help materials can be printed off for use with patients.

Delivering SPIRIT

The project has three stages:
- *Step 1: Identify the trainers* These are the skilled practitioners who deliver the training to the clinical teams. The individuals selected have clinical credibility, training in psychosocial interventions (not always CBT) and importantly possess skills in small group skills-based training and clinical supervision.
- *Step 2: Training the trainers course* Chris Williams and Anne Garland (Nurse Consultant in Psychological Therapies, Nottingham – email Anne.Garland@nhc-tr.trent.nhs.uk) have trained eight local trainers in Glasgow to train others in how to offer the SPIRIT course.
- *Step 3: Training delivery* The trainers are responsible for the training delivery within the chosen clinical teams (community and linked inpatient staff) and for sustainability of the gains of this training.

The SPIRIT training course is being offered to all adult and elderly teams throughout Glasgow. The training is multidisciplinary by choice and is offered to teams rather than to individuals. This was based on the observation that when individuals do such training it often proves difficult for them to make changes in their own clinical work setting. A related difficulty is that clinical staff often work only within specific parts of the clinical service. The danger for staff is that they sometimes fail to make the links between their own particular work setting and other aspects of the same sector service. The SPIRIT training therefore has by choice offered team-based training to staff working in all components of the same clinical service so as to include both community and inpatient staff. Sessions are deliberately multidisciplinary and multi-agency to enhance this, and trainers are chosen from different practitioner backgrounds. The purpose is to break down boundaries, enhancing the team-based approach and developing a common language of assessment, thereby encouraging collaborative team working.

How many staff will benefit?

Eight trainers have been trained and work in pairs (multidisciplinary by choice) to deliver the training. They offer the ten sessions of training over approximately a three-month period and, at the end of the formal training, fortnightly supervisions sessions are offered for a further three months to support changes by the individual and the team. By offering this course three times each year, with up to 18 staff attending each course (as a closed group including up to 4 inpatient staff – for whom agency cover is provided, and 12 to 16 community team members) a total of 214 staff have received training and ongoing supervision during the first year of the training. A certificate of completion is offered to staff who achieve more than 70 per cent attendance.

Is the teaching effective?

The teaching is being offered to all adult and elderly teams throughout Glasgow. An evaluation of the training examines the impact on subjective and objective knowledge and skills, team functioning, and also adherence to the training content of the course by the trainers together with the measures of the acceptability and content of training. This has confirmed high acceptability of the training, as well as confirming gains in each of the key knowledge/skills areas. Follow-up has confirmed increasing use of the skills over time.

The challenge of how to achieve sustainable and relevent change is not to be underestimated. Previous research has confirmed the great difficulties in both bringing about change in staff knowledge, attitudes and skills, and in maintaining any such change and confirming an impact on patient care (King *et al.*, 2002). The next stage of the project includes an analysis of the impact on staff care delivery and on patient outcomes.

References

Beck, A.T., Rush, J.A., Shaw, B.F. and Emery, G. (1979). *Cognitive Therapy of Depression*. New York: Guilford Press.

Cole, F., Hardy, J., Ditchburn, V. (2001). *Psychological Skills Training of Primary Care Practitioners: Report of a pilot project developed by Calderdale and Kirklees Health Authority*. Data presented at the annual conference of the British Association for Behavioural and Cognitive Psychotherapies (BABCP), Glasgow.

Cuijpers, P. (1997) Bibliotherapy in unipolar depression: a meta-analysis. *Journal of Behavioural Therapy & Experimental Psychiatry*, **28**: 2: 139–47.

Department of Health (2001). *Treatment Choice in Psychological Therapies and Counselling*. London: HMSO.

Gould, R.A. and Clum, A.A. (1993). Meta-analysis of self-help treatment approaches. *Clinical Psychology Review*, **13**: 169–86.

Glasgow, R. and Rosen G. (1978). Behavioural bibliotherapy: a review of self-help behaviour therapy manuals. *Psychological Bulletin*, **85**: 1–23.

Haaga, D.A.F. (2000). Introduction to the special section on stepped care models in psychotherapy. *J. Consult. Clin. Psychol.*, **68**: 547–8.

Jorm, A.F., Korten, A.E., Jacomb, P.A., Rodgers, B., Pollitt, P., Christensen, H. and Henderson, S. (1997). Helpfulness of interventions for mental disorders: beliefs of health professionals compared with the general public. *British Journal of Psychiatry*, **171**: 233–7.

Keeley, H., Williams, C.J. and Shapiro, D. (2002). A United Kingdom survey of accredited cognitive behaviour therapists' attitudes towards and use of structured self-help materials. *Behavioural and Cognitive Psychotherapy*, **30**: 191–201.

King, M., Davidson, O., Taylor, F., Haines, A., Sharp, D. and Turner, R. (2002). Effectiveness of teaching general practitioners skills in brief cognitive behaviour therapy to treat patients with depression: randomised controlled trial. *British Medical Journal*, 20 April, **324**: 947.

Lovell, K. and Richards, D. (2000). Multiple Access Points and Levels of Entry (MAPLE): ensuring choice, accessibility and equity for CBT services. *Behavioural and Cognitive Psychotherapy*, **28**: 379–91.

Marrs R. (1995). A meta-analysis of bibliotherapy studies. *Am. J. Community Psychol.*, **23**: 843–70.

Quackenbush, R.L. (1991). The prescription of self-help books by psychologists: a bibliography of selected bibliotherapy resources. *Psychotherapy*, **28**: 4: 671–7.

Richards, A., Barkham, M., Cahill, J., Richards, D., Williams C. and Heywood, P. (2003). PHASE: Assessing Self-Help Education in Primary Care: A Randomised Controlled Trial. *British Journal of General Practice* 53: 495: 764–71.

Richards, D.A., Richards, A., Barkham, M., Cahill, J. and Williams, C. (2002). PHASE: a health technology approach to psychological treatment in primary mental health care. *Primary Health Care Research and Development*, 3: 159–68.

Scogin, F., Bynum, J., Stephens, G. and Calhoon, S. (1990). Efficacy of self-administered programs: meta-analytic review. *Professional Psychology: Research and Practice*, **21**: **1**: 42–7.

Whitfield, G., Williams, C.J. and Shapiro, D. (2001). An evaluation of a self-help room in a general adult psychiatry service. *Behavioural and Cognitive Psychotherapy*, **29**: **3**: 333–43.

Whitfield, G. and Williams, C.J. (2003). The evidence base for CBT in depression: delivering CBT in busy clinical settings. *Advances in Psychiatric Treatment*, 9: 21–30.

Williams, C.J. (2001). Ready access to proven psychosocial interventions? The use of written CBT self-help materials to treat depression. *Advances in Psychiatric Treatment*, 7: 233–40.

Williams, C.J. and Whitfield, G. (2001). Written and computer-based self-help treatments for depression. *British Medical Bulletin*, 57: 133–44.

Additional self-help resources

A range of other five areas materials are available.

Written self-help workbooks

Overcoming Depression: A Five Areas Approach, by Chris Williams, published by Arnold (2001). ISBN 0–340–76383–3.

I'm not supposed to feel like this: A Christian self-help approach to depression and anxiety, by Chris Williams, Paul Richards and Ingrid Whitton, published by Hodder & Stoughton (2002). ISBN 0–340–78639–6.

Computer self-help CD-Rom-based self-help programmes

1 *Overcoming Depression*
2 *Overcoming Bulimia*

Both are published by Media Innovations (www.calipso.co.uk), who act on behalf of the University of Leeds.

In addition, two CD Roms that aim to train practitioners in the use of the *Overcoming Anxiety* and *Overcoming Depression* resources are available.

Contact details: Mr Stephen Taylor-Parker, Media Innovations, 3 Gemini Business Park, Sheepscar Way, Leeds, LS7 3J
Email: s.taylor-parker@media-innovations.ltd.uk
Tel: 0113 284 9222

Index